Ranadhir Barua

Tumours of the Female Lower Genital Tract

Classification and Pathology

With 141 Figures and 2 Tables

Springer-Verlag
Berlin Heidelberg New York
London Paris Tokyo
Hong Kong Barcelona

RANADHIR BARUA, M.D., F.R.C.P.A., M.I.A.C.
Senior Consultant
Department of Histopathology and Cytopathology
The Queen Elizabeth Hospital
Woodville, South Australia 5011
Australia

Address for correspondence:
6, Airport Rd, Brooklyn Park 5032
South Australia

ISBN 3-540-51277-2 Springer-Verlag Berlin Heidelberg New York
ISBN 0-387-51277-2 Springer-Verlag New York Berlin Heidelberg

Library of Congress Cataloging-in-Publication Data. Barua, Ranadhir, 1928–Tumours of the female lower genital tract : classification and pathology / Ranadhir Barua. p. cm. Includes bibliographical references. 1. Generative organs, Female–Tumors–Classification. 2. Generative organs, Female–Tumors –Histopathology. I. Title. [DNLM: 1. Vaginal Neoplasms–classification. 2. Vaginal Neoplasms–pathology. 3. Vulvar Neoplasms–classification. 4. Vulvar Neoplasms–pathology. WP 15 B295t] RC280.G5B38 1990 616.99'267–dc20 DNLM/DLC for Library of Congress 90–9761 CIP

2121/3130-543210 – Printed on acid-free paper

Preface

Classifications of vulval and vaginal tumours, like those of tumours of many other areas of the human body, are incomplete. There is an ever-increasing number of reports of newly identified tumours arising at unexpected sites. With our new knowledge, many tumours have been regrouped, put into different or altogether new categories, or their nature and histogenesis questioned. Some tumours still defy classification.

During the past decade, a number of uncommon tumours and tumour-like conditions have been reported from this area of the female genital tract. I have not seen any recent classification including all these lesions. Thus, I have attempted here to organise them, with the more familiar common tumours, into a classification which, given the information available today, is fairly elaborate. The histogenesis of some tumours is still a matter of controversy, and it may be some time before these controversies are finally resolved. Paget's disease of the vulva, mixed tumours and mesonephric papilloma of the vagina are but a few examples.

Vulval dystrophies have always been an interesting subject for students and clinicians. I have included a separate chapter on this topic at the end of the section on the vulva.

I was privileged to be part of a discussion group during the gynaecological ward rounds for some 20 years. It became increasingly obvious to me that a pathologist's participation in patient care remains incomplete unless he or she takes into account the clinical condition underlying the morphological changes and looks beyond the tissue slides, considering the patient's medical background and history with a clinical awareness which can only be developed through constant discussion and reading. Keeping this in mind, I have included the clinical features and outlines of treatment.

I am greatly indebted to Professor L.W. Cox, now Professor Emeritus, Department of Obstetrics and Gynaecology, University of Adelaide, for his constant support, guidance and encouragement over the two decades I worked under him in the University's Gynaecological Pathology and Cytopathology Laboratory. I remember with gratitude the late Dr. J.A. Kirkland, former Pathologist-in-Charge of the Laboratory, whose advice and guidance were invaluable in my development as a pathologist. I am thankful to Dr. R.N. Munday, the Visiting Senior Gynaecologist, whose keen interest in gynaecological pathology has always been stimulating. I am also grateful to Professor C.D. Mathews, Department of Reproductive Medicine, for his encouragement in my work over the years. I acknowledge the co-operation and help of some former colleagues during my early years in the Department of Obstetrics and Gynaecology who have now either retired or left the department.

I am, indeed, thankful to Drs. P.W. Allen and R.B. Dymock and other colleagues in my present department for their tolerance, professional help and advice. Thanks are also due to my younger colleagues, whose questions and inquisitiveness have always been a source of stimulus. I appreciate the help of Dr. I. Strung, who translated several articles from the German literature for this work. I also thank Dr. A.J. Bourne of Adelaide Children's Hospital for providing two slides for this book.

I appreciate the opportunity for using some slides from the departmental files for this work.

I thank the technical staff of the former Gynaecological and Cytopathology Laboratory and Histopathology Laboratory for their assistance. My gratitude is also due to S. Rockliff and B. Duquen for their very valuable help in the MEDLARS searches, and to Mrs. K. Alexopoulos and J. Humby for secretarial assistance.

Finally, preparation of the book would have been impossible without the understanding and tolerance shown by my family. No words suffice to express my gratitude to them.

December 1989 R. Barua

Contents

Part I: The Vulva

1 Classification of the Tumours and Tumour-like Conditions of the Vulva

I. Cysts, Tumours and Tumour-like Conditions of the Epidermis and Adnexae

Cysts and tumours
Epidermal cysts
Pilar cysts
Seborrheic keratosis
Keratoacanthoma
Angiokeratoma
Warty dyskeratoma
Verruciform xanthoma
Hidradenoma
Syingoma
Syringocystadenoma papilliferum
Chondroid syringom
Pilar tumour
Trichoepithelioma

Tumour-like conditions
Skin tag
Verruca vulgaris
Senile sebaceous hyperplasia
Nodular amyloidosis
Isolated epidermolytic acanthoma

II. Developmental Cysts and Tumours

Mesonephric cysts
Paramesonephric cysts
Cysts of canal of Nuck

III. Cysts, Tumours and Tumour-like Conditions of the Vestubular Glands

Cysts and tumours
Bartholin's duct cysts
Bartholin's gland adenoma
Mixed tumours of Bartholin's gland (benign and, malignant)

Tumour-like condition
Malakoplakia of Bartholin's gland

IV. Tumours and Tumor-like Conditions of Ectopic Tissues

Normal breast tissue
Vulval breast
Vulval lactating breast

Breast cyst
Milk cyst

Ectopic breast tumours
Fibroadenoma
Intraduct papilloma

Tumour-like conditions
Endometriosis
Deciduoma
Choriostoma

V. Intraepithelial Neoplasia and Invasive Carcinomas of Squamous Cell Origin

Intraepithelial neoplasia
Superficially invasive (stage 1a) carcinoma
Invasive carcinoma
Verrucous carcinoma

VI. Basal Cell Carcinoma

VII. Adenocarcinomas

Arising in sweat glands
Apocrine glands
Eccrine glands

Arising in sebaceous glands

Arising in paraurethral glands

Arising in major and minor vestibular glands

Arising in ectopic tissue
Breasts
Endometriosis

Arising in misplaced cloacal tissue

VIII. Paget's Disease

IX. Naevi and Melanoma

X. Tumours of Mesenchymal and Neural Origin

Benign
Fibroma
Lipoma
Neurofibroma
Granular cell tumour
Neurilemmoma
Leiomyoma
Rhabdomyoma
Fibrous histiocytoma
Haemangioma
Lymphangioma
Glomus tumour
Myxoma
Ganglioneuroma

Malignant
Leiomyosarcoma
Malignant fibrous histiocytoma
Fibrosarcoma
Liposarcoma
Epithelioid sarcoma
Malignant schwannoma
Rhabdomyosarcoma
Angiosarcoma
Kaposi's sarcoma
Alveolar soft part sarcoma
Dermatofibrosarcoma protuberans
Aggressive angiomyxoma
Haemangiopericytoma
Desmoid tumour

Tumour-like conditions
Benign enlargement of the labia
Benign enlargement of the clitoris
Tumoral calcinosis
Nodular fasciitis
Traumatic neuroma
Lymphoid hyperplasia
Fibrohistiocytic proliferative lesions

XI. Lymphomas

XII. Merkel Cell and Amphicrine Tumour

XIII. Germ Cell Tumour: Endodermal Sinus Tumour

XIV. Histiocytosis X

XV. Inflammatory Conditions Which May Simulate Tumours

Specific
Human papilloma virus infections –
condylomata acuminata, squamous papilloma
Herpes simplex virus infection
Tuberculous lesion
Syphilis (tertiary)
Granuloma venereum
Lymphogranuloma inguinale
Chancroid
Molluscum contagiosum
Amoebic ulcers
Schistosomiasis
Filariasis
Loxosceles recusa spider bite

Non-specific
Granulation tissue
Granuloma pyogenicum
Hidradenitis suppuritivum
Pilonidal sinus
Sclerosing lipogranuloma
Crohn's disease
Malakoplakia

XVI. Secondary Tumours

2 Cysts, Tumours and Tumour-like Conditions of the Epidermis and Adnexae

2.1 Cysts and Tumours

2.1.1 Epidermal Cyst

The epidermal cyst is one of the most common cysts occurring in the labia. It is believed to develop from the inclusion of squamous epithelium in the dermis during embryological reorganisation or from misplaced squamous epithelium due to trauma. It presents as an asymptomatic, stationary or gradually enlarging, round, firm subcutaneous swelling a few millimeters to a few centimeters in size. Multiple epidermal cysts may sometimes be associated with Gardner's syndrome (osteoma, gastrointestinal polyposis usually of malignant variety; Knox and Freeman 1965). Post-circumcisional epidermal cysts of the clitoris are reported to be common complications in some parts of Nigeria (Ofadile et al. 1979).

2.1.1.1 Microscopical Appearance

The wall is formed by several layers of squamous cells with intercellular bridges and granular cells (Fig. 2.1). Foreign body-type giant cell rections can be seen in the wall and surrounding areas when the cyst ruptures.

2.1.2 Pilar Cyst (Sebaceous Cyst)

The pilar cyst commonly occurs on the scalp but can also appear on the vulva. Grossly, the cyst is similar to an epidermal cyst but may, on rare occasions, be very large, weighing up to 6 kg (Sackdeva and Narang 1968).

Microscopically, the cyst wall consists of several layers of squamoid cells without intercellular bridges and is devoid of granular layer (Fig. 2.2). The peripheral outermost layer displays a palisading arrangement not seen in epidermal cysts. The cyst content is eosinophilic amorphous material, which unlike that of an epidermal cyst tends frequently to be calcified. Giant cell reactions within and around the cyst occur when its wall ruptures.

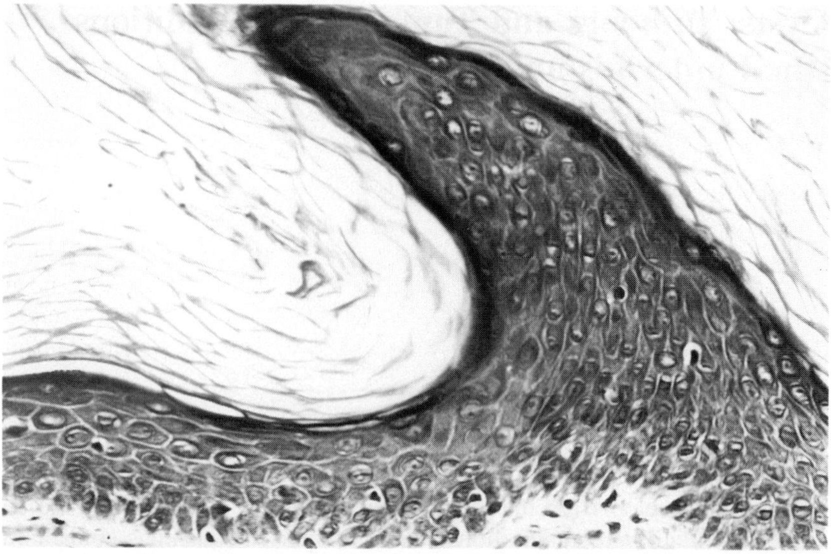

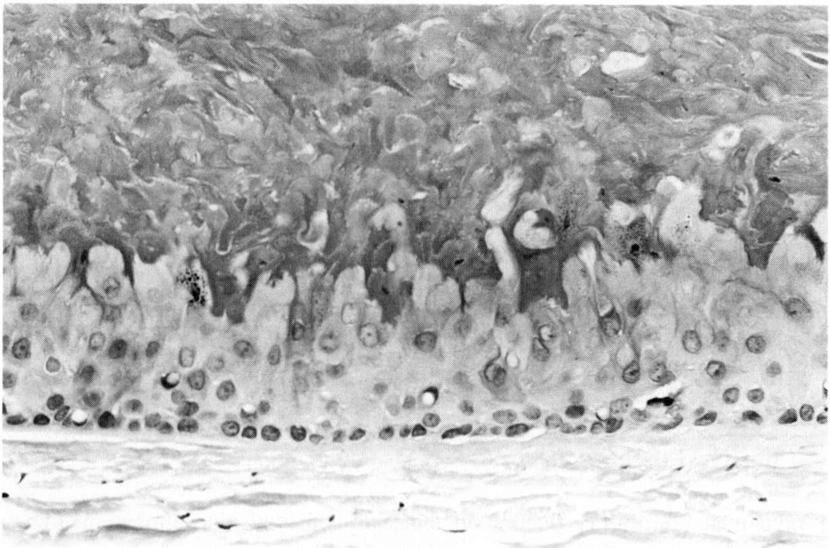

Fig. 2.1. Wall of an epidermal cyst formed by layers of squamous cells

Fig. 2.2. Wall of a pilar cyst consisting of squamoid-type cells

2.1.2.1 Treatment

Malignant changes are rare in these cysts. Unless fibrous adhesions result from rupture or infection, the cysts can be shelled out without difficulty.

2.1.3 Seborrhoeic Keratosis

Seborrhoeic keratosis, also known as basal cell papilloma, is very common. The lesions do not occur on the palm and sole and are infrequent on the vulva. The gross appearance is of light brown, black to flesh-coloured, sharply demarcated, macular, papular or somewhat greasy, polypoid lesions varying in size from minute papules to tumours of several millimeters. The surface may show papillary lobulations (Knox and Freeman 1965). A sudden increase in the number and size of seborrhoeic keratotic lesions known as the Leser-Trélat sign, may be an indication of occult internal malignancy (Holdiness 1986). Ovarian, uterine and cervical malignancies have been reported with this sign (Holguin et al. 1986).

2.1.3.1 Microscopical Appearance

The basic freatures of these tumours are hyperkeratosis, acanthosis and papillomatosis. The small and dark cells which are the major constituent cells of the lesion seem like basal cells of the epidermis. These cells are admixed in various proportions with the larger keratinocytes containing abundant cytoplasm and round vesicular nuclei. Characteristically, the horn cysts containing keratin material are distributed at all levels of the tumour (Fig. 2.3). The base of the seborrheic keratosis is generally in the same plane as the adjacent normal skin. Variations in the microscopical features occur, and accordingly the lesions have been described as solid or acanthotic, reticular or adenoid, and irritated types. In the last type, the mature squamous cells are arranged in whorls or eddies. Melanin pigments in variable amount may be present in the cytoplasm of basaloid cells.

2.1.3.2 Treatment

These tumours are benign, and simple excision is adequate.

2.1.4 Keratoacanthoma

Once known as molluscum sebaceum (McCormac and Scarff 1936), keratoacanthomas commonly occur on exposed sites as small nodules which rapidly grow to their maximum size in 6–8 weeks. When fully developed they appear as cup-shaped lesions 1–3 cm in diameter, containing keratin plugs in the centre, and resemble squamous cells carcinoma. Keratoacanthomas involute spontaneously in a few months (usually within 6 months). An increased incidence of these lesions has been noticed in immunosuppressed patients (Sullivan and Colditz 1979)

Keratoacanthomas are rare on the vulva, where they appear as lumps and are often mistaken for squamous cell carcinoma (Rhatigan and Nuss 1985). They are non-tender and usually not associated with pruritus.

2.1.4.1 Microscopical Appearance

Keratoacanthomas are well-demarcated, cup-shaped lesions with a sharp angular shoulder formed by the proliferating squamous epithelium and adjacent normal epidermis (Fig. 2.4). The central crater is filled with keratin, and the base is formed by irregularly proliferating squamous cells which may display disturbing features of atypia and mitoses. The early phase of the lesion is characterised by the invagination of the epidermis into the dermis, forming irregular strands of squamous cells which protrude from the base and create a pushing margin. This is followed by the formation of keratin plugs which are finally extruded to the central crater. Chronic inflammatory cells and foreign body type giant cells are frequently present at the base of the lesion.

Differentiation in the early stage from squamous cell carcinoma may be difficult. The presence of an angulated shoulder, absence of invasion at the base and clinical history are helpful in establishing the ultimate diagnosis.

The aetiology of these lesions is not known. Immunosuppression seems to be an important predisposing factor. Viral aetiology has not been confirmed. The aggressiveness of keratoacanthomas or their sudden appearance in crops may indicate immunological incompletence or internal malignancy (Fathizadeh et al. 1982).

2.1.4.2 Treatment

Keratoacanthomas are benign. Whether an occasional metastasising lesion is in fact a squamous cell carcinoma is not settled (Piscioli et al. 1984).

Complete excision and histological assessment of the margins are essential.

2.1.5 Angiokeratoma

Angiokeratomas are probably not as rare as the literature suggests (Novick 1985). The lesions are bright red to black-coloured, papular, warty nodules of 5 mm average diameter. Sometimes the lesions are extensive and confluent (Clark and Wheelock 1988). Some 68% of the patients with vulal lesions are in the reproductive age group, and 50% of them have onset during pregnancy (Imperial and Helwig 1967). The lesions are, however, not infrequent in old age (Verbov and Manglabruks 1978). They occur mostly on the labia majora and are usually asymptomatic. Occasionally, the patients may present with bleeding, pruritus, slowly growing tumour and pain. Clinical differentiation of the asymptomatic bleeding nodules from haemangiomata or even melanoma (Uhlin 1980) may be difficult. In some patients, the lesions are aggravated by pregnancy. Increased venous pressure and primary degeneration of elastic tissue with secondary dilatation of the vessels have been suggested to be

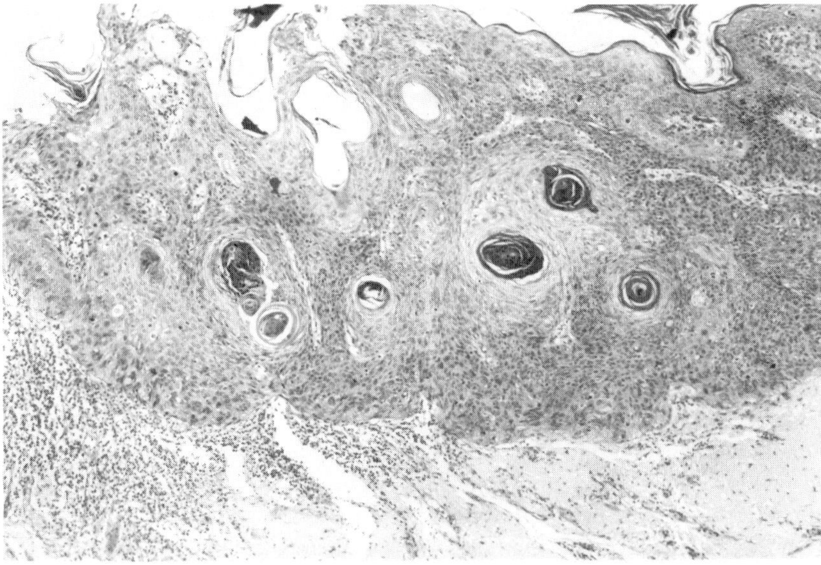

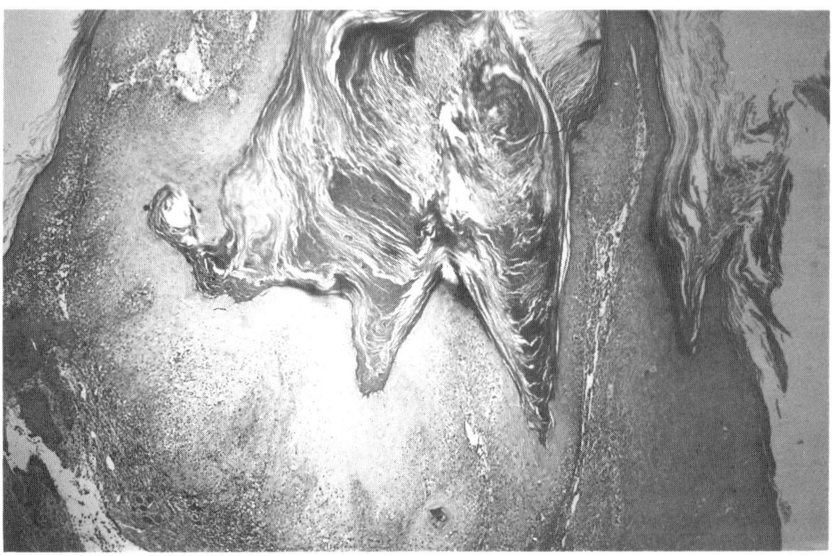

Fig. 2.3. Seborrhoeic keratosis: thick layer of basaloid cells containing horny cysts

Fig. 2.4. Keratoacanthoma: cup-shaped lesion with angular shoulder

pathogenetic factors. Angiokeratomas have been noticed in association with varicose conditions of the vulva (Blair 1970).

Microscopically, the lesions consist of dilated capillaries of various sizes covered by acanthotic epidermis (Fig. 2.5). Dilated capillaries lined by flattened endothelial cells are also seen in the upper dermis.

2.1.5.1 Treatment

The treatment is surgical excision. Electrocautery (Novick 1985) and argon laser are now being used with success (Dotters et al. 1986).

2.1.6 Warty Dyskeratoma

Although warty dyskeratomas commonly occur in sun-expsoed areas, they can occasionally be seen in unexposed areas. The vulval lesion commonly appears as a single, sharply demarcated, tan to pale pink, keratotic nodule on the labia majora. The patients are usually in their 30s of 40s (Duray et al. 1983). In spite of the histological similarities, warty dyskeratomas are not considered to be related to Darier's disease, which is inherited as an autosomal dominant gene.

2.1.6.1 Microscopical Appearance

Warty dyskeratomas consist of a characteristic, cup-shaped, epidermal invagination in the dermis. The base of the cup is formed by the upward villous projections of the dermal papillae which are lined by one to two layers of basal cells, while the cap itself is filled with many acantholytic and dyskeratotic cells (corps ronds) and keratin debris (Fig. 2.6). The lesion is to be differentiated from other acantholytic dermatoses such as Darier's disease (Keratosis follicularis) and benign familial pemphigus. Darier's disease is slowly progressive with more extensive bullous or vesicular lesions rather than a single nodule. Histologically, Darier's disease also shows suprabasal acantholysis forming clefts and lacunae, corps ronds and rather more tortuous villi. In the familial benign pemphigus which is inherited as an autosomal dominant trait, suprabasal separation forming bullae are larger, acantholysis and corps ronds are pronounced, and villi are more elongated.

2.1.6.2 Treatment

The treatment consists of excision of the nodule.

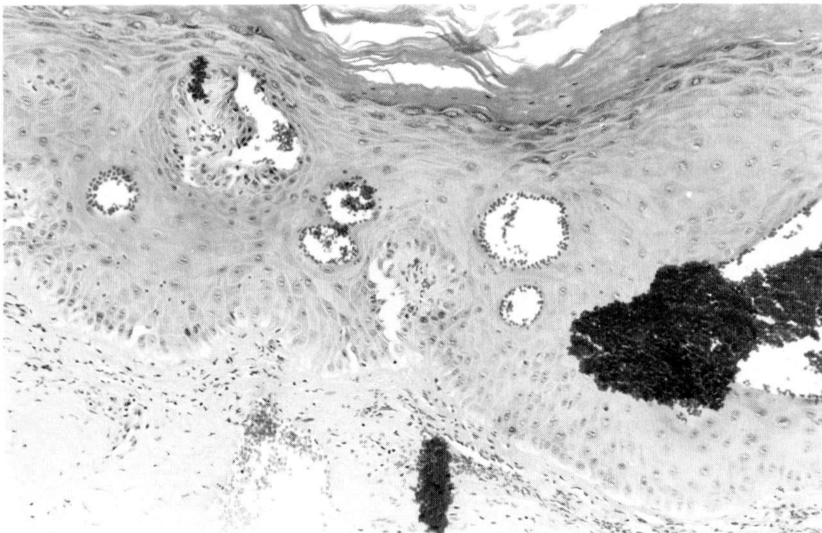

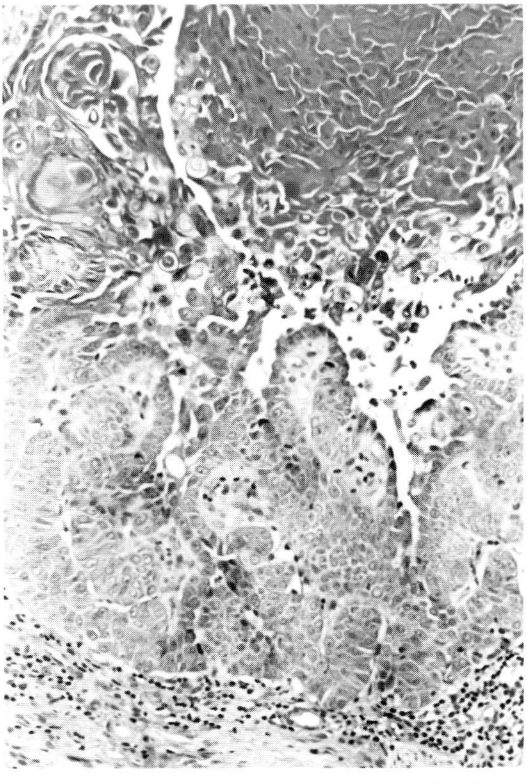

Fig. 2.5. Angiokeratoma: dilated capillaries at the upper dermis

Fig. 2.6. Warty dyskeratoma: upward villous projection from the base of a cup-shaped depression

2.1.7 Verruciform Xanthoma

Until recently it was believed that verruciform xanthoma occurs exclusively in the oral cavity. However, Santa-Cruz and Martin (1979) reported two cases with vulval lesions and emphasised the importance of recognition of the condition which might be clinically misdiagnosed as carcinoma. The histological appearance is of a verrucous lesion consisting of hyperkeratosis, parakeratosis, acanthosis and elongation of rete pegs with collections of histiocytic foam (xanthoma) cells in the dermis between the rete pegs.

The nature of the condition is unknown.

2.1.7.1 Treatment

The treatment is excision of the lesion.

2.1.8 Hidradenoma Vulvae

Hidradenoma vulvae, also known as apocrine adenoma of the vulva, presents as an asymptomatic intradermal or subcutaneous tumour of the labium majus. It also occurs in the paralabial tissue and less commonly in the perineum (Cox 1954). Whether the tumour arises from the apocrine or eccrine gland has been debated for a long time. The general belief is that the tumour is of apocrine gland origin (Chung 1958; Meeker et al. 1962), although Woodworth et al. (1971) in a series of 69 cases of papillary hidradenoma found 18 cases arising in the labia minora where apocrine glands are not present. The sweat glands in these locations, according to these authors, are neither apocrine nor accrine, but an intermediate type with the attributes of both.

The tumour does not occur before puberty. The age of the patient varies from 19 (Deacon and Taylor 1952) to 77 years old (Danforth 1943). The tumour is usually discovered as an incidental finding during pelvic examination, although occasionally a patient may seek medical advice for a vulval tumour.

2.1.8.1 Gross Appearance

The tumour is a reddish-brown, freely mobile, well-circumscribed, cystic mass averaging 1.0–2.0 cm in diameter. It can be larger and measure up to 8 cm in diameter (Kaufmann et al. 1987). Generally, the tumour is signle but may occasionally be multiple. The skin overlying the lesion may ulcerate and bleed, leading to a mistaken diagnosis of carcinoma of the vulva (Nielsen 1973).

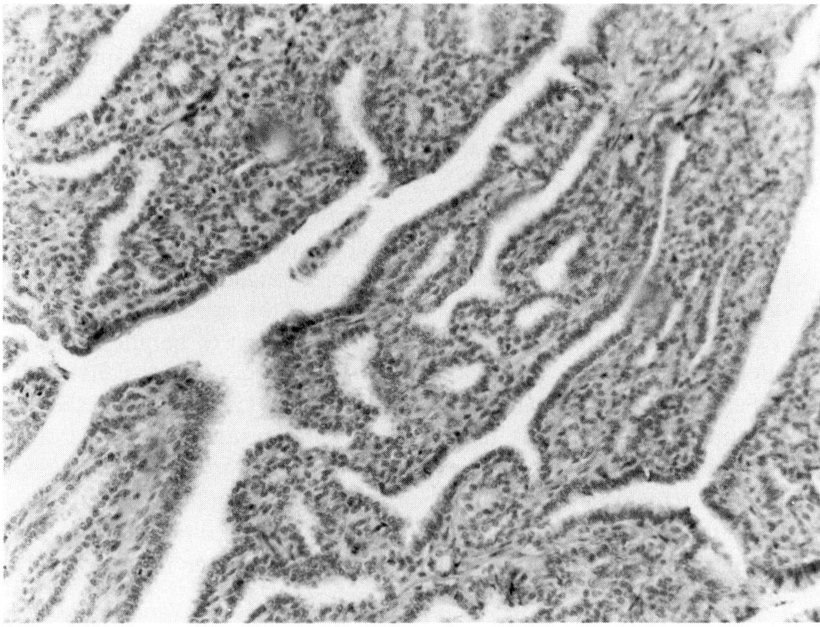

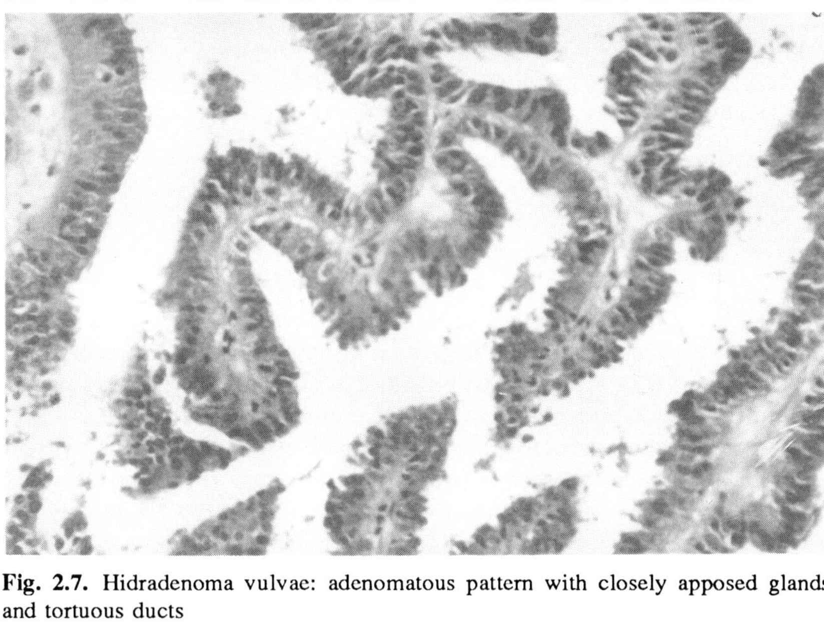

Fig. 2.7. Hidradenoma vulvae: adenomatous pattern with closely apposed glands and tortuous ducts

Fig. 2.8. Hidradenoma vulvae: papillae lined by cuboidal and columnar cells

2.1.8.2 Microscopical Appearance

The solid tumour, which is less common than the cystic type, displays predominantly an adenomatous pattern composed of closely opposed glands and ducts (Fig. 2.7) lined by two layers of cells, the luminal layer of cuboidal or columnar cells with eosinophilic cytoplasm and basal vesicular nuclei, and the deeper layer of spindle or low cuboidal cells with a small amount of cytoplasm and small, dark nuclei. The cystic variety shows tubules as well as complex, interwoven, papillary structures supported on variable, stromal connective tissue. The cells lining the papillae are cuboidal to columnar in shape, arranged either stratified or in a single layer (Fig. 2.8). Secretory activities present at the apical part of the cells are known as the decapitation phenomenon and are thought to be artefactual due to dehydration and shrinkage (Ioannides 1966). Small foci of clear cells (Ioannides 1966) and squamous cells due to squamous metaplasia (Woodruff and Seeds 1962) may occasionally be seen. The tumour bears close histological similarities with papillary hidradenoma and breast papilloma. Whether these two lesions are similar in histogenesis remains a subject of speculation (Novak and Stevensen 1945).

Ultrastructural studies of the tumour showed the presence of secretory granules, well-developed Golgi apparatus, decapitation secretion and myoepithelial cells, which all support apocrine differentiation (Hashimoto 1973).

The tumour is benign. Although a malignant variety has been reported (McDonald 1941), such tumours are, indeed, very rare (Novak and Stevenson 1945).

2.1.8.3 Treatment

Simple excision is adequate. Recurrence after the excision is very rare.

2.1.9 Syringoma

Syringomas are soft, firm, skin-coloured, slightly raised nodules 1–2 cm in diameter arising from the ductal cells of the accrine sweat glands (Carneiro et al. 1971; Zalla and Perry 1971). Although only eight cases of vulval syringoma have been reported in the English literature up to 1982 (Ghirardini 1982), these lesions may not be as uncommon as generally thought (Carneiro et al. 1971). Vulval syringomas can be seen in patients between 9 (Brown and Freeman 1971) and 74 years old (Ghirardini 1982). They become manifest usually at or shortly after puberty (Ridley 1975). Syringomas commonly occur on one of the labia majora but display a strong tendency to be bilateral and symmetrical in distribution (Isaacson and Turner 1979; Thomas et al. 1979). The tumours are mostly asymptomatic and discovered accidentally. Occasionally the lesions are associated with mild pruritus (Young et al. 1980). Patients with Down's syndrome have been reported to be thirty times more prone to develop these lesions than the normal population (Butterworth et al. 1964). The lesions have also been noticed in association with familial benign pemphigus (King et al. 1978).

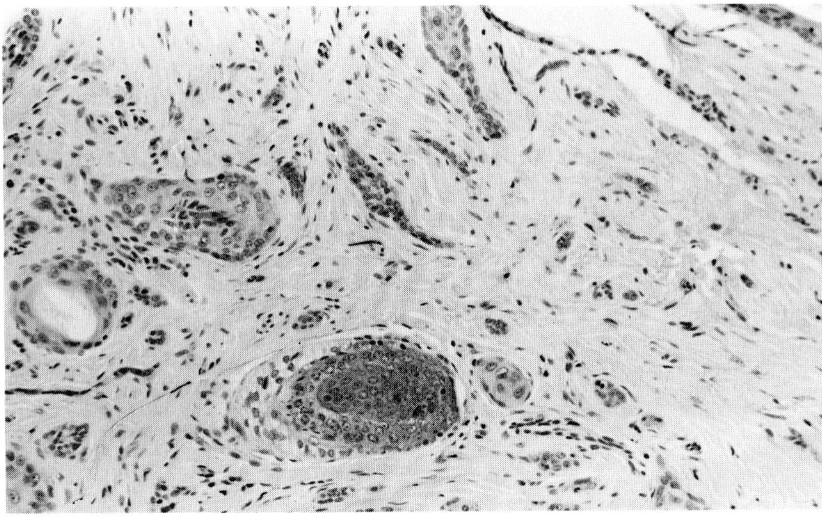

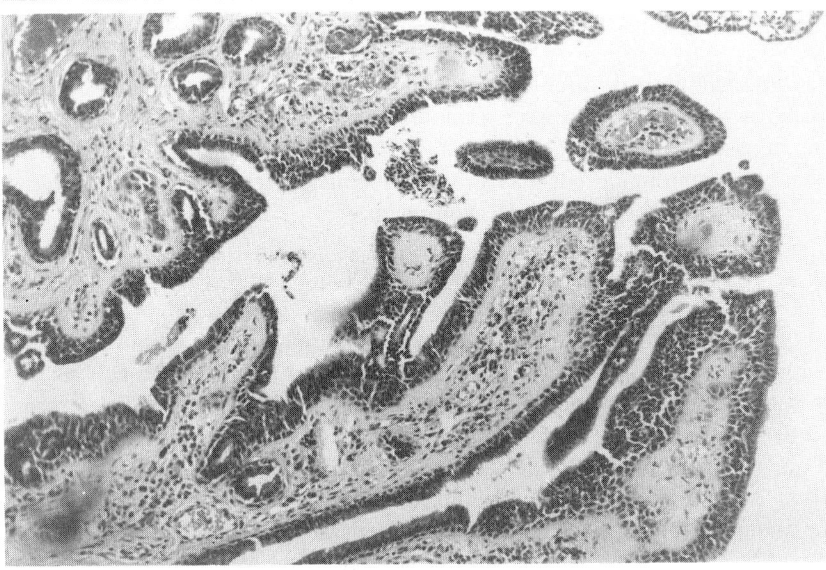

Fig. 2.9. Syringoma: elongated and curved eccrine structures of basaloid cells

Fig. 2.10. Syringocystadenoma papilliferum: papillary structures lined by two layers of cells, fibrous core contains many plasma cells

2.1.9.1 Microscopical Appearance

The lesions consist of numerous small cystic ducts with comma-like ends scattered in the dense fibrous stroma of the dermis (Fig. 2.9). They may also be composed of tadpole-shaped, solid structures made of basaloid epithelial cells. The ducts are lined by two layers of flattened cells; the inner layer may be clear and vacuolated. A clear cell variant which is composed of circumscribed masses of clear cells and not otherwise distinct from the classic type has also been described (Furue et al. 1984). The lumen may be filled with dense, colloid secretions. Trichoepitheliomatous elements can be noticed occasionally in these lesions (Guindi et al. 1974).

2.1.9.2 Treatment

Treatment is usually not necessary, but the tumours may be excised for symptoms or cosmetic reason.

2.1.10 Syringocystadenoma Papilliferum

Syringocystadenoma papilliferum is a benign tumour of apocrine duct origin and infrequent on the vulva. It occurs commonly as a small papillomatous lesion on the labium majus and clitoris (Woodruff and Seeds 1962). The tumour is slow-growing and usually asymptomatic but may produce itchiness, irritation and discharge. Ulceration and bleeding are infrequent complications.

2.1.10.1 Microscopical Apperance

The tumour shows cystic or funnel-shaped epidermal invaginations in the dermis, with numerous, duct-like, tubular structures and papillary projections at the deeper part. Both tubular and papillary structures are lined by two layers of cells (Fig. 2.10). The luminal layer is formed of tall columnar cells with eosinophilic cytoplasm and pale nuclei, while the deeper layer is composed of cuboidal cells containing a moderate amount of cytoplasm and vesicular nuclei. Abundant connective tissue stroma support the paillae and separate the ductal structures. Plasma cells are characteristically numerous in the stroma, particularly of the papillae. Occasionally, small group of squamous cells may be seen at the top of the papillae. The epidermis adjacent to the tumour may be acanthotic.

2.1.10.2 Treatment

Syringocystadenoma papilliferum is a benign tumour which rarely becomes invasive (Dissanayake and Salm 1980). The lesion should be completely excised.

2.1.11 Pleomorphic Adenoma (Chondroid Syringoma)

Pleomorphic adenoma, as it is known in the gynaecological literature, also has other eponyms such as mixed tumours and chondroid syringoma: the latter term is widely accepted. This tumour is commonly seen in the head and neck region and infrequently on the vulva. When it occurs at this site, one of the labia majora is usually affected (Rorat and Wallace 1984). Bartholin's glands have also been thought as the possible site of origin (Ordonez et al. 1981).

2.1.11.1 Gross Appearance

The tumour occurs as an unencapsulated, lobulated, discrete nodule averaging 1.5 in size.

2.1.11.2 Microscopic Appearance

The tumour is composed of tubular structures of various sizes lined by two layers of cells (Fig. 2.11). The luminal layer is low cuboidal whereas the outer layer consists of flattened myoepithelial cells. The stroma is abundant with areas of mucoid changes and cartilagenous foci. The mucoid areas show positive staining reactions with alcian blue, periodic acid-Schiff (PAS) and aldehyde fuchsin. The alcian blue reaction is not altered by pretreatment with hyaluronidase. The reported tumours of the labium majus consisted predominantly of myoepithelial cells with abundant mucoid stroma containing many pseudocartilaginous foci (Wilson and Woodger 1974), areas of bone and apocrine epithelium (Lennox 1954).

Malignant chondroid syringoma is very rare, and only nine cases have so far been reported from all sites (Ishimura et al. 1983). The malignant variant displays pleomorphism, high rate of mitotic activity and sparse alveolar and ductal structures (Redono et al. 1982). The tumour is composed of nests and cords of pleomorphic, cuboidal and spindle cells with abundant myxoid strome. Extension outside the main tumour mass is often evident (Redono et al. 1982; Ishimura et al. 1983). Metastases, albeit rare, can occur both by the lymphatic system and blood stream.

The origin of the vulval tumour is thought to be from the sweat glands (Wilson and Woodger 1974) but according to Hertig and Gore (1960), the paravestibular glands are a possible source.

2.1.11.3 Treatment an Biological Behaviour

These tumours are generally benign and can be excised with adequate free margins. Rare reccurrences (Botha and Kahn 1978) and metastases (Hilton and Blackwell 1973) have been reported. One of the vulval mixed tumours reported by Ordonez et al. (1981) was malignant and metastasised to the lungs. The tumour displayed areas of pleomorphic adenoma, adenocystic and undifferentiated carcinoma with many mitoses.

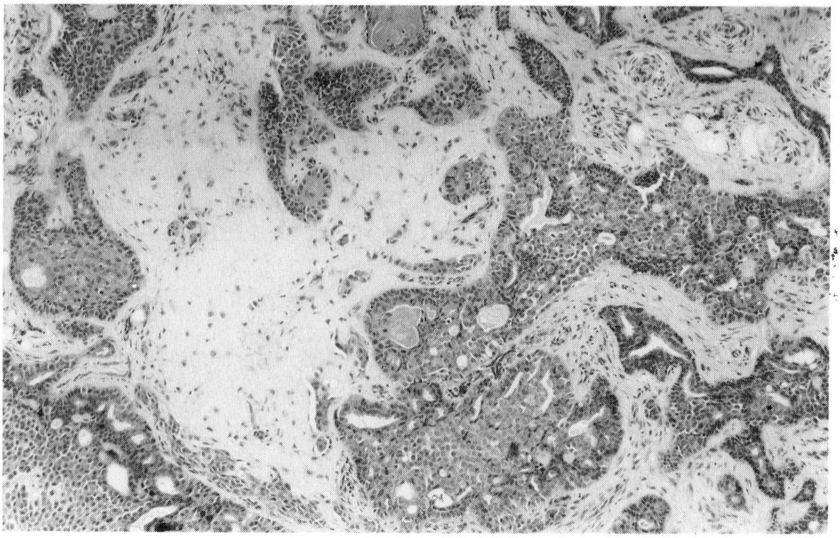

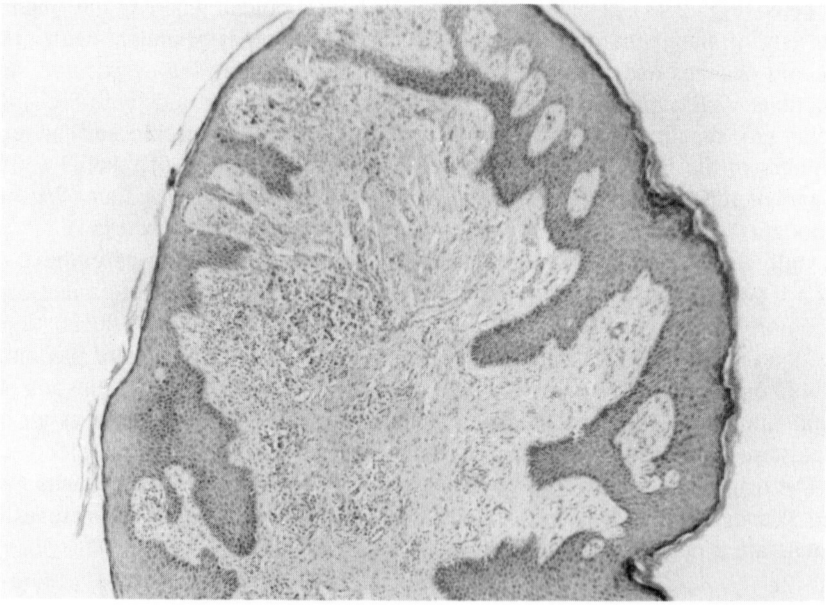

Fig. 2.11. Pleomorphic adenoma: solid tubular and chondroid area

Fig. 2.12. Skin tag: polypoid mass of connective tissue covered by thickened layer of squamous cells

2.1.12 Pilar Tumour

Also known as pilomatrixoma and calcifying epithelioma, pilar tumours occur commonly on the skin of the extremities, face and scalp. The tumour is believed to originate from the anterior root hair sheath (Holmes 1968). According to Dabska (1971), the pilar tumours are distinct from pilomatrixomas and should be differentiated by their larger size, infiltrative character and lack of metastatic potential. They may recur when incompletely excised. The pilar tumours are rare on the vulval skin but can nevertheless occur at this site (Buchler et al. 1978).

Clinically, these tumours may appear as nodules which can ulcerate and are erroneously diagnosed as carcinoma.

2.1.12.1 Microscopical Appearance

They are dermal tumours composed of lobules of squamous cells with varying degrees of maturation from the periphery toward the centre where keratins are formed. The squamous cells do not display atypia or mitoses. The peripheral margins may be irregular with small tongues of benign-looking sequamous cells. Cystic changes and foci of calcifications are common. Chronic inflammatory cell infiltrations can be seen in the stroma around the tumour.

2.1.12.2 Treatment

The tumour is benign, and adequate excision is curative.

2.1.13 Trichoepithelioma

Trichoepithelioma, also known as epithelioma adenoides cysticum, is a benign tumour of the hair follicle. Two types of tumours are known: a multiple, autosomal dominant type and a solitary type which does not show any definite mode of transmission. The hereditary multiple type commonly appears in childhood on the face, gradually becomes numerous (Gray and Helwig 1963) and spreads to forehead, scalp, neck and trunk. Grossly, they are skin-coloured, rounded or dome-shaped nodules 2–8 mm in diameter. Skin covering the nodules remains intact, but the long-standing lesions which gradually become confluent and large tend to ulcerate (Ziprkowski and Schewach-Miller 1956). The solitary variant is more common than the hereditary type. The face is the common site of occurrence, but other areas may also be affected. The nodule is usually larger than the nodules of the hereditary type (Muller-Hess and Delacrelaz 1973). The genital area is rarely involved by either type. The two patiens with vulval lesion reported were 60 and 66 years old (Cho and Woodruff 1988). In both patients the lesions were solitary and located close to the clitoris.

2.1.13.1 Microscopical Appearance

Both solitary and multiple types display similar histological features. They are composed of irregular masses of small, dark cells with scant cytoplasm and oval nuclei which appear similar to the cells of basal cell carcinoma. The cells surround keratin-filled horn cysts, which are a prominent feature of this lesion and may be numerous. Structures simulating abortive hair follicles can also be noticed. In the solitary type, the solid masses of small cells with peripheral palisading are hardly distinguishable from a basal cell carcinoma. Both solitary (Brownstein and Shapiro 1976) and multiple desmoplastic trichoepitheliomas (Lazorik and Wood 1982) are composed of small nests of basaloid cells embedded in dense fibrous tissue.

2.1.13.2 Treatment

Excision of the lesion is adequate.

2.2 Tumour-like Conditions

2.2.1 Skin Tag

The skin tags, also known as fibroma molle and fibroepithelial polyps, are sessile or pedunculated, soft, wrinkled, polypoid masses, a few millimeters to a few centimeters in size. They are quite common on the vulva and perineum. Their aetiology is unknown. Such skin tags are occasionally extraintestinal manifestations of Crohn's disease (Fielding 1972; Holohan et al. 1988). They should therefore be subjected to histological examination for the presence of granulomas.

Histologically, the skin tags consist of polypoid masses of fibrovascular connective tissue covered by thickened and wrinkled squamous epithelium (Fig. 2.12). Malignant changes in the covering epithelium is rare, although in situ carcinoma can occasionally be seen in association with human papillomavirus infections.

2.2.1.1 Treatment

The Treatment is simple excision.

2.2.2 Verruca Vulgaris

Verruca vulgaris lesions are a few millimeters to a few centimeters in size, occurring as single or in groups of warty polypoid lesions on the vulval skin. Human papillomavirus (HPV) is thought to be the aetiological agent. HPV capsid antigen and type 2 genomes have been demonstrated in these lesions (Eversole et al. 1987).

2.2.2.1 Microscopical Appearance

The epidermal changes consist of hyperkeratosis, parakeratosis, papillomatosis and elongation of rete pegs. The stratum malpighii and granular layer show foci of large, vauolated cells containing intranuclear and intracytoplasmic eosinophilic inclusion bodies (Fig. 2.13). The granular cells are usually absent over the papillomatous crests.

2.2.2.2 Treatment

Verrucae disappear spontaneously in 50% or more of cases. Electrocauterisation is commonly used when treatment is necessary.

2.2.3 Sebaceous Gland Hyperplasia

The common sites of sebaceous gland hyperplasia are the face and forehead. Hyperplastic sebaceous glands are occasionally seen on the vulval skin of women past middle age as punctate yellow papules (Rocamora et al. 1986). Histologically, the lesions consist of an increased number of mature sebaceous glands and ducts arranged in lobules (Fig. 2.14). Some of the ducts may be dilated. The openings of the main ducts to the skin surface correspond to the punctations of papules. Hair follicles of the area do not take part in these changes. Diagnosis of sebaceous gland hyperplasia is most often made after excision (Knox and Freeman 1965).

The lesions are to be differentiated from sebaceous adenomas, which are well-circumscribed due to compression of the surrounding collagen and composed of lobules of sebaceous glands in varying stages of maturity. Basaloid and transitional cells may be seen at the periphery of the lobules (Rulon and Helwig 1974).

2.2.3.1 Treatment

Treatment is excision.

2.2.4 Fox-Fordyce Disease

Fox-Fordyce disease is characterised by multiple, firm, pruritic papules occurring in the pubic and perianal region. The papules are formed due to obstruction of the apocrine ducts following excessive hyperkeratosis. As the apocrine glands are not functional before puberty, the disease rarely manifests earlier. The lesions occur in groups of discrete macules 1–3 mm in diameter in the apocrine gland-bearing areas – axillae, nipples and perineum. It is a chronic disease persisting for many years with pruritic exacerbation during menstruation. There is some improvement of symptoms during pregnancy and when the patient is on oral contraceptives, suggesting a strong association with hormonal factors. Fox-Fordyce disease appears

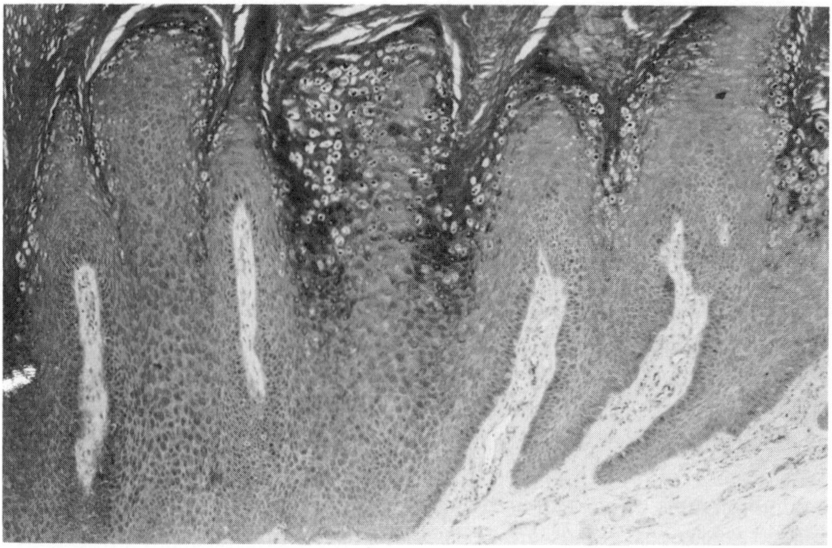

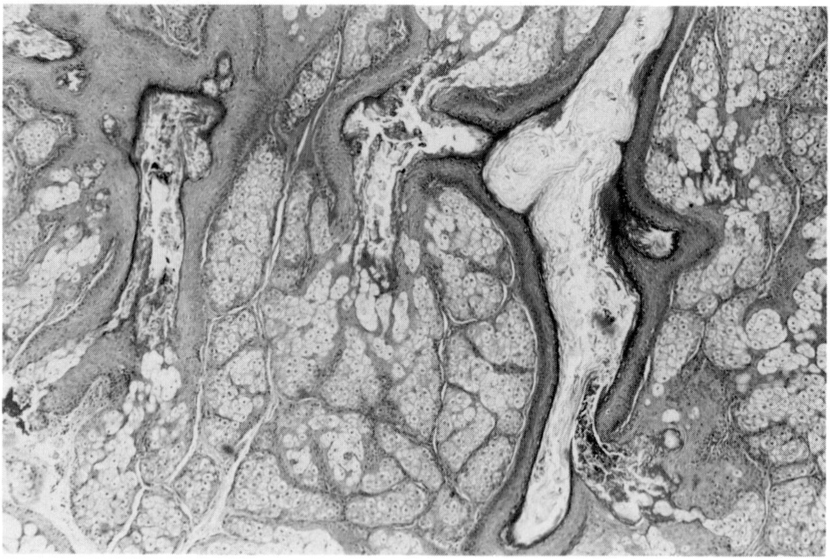

Fig. 2.13. Verruca vulgaris: hyperkeratosis, papillomatosis and large, vacuolated cells in the stratum malpighii

Fig. 2.14. Sebaceous gland hyperplasia: lobules of hyperplastic sebaceous glands

to be a systemic lesion due to dysfunction of the apocrine glands (Montes et al. 1959).

2.2.4.1 Microscopical Appearance

The terminal intra-epidermal apocrine ducts are obstructed by hyperkeratotic plugs, leading to the formation of retention vesicles which are diagnostic of the condition (Shelley and Levy 1956). The vesicles are usually small and missed in the histological sections unless serial sections are made (MacMillan and Vickers 1971). The dilated and distended ducts filled with inspissated secretion of mucoprotein rupture with excitatiaon of local inflammatory reactions.

2.2.4.2 Treatment

Beneficial results have been reported with oestrogen therapy (Kronthal et al. 1965).

2.2.5 Nodular Amyloidosis

Amyloidosis denotes a group of diseases characterised by deposition of diverse, abnormal, fibrillar proteins in the extra- and intracellular spaces (Castano and Frangione 1988). The fibrillar proteins, although looking structurally similar, are derived from different sources in different diseases. The fibrillar proteins of multiple myeloma are formed from a light chain of immunoglobulin produced by the myeloma cells; in medullary carcinoma of thyroid they are derived from the polypeptide hormone; and in inflammatory conditions the proteins are formed of the N-terminal two-thirds of acute phase proteins manufactured by the hepatic cells.

Clinically, amlyoidosis is classified into primary, secondary and localised forms. In primary amyloidosis, which occurs usually in the connective tissue, the fibrils are made of AL protein consisting of fragments or intact light chain or both of an immunoglobulin (Glenner et al. 1971). In secondary or reactive amyloidosis, which affects epithelial cells chiefly, the fibrils are composed of protein (AA protein) not related to any of the known immunoglobulins but rather to the N-terminal two-thirds of serum protein. Protein AA has a serum precursor (SAA, serum amyloid A protein), which is an apoprotein of high density lipoprotein and present in the serum of normal individuals (Benditt and Eriksen 1977). The fibrils of nodular amyloidosis of skin have been found to be composed of AL protein (Husby et al. 1981). However, the precise character of the structural protein of localised cutaneous amlyoidosis has not yet been clearly defined (Mashu et al. 1981; Ann et al. 1988). The epidermal keratinocytes have been suggested to be the source of cutaneous amyloid which is formed through several sequential stages of ultrastructural changes in these cells. Initially, there are fibrillar changes in the cytoplasm followed by formation of bundles of tonofilaments with the degeneration of cell organelles, filamentous degeneration of the tonofilaments converting them into tightly packed whorls and bundles, formation of filamentous masses, early accumulation of amyloid in the upper dermis and finally in the deeper dermis (Kumakiri and Hashimoto 1979).

The vulval skin can be affected by primary, secondary and localised amyloidosis. It is usually the primary amyloidosis which tends to manifest with a primary skin lesion; involvement of the skin in the secondary type is infrequent (Danielsen et al. 1970). Cutaneous, localised amyloidosis can be either nodular, lichenoid or macular. The nodular form of primary amyloidosis may affect the face, trunk, extremities and genitalia. The vulva is only rarely affected (Northcutt and Vanover 1985).

Clinically, the patients are elderly (in their 50s) and present with multiple, shiny, pinkish to brownish nodules averaging 0.5 cm in size on the vulva. When the nodules ulcerate, a mistaken diagnosis of malignancy may be made.

2.2.5.1 Microscopical Appearance

The amyloid nodules occupy the entire dermis, extending up to the subcutaneous fat. Deposition may also be noticed in the wall of the blood vessels, sweat glands and fat cells (Lindemayr and Partsch 1970). The nodules are composed of hyaline, amorphous, eosinophilic material which displays light-green birefringence with Congo red, purple blue with crystal violet and fluorescence with thioflavin-T. Ultrastructurally, all types of amyloid, irrespective of origin, consist of parallel arrays of non-branching filaments of variable length, and all of them have a characteristic diameter of 7–10 nm (Shirahama and Cohen 1967). In X-ray diffraction studies, the fibrils exhibit crossed B-pleated sheet structure (Kisilevsky 1983).

At the periphery of amyloid, a variable number of chronic inflammatory cells with predominant plasma cells can be seen in the majority of skin lesions.

Nodular amyloidosis of the skin is to be differentiated from lichenoid and macular amyloidosis by its large mass involving the entire dermis, whereas in the latter two conditions amyloids involve only the papillary dermis. In the lichenoid type the peidermis is acanthotic and hyperkeratotic, whereas in the macular type the epidermis is normal; in nodular amyloidosis the epidermis is atrophic and may ulcerate.

2.2.5.2 Treatment

As some patients with localised amyloidosis later develop systemic disease (Brownstein and Helwig 1970), follow-up of the patients by gingival and rectal biopsy and evaluation of immunoglobulin is necessary (Northcutt and Vanover 1985). At present no satisfactory treatment of amyloidosis seems to be available.

2.2.6 Isolated Epidermolytic Acanthoma

Isolated epidermolytic acanthoma appears as a light-pink, oval nodule with a shiny or rough surface and is about 1.0 cm in diameter (Lindgren and Neumann 1973). The lesion usually occurs on the eyelids, cheeks, extremities and genital region and clinically may simulate a soft fibroma, molluscum contagiosum or warts (Shapiro and Baraf 1970). It is rare on the vulva. The patient reported by Coninck et al. (1986) was a 60-year-old woman who presented with vulval pruritis for several years. On examination the lesion was found to consist of four, verrucoid, light-brown nodules averaging 5 mm in diameter on the left labium majus.

The essential histological features are epidermolytic hyperkeratosis (Frost et al. 1966), also described as granular degeneration (Ishibashi and Klingmuller 1968). The epidermis is thickened, and there are compact hyperkeratosis, conspicuous, clear spaces around the nuclei of stratum malpighii and granulosum, indistinct cell boundaries due to lightly staining amphophilic material and a thickened granular zone containing an increased number of keratohyaline-like bodies (Ackerman 1970). Although a few congenital or heriditary conditions share these histological festures, isolated epidermolytic acanthoma is not congenital or familial (Shapiro and Baraf 1970).

References

Epidermal Cysts

Knox JM, Freeman RG (1965) Epidermal tumors. Clin Obstet Gynecol 8:925–937

Ofadile FA, Oluwasanmi JO (1979) Post circumcisional epidermal cysts of the clitoris. Plast Reconstr Surg 63:485–486

Pilar Cyst

Sachdeva HS, Narang R (1968) Sebaceous cyst vulva. A case report. Am Surg 34:461–462

Seborrheic Keratosis

Holdiness MR (1986) The sign of Leser-Trelat. Int J Dermatol 25:564–572

Holguin T, Padilla RS, Ampuere F (1986) Ovarian adenocarcinoma presenting with sign of Leser-Trelat. Gynecol Oncol 25:128–132

Knox JM, Freeman RG (1965) Epidermal tumors. Obstet Gynecol 8:925–937

Keratoacanthoma

Fathizadeh A, Medenica MM, Sultani K et al. (1982) Aggressive keratoacanthoma and internal malignant neoplasm. Arch Dermatol 118:112–114

McCormac H, Scarff RW (1936) Molluscum sebaceum. Br J Dermatol 48:624–626

Piscioli F, Boi S, Zumiani G et al. (1984) A gigantic metastasising keroacanthoma: report of a case and discussion on classification. Am J Dermatopathol 6:123–129

Rhatigan RM, Nuss RC (1985) Keratoacanthoma of the vulva. Gynecol Oncol 21:118–123

Sullivan JJ, Colditz GA (1979) Keratoacanthoma in a subtropical climate. Aust J Dermatol 20:34–42

Angiokeratoma

Blair C (1970) Angiokeratoma of the vulva. Br J Dermatol 83:409–411

Clark JR, Wheelock JR (1988) Angiokeratoma of the vulva: a case report. J Reprod Med 33:473–474
Dotters DJ, Fowler WC Jr, Powers SK et al. (1986) Argon laser therapy of vulvar angiokeratoma. Obstet Gynecol 68 [Suppl]:56–59
Imperial R, Helwig EB (1967) Angiokeratoma of the vulva. Obstet Gynecol 29:307–312
Novick L (1985) Angiokeratoma vulvae. J Am Acad Dermatol 12:561–563
Uhlin SR (1980) Angiokeratoma of the vulva. Arch Dermatol 116:112–113
Verbov J, Manglabruks K (1978) Angiokeratoma of the vulva. Dermatologica 156:296–298

Warty Dyskeratoma
Duray PH, Merino HJ, Axiotis C (1983) Warty dyskeratoma of the vulva. Int J Gynecol Pathol 2:286–293

Verruciform Xanthoma
Santa-Cruz DJ, Martin SA (1979) Verriciform xanthoma of the vulva. Am J Clin Pathol 71:224–228

Hidradenoma Vulvae
Chung JT (1958) Hidradenoma of the vulva. Am J Obstet Gynecol 75:310–318
Cox EA (1954) Hidradenoma of the perineum. Am J Surg 88:789–792
Danforth WC (1943) Hidradenoma vulvae. Am J Obstet Gynecol 45:329–333
Deacon AL, Taylor CW (1952) Hidradenoma of the vulva. J Obstet Gynaecol Br Emp 59:64–66
Hashimoto K (1973) Hidradenoma pepilliferum: an electron microscopic study. Acta Derm. Venereol (Stockh) 53:22–30
Ioannides G (1966) Hidradenoma papilliferum. Am J Obstet Gynecol 94:849–853
Kaufmann T, Pawi NO, Sohfer I et al. (1987) Cystic papillary hidradenoma of the vulva: a case report and review of the literature. Gynecol Oncol 26:240–245
McDonald JR, Lovelady SB, Waugh JM (1941) Adenocarcinoma of the vulva. Am J Obstet Gynecol 42:304–309
Meeker JH, Neubecker RD, Helwig EB (1962) Hidradenoma papilliferum. Am J Clin Pathol 37:182–195
Nielsen NC (1973) Hidradenoma of the vulva. Acta Obstet Gynecol Scand 52:387–389
Novak E, Stevenson RR (1945) Sweat gland tumors of the vulva: benign (hidradenoma) and malignant (adenocarcinoma). Am J Obstet Gynecol 50:641–659
Woodruff JD, Seeds AE Jr (1962) Benign and malignant adenomatous lesions of the vulva: summaries of six cases. Obstet Gynecol 20:690–695
Woodworth H Jr, Dockerty MB, Wilson RB et al. (1971) Papillary hidradenoma of the vulva: a clinicopathological study of 69 cases. Am J Obstet Gynecol 110:501–506

Syringoma
Brown SM, Freeman RG (1971) Syringoma limited to the vulva. Arch Dermatol 104:331
Butterworth T, Strean LP, Beerman H et al. (1964) Syringoma and mongolism. Arch Dermatol 90:483–487
Carneiro SGC, Gardner HL, Knox JM (1971) Syringoma of the vulva. Arch Dermatol 103:494–496
Furue M, Hori Y, Nakabayashi Y (1984) Clear cell syringoma associated with diabetes mellitus. Am J Dermatopathol 6:131–150
Ghirardini G (1982) Syringoma of the vulva in postmenopausal age. Diagn Gynecol Obstet 4:325–326
Guindi SF, Silberberg BK, Evans TN (1974) Multifocal mixed adnexoid tumors of the vulva. In J Gynecol Obstet 12:138–140
Issacson D, Turner ML (1979) Localised vulvar syringoma. J Am Acad Dermatol 1:352–356

King DT, Hirose M, King LA (1978) Simultaneous occurrence of familial pemphigus (Heiley-Heiley disease) and syringoma of the vulva. Arch Dermatol 114:801

Ridley CM (1975) The vulva: major problems in dermatology. Saunders, London, pp 224–225

Thomas J, Majumdar B, Gorelkin L (1979) Syringoma localised to the vulva. Arch Dermatol 115:95–96

Young AW Jr, Herman EW, Tovell HMM (1980) Syringoma of the vulva: incidence, diagnosis and cause of pruritus. Obstet Gynecol 55:515–518

Zalla JA, Perry HO (1971) An unusual case of syringoma. Arch Dermatol 103:215–217

Syringocystadenoma Papilliferum

Dissanayake EVP, Salm R (1980) Sweat gland carcinoma: prognosis related to histological types. Histopathology 4:445–466

Woodruff JD, Seeds AE Jr (1962) Benign and malignant adenomatous lesions of the vulva: summaries of six cases. Obstet Gynecol 20:690–695

Pleomorphic Adenoma

Botha JBC, Kahn LB (1978) Aggressive chondroid syringoma. Arch Dermatol 114:954–955

Hertig AT, Gore H (1960) Atlas of tumor pathology: tumors of the female sex organs, pt 2. Armed Forces Institute of Pathology, Washington DC, pp 68–69

Hilton JMN, Blackwell JB (1973) Metastasising chondroid syringoma. J Pathol 109:167–170

Ishimura E, Iwamoto H, Kobashi Y et al. (1983) Malignant chondroid syringoma: report of a case with widespread metastasis and review of pertinent literature. Cancer 52:1966–1973

Lennox B (1954) The superficial hidradenomata. J Pathol Bacteriol 67:553–562

Ordonez NG, Manning AT, Luna MA (1981) Mixed tumors of the vulva: a report of two cases probably arising in Bartholin's gland. Cancer 48:181–185

Redono C, Rocamora A, Villoria F et al. (1982) Malignant mixed tumor of the skin: malignant chondroid syringoma. Cancer 49:1690–1696

Rorat E, Wallace RC (1984) Mixed tumors of the vulva: clinical outcome and pathology. Int J Gynecol Pathol 3:323–328

Wilson D, Woodger BA (1974) Pleomorphic adenoma of the vulva. J Obstet Gynaecol Br Commonw 81:1000–1002

Pilar Tumour

Buchler DA, Sun F, Chuprevich T (1978) Pilar tumor of the vulva. Gynecol Oncol 6:479–486

Debska M (1971) Giant hair matrix tumor. Cancer 28:701–706

Holmes EJ (1968) Tumors of lower hair sheath. Cancer 21:234–248

Trichoepithelioma

Brownstein MH, Shapiro L (1976) Desmoplastic trichoepithelioma. Arch Dermatol 112:1782

Cho D, Woodruff JD (1988) Trichoepithelioma of the vulva: report of two cases. J Reprod Med 33:317–319

Gray HR, Helwig EB (1963) Epithelioma adenoides cysticum and solitory trichoepithelioma. Arch Dermatol 87:102–114

Lazorik FC, Wood MG (1982) Multiple desmoplastic trichoepitheliomas. Arch Dermatol 118:361–362

Muller-Hess S, Delacrelaz J (1973) Trichoepitheliom mit Strukturen eines apocrinen Adenoms. Dermatologica 146:170–176

Ziprkowski L, Schewach-Miller M (1956) Multiple trichoepithelioma in a mother and two children. Dermatologica 132:248–256

Skin Tag

Fielding JF (1972) Perianal lesions in Crohn's disease. J R Coll Surg Edinb 17:32–37

Holohan M, Coughlan M, O'Loughlin S et al. (1988) Crohn's disease of vulva: case report. Br J Obstet Gynaecol 95:943–945

Verruca Vulgaris

Eversole LR, Laipis PJ, Green TL (1987) Human papillomavirus virus type 2 DNA in oral and labial verruca vulgaris. J Cutan Pathol 14:319–325

Sebaceous Gland Hyperplasia

Knox JM, Greeman RC (1965) Epidermal tumors. Clin Obstet Gynecol 8:925–937

Rocamora A, Santonja C, Vives R et al. (1986) Sebaceous gland hyperplasia of the vulva: a case report. Obstet Gynecol 68 [Suppl]:63–65

Rulon DB, Helwig EB (1974) Cutaneous sebaceous neoplasm. Cancer 33:82–102

Fox Fordyce Disease

Kronthal HL, Pomeranz JR, Sitomer G (1965) Fox-Fordyce disease. Arch Dermatol 91:243–245

MacMillan DC, Vickers HR (1971) Fox Fordyce disease. Br J Dermatol 84:181

Montes LF, Cortes A, Baker BL et al. (1959) Fox-Fordyce disease. Arch Dermatol 80:549–553

Shelley WB, Levy DJ (1956) Apocrine sweat retention in man. II. Fox-Fordyce disease (apocrine milaria). Arch Dermatol 73:38–49

Nodular Amyloidosis

Ann CC, Lin C-S, Wong C-K (1988) Nodular amyloidosis. Clin Exp Dermatol 13:20–23

Benditt EP, Eriksen N (1977) Amyloid protein SAA is associated with high density lipoprotein from human serum. Proc Natl Acad Sci USA 74:4025–4028

Brownstein M, Helwig E (1970) The cutaneous amyloidosis: localised forms. Arch Dermatol 102:8–19

Castano EM, Frangione B (1988) Human amyloidosis, Alzheimer disease, and related disorders. Lab Invest 58:122–132

Danielsen L, Christensen HE, Wanstrup J (1970) Cutaneous amyloidosis: classification, pathogenesis and relation to collagen disease. Acta Pathol Microbiol Scand [A] 78:335–344

Glenner GG, Terry W, Harada M et al. (1971) Amyloid fibril proteins. Proof of homology with immunoglobulin light chains by sequence analyses. Science 172:1150–1151

Husby G, Sletten K, Blumenkrantz N et al. (1981) Characterisation of an amyloid fibril protein from localised amyloidosis of the skin as lamda immunoglobulin light chains of variable subgroup I (A lamda I). Clin Exp Immunol 45:90–96

Kisilevsky R (1983) Amyloidosis: a familiar problem in the light of current pathogenetic developments. Lab Invest 49:381–390

Kumakiri M, Hashimoto K (1979) Histogenesis of primary localised cutaneous amyloidosis. J Invest Dermatol 73:150–152

Lindemayr W, Partsch H (1970) Plattenartig infiltrierte localisierte Hautamyloïose. Hautarzt 2:104–107

Mashu S, Hosokawa M, Seiji M (1981) Amyloid in cutaneous amyloidosis: immunofluorescence studies with antikeratin antiserum especially concerning the difference between systemic and cutaneous amyloidosis. Acta Derm Venereol (Stockh) 61:381–384

Northcutt AD, Vanover MJ (1985) Nodular cutaneous amyloidosis involving the vulva: case report and literature review. Arch Dermatol 121:518–521

Shirahama T, Cohen AS (1967) High resolution electron microscopic analysis of the amyloid fibril. J Cell Biol 33:679–708

Isolated Epidermolytic Acanthoma

Ackerman AB (1970) Histopathological concept of epidermolytic hyperkeratosis. Arch Dermatol 102:220–223

Coninck AD, Willemsen M, Dobbeleer GD et al. (1986) Vulvar localisation of epidermolytic acanthoma: a light and electron microscopic study. Dermatologica 172:276–278

Frost P, Weinstein GD, van Scott EJ (1966) The ichthyosiform dermatosis. II Autoradiographic studies of epidermal proliferation. J Invest Dermatol 47:561–567

Ishibashi Y, Klingmuller G (1968) Erythroderma ichthyoseformis congenita bullosa. Arch Klin Exp Dermatol 232:205–224

Lindgren AGH, Neumann E (1973) Some evidence concerning the sweat duct origin of clear cell acanthoma. Acta Derm Venereol (Stockh) 53:511–514

Shapiro L, Baraf S (1970) Isolated epidermytic acanthoma. Arch Dermatol 101:220–223

3 Developmental Cysts and Tumours

3.1 Paramesonephric Cyst, Mesonephric Cyst, Mucinous Ciliated Cyst, Urogenital Sinus Cyst

Controversies still surround the issue of origin of the vulval cysts lined by mucinous and ciliated epithelium. While the views are conflicting, it appears that because of the pleuripotentiality of the urogenital sinus epithelium and close proximity of several embryological structures in this area cysts may develop from any of these structures. According to Janovski (1962), these cysts develop from the paramesonephric epithelium which was displaced into the urogenital sinus during embryological development. Thus, one finds in the cysts the endocervical type mucinous and fallopian tube-type ciliated epithelium. This view has been supported in other reports (Hart 1970). The other view favouring a mesonephric duct origin was pur forward by Evans and Paine (1965), who held that the vestigial remnants of mesonephric ducts could be traced to the vestibule, and cysts could develop from these vestiges. It was also expressed that the paramesonephric mesoderm was not involved in the formation of the vestibule (Hamilton et al. 1972), which has been defined as that protion of the genital tract internal to the labia minora and external to the hymenal ring (Friedrich and Wilkinson 1973). Robboy et al. (1978), on the other hand, maintain that these cysts develop from the normal gland constituents of the vestibule, which are urogenital sinus derivatives. The mucinous type glands can be demonstrated regularly in this area at autopsy. They argue that adenosis and clear cell adenocarcinoma, which are known to occur in the vagina, a paramesonephric organ, of exposed to DES (diethylstilboestrol) women are almost unknown in the vulva. There is now a general tendency to include all these cysts in the category of mucinous cysts or ciliated mucinous cysts of the vulva. Novak and Woodruff (1979) favour the term mucinous cysts; these, according to them, develop from the aberrant mucinous epithelium displaced at the time of division of the cloaca by the urorectal fold. While it is convenient to follow a working rule, it is conceivable that this area of complex embryological development can harbour the vestiges of several embryological tissues, all of which may provide a source for the development of cysts or tumours.

The patients are usually asymptomatic but may present with gradually enlarging unilateral cysts on the labia minora, periclitoral tissue and vestibule. The size varies from a few millimeters to 10 cm. The cysts may be pedunculated when large and, depending on location, may cause dyspareunia und urinary symptoms. Occasionally, they may protrude into the introitus. The cysts are seldom noticed before puberty. Hormones (Friedrich and Wilkinson 1973) and pregnancy seem to exert stimulating effects on their growth.

The cysts are round and ovoid in shape, with a smooth and shiny external surface. The walls are thin, and the contents are either mucinous or watery.

3.1.1 Microscopical Appearance

Three types of epithelium may be identified in the lining of the cysts: (a) picket cell type of ednocervix, which are tall, columnar cells containing mucous-secreting pale cytoplasm, basal nuclei and prominent basement membrane (Fig. 3.1), (b) tubal type epithelium with ciliated, intercalated and secretory cells (Fig. 3.2) and (c) squamous cells. According to Janovski (1962), these cysts can be classified into the paramesonephric and mesonephric groups on the basis of histochemical reactions. The paramesonephric epithelium contains mucin, as demonstrated by PAS/D and alcian blue stains. The mesonephric cysts are lined by non-ciliated, low columnar, cuboidal (Fig. 3.3) or stratified squamous cells (Radman 1966). The wall of the mesonephric cyst contains smooth muscle fibres, and the lining epithelium is mucin negative (Janovski 1962). It is, nevertheless, true that even by elaborate histochemical stains such differentiation sometimes cannot be made with absolute certainty.

Ultrastructurally, the epithelial cells of a mucinous cyst display microvilli, secretory vacuoles indistinguishable from the mucus-producing cells of the gastrointestinal tract, Bartholin's glands, endocervical cells (Friedrich and Wilkinson 1973) and also paraurethral glands which are derived from the urogenital sinus (Oi and Munn 1982).

3.1.2 Treatment

In most cases these cysts can be excised. When the cysts insinuate in the parametrium or pelvis, wider exploration may be necessary to guard against damage to the urethra, bladder and ureter.

3.2 Cyst (Hydrocoele) of the Canal of Nuck

Cyst of the canal of Nuck, also known as hydrocoele of the canal of Nuck, is a collection of fluid in the rudimentary peritoneal recess along the course of the round ligament and is similar to the vaginal hydrocoele in the male. The canal is obliterated early in embryonic life. Incomplete obliteration at any level from the internal inguinal ring to the labium majus may lead to the accumulation of fluid in the sac with formation of uni- or multilocular cystic swelling. The average size

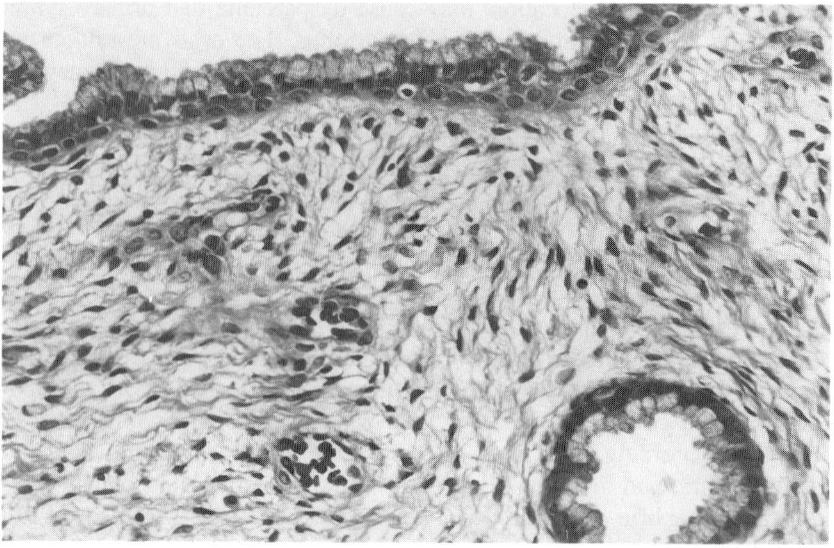

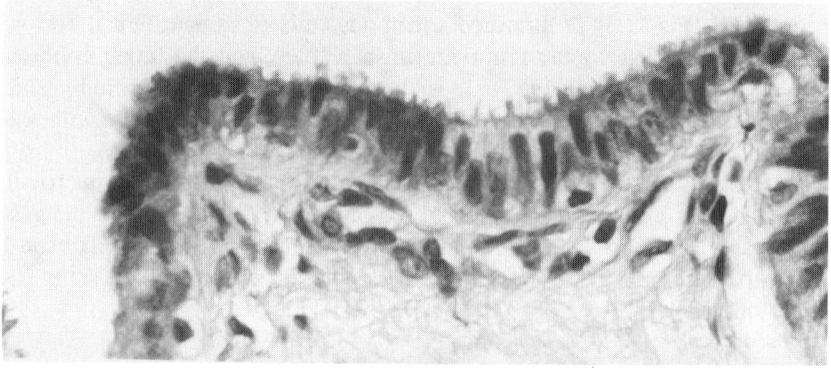

Fig. 3.1. Paramesonephric cyst: the cyst is lined by mucus-secreting columnar cells with basal nuclei

Fig. 3.2. Paramesonephric cyst: the cyst is lined by tubal type, ciliated epithelium

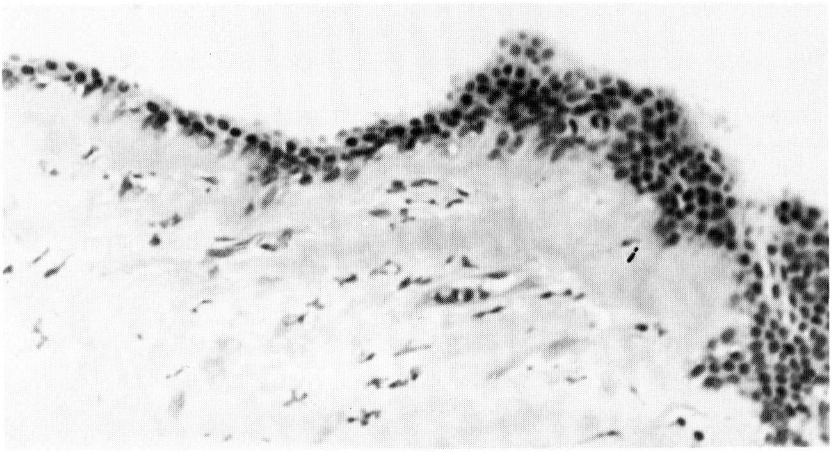

Fig. 3.3. Mesonephric cyst: the cyst is lined by cuboidal epithelium

of these cysts varies from 3 to 5 cm in diameter. On rare occasions, the cyst is large and extends to the retroperitoneal space (McCune 1948). The inner wall is smooth and lined by a single layer of flattened epithelium (mesothelium). Smooth muscle fibres may be present in the wall but are inconstant features (McElfatrick and Condon 1975). Inflammation and fibrosis may occasionally complicate the cyst. Inguinal hernia can be associated in one-third of all patients (Kucera and Glazer 1985).

The condition is to be differentiated from other swellings in the area, namely, hernia, other vulvovaginal cysts, adenomyosis and endometriosis (Block 1975). Endometriosis, on rare occasions, may occur within the canal of Nuck (Mesko et al. 1988).

3.2.1 Treatment

The cysts are usually asymptomatic and are removed when they are painful, tender, produce discomfort or cosmetic problems. Before excision, inguinal hernia should be excluded and if discovered, should be repaired (Schwartz and Peyser 1975).

References

Paramesonephric Cyst, Mesonephric Cyst, Mucinous Ciliated Cyst, Urogenital sinus Cyst

Evans DMD, Paine CG (1965) Benign cysts and tumors of developmental origin. Clin Obstet Gynecol 8:997–1019

Freidrich EG, Wilkinson EG (1973) Mucous cysts of the vulvar vestibule. Obstet Gynecol 42:407–414

Hamilton WJ, Boyd JD, Mossman HW (1962) Human embryology. Williams and Wilkins, Baltimore, p 298

Hart WR (1970) Paramesonephric mucinous cysts of the vulva. Am J Obstet Gynecol 107:1079–1084

Janovski NA (1962) Dysontogenetic cyst of the vulva: report of a case with reference to etiologic classification of vulvar cysts. Obstet Gynecol 20:227–231

Novak ER, Woodruff JD (1979) Gynecologic and obstetric pathology. Saunders, Philadelphia, p 26

Oi RH, Munn R (1982) Mucous cysts of the vulvar vestibule. Hum Pathol 13:584–586

Radman HM (1966) Wolffian duct cyst of the vulva. Pac Med Surg 74:170–171

Robboy SJ, Ross JS, Prat J et al. (1978) Urogenital sinus origin of mucinous and ciliated cysts of the vulva. Obstet Gynecol 51:347–351

Cyst of Canal of Nuck

Block RE (1975) Hydrocele of the canal of Nuck: report of a case. Obstet Gynecol 45:464–466

Kucera PR, Glazer J (1985) Hydrocele of the canal of Nuck: a case report of four cases. J Reprod Med 30:439–442

McCune WS (1948) Hydrocele of the canal of Nuck with large cystic retroperitoneal extension. Ann Surg 127:750–753

McElfatrick RA, Condon WB (1975) Hydrocele of the canal of Nuck. Rocky Mount Med J 72:112–113

Mesko JD, Gates H, McDonald TW et al. (1988) Clear cell (mesonephroid) adenocarcinoma of the vulva rising in endometriosis: a case report. Gynecol Oncol 29:385–391

Schwartz A, Peyser MR (1975) Nuck's hydrocele (hydrocele Muliebris). Int Surg 60:91–92

4 Cysts and Tumours of the Vestibular Glands

4.1 Major Vestibular Glands

4.1.1 Bartholin's Duct Cyst (Bartholin's Cyst)

Bartholin's duct cyst is a sequel of occlusion of the main duct leading to the accumulation of secretion. It presents as a slightly tender, round to ovoid swelling at the lower part of labium majus. The size usually varies from 3 to 6 cm with an average of 5 cm. A larger cyst attaining 12.5 cm and weighing up to 183 g has been described (Aborjaily et al. 1958). The cyst is more commonly unilateral, but bilateral cysts are sometimes seen. Depending on whether the main or smaller ducts are obstructed, the cyst may be uni- or multilocular; the unilocular cyst usually results from main duct obstruction. A collar-button-type distension generally occurs proximal to the obstruction of the main duct (Tancer 1965). The common cause of obstruction is Bartholin adenitis due to gonococcal infections. Infections by other organisms have also been incriminated. Mechanical trauma can cause distortion of the duct and thereby hindrance to the outflow of secretions. Rarely, malignancy of the organ can manifest as a cystic swelling in elderly women. The posterior third of vulva is the usual site for these cysts.

4.1.1.1 Microscopical Appearance

The cyst may be lined by transitional, squamous (Fig. 4.1) or both types of epithelium. When the acini are distended, the lining is formed by low columnar and cuboidal cells (Fig. 4.2). Variable chronic inflammatory cells and fibrosis are always evident around some ducts, acini and the cyst. Occasionally, a collection of mucin within the ducts and stroma gives rise to a swelling similar to the mucocoele of the minor salivary glands. This is often the result of disruption of the ductal system with extravasation of mucin to the surrounding stroma accompanied by chronic inflammatory cells particularly mucinophages (Freedman and Goldman 1978).

Ultrastructural studies of the lining cells demonstrated lysosomes and phagosome-rich microvilli, apical pinocytic vesicles in the superficial cells and a stratified cell population poor in organelles but rich in tonofilaments, free ribosomes and dilated intercellular spaces imparting a close semblance to the transitional cell of the urinary tract, Brenner tumours and Walthard's cell rests (Rorat et al. 1975).

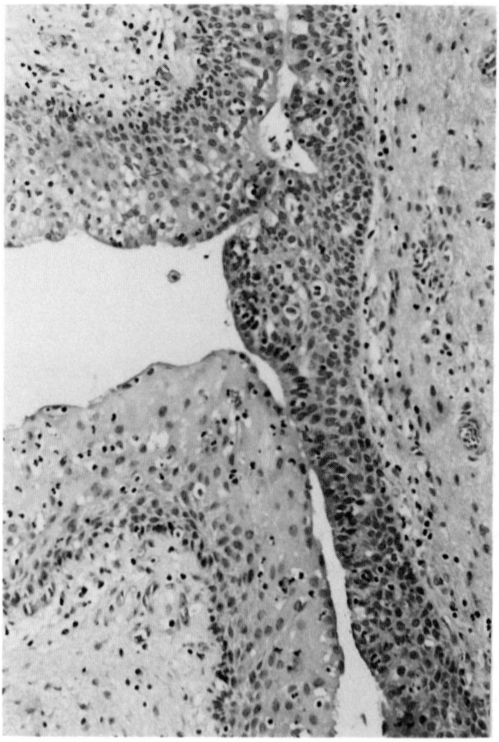

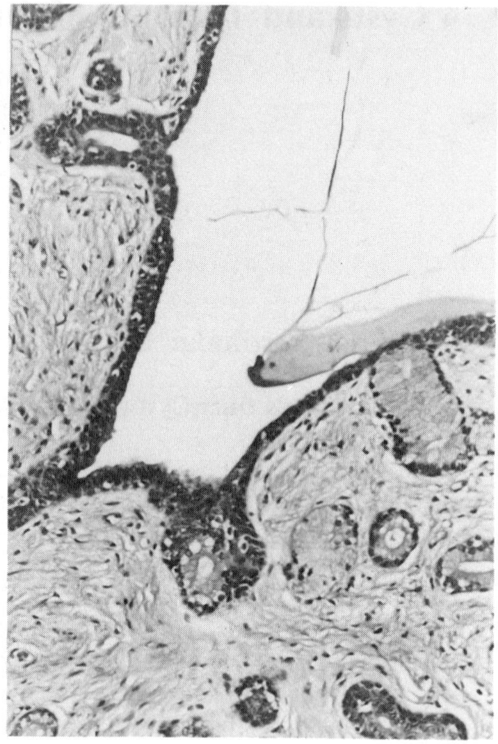

Fig. 4.1. Bartholin's cyst: the cyst is lined by squamous epithelium

Fig. 4.2. Bartholin's cyst lined by 2–3 layers of cuboidal cells

4.1.1.2 Treatment

Fluid aspirated preoperatively can be conveniently used for bacteriological culture and cytological examination to exclude malignancy. Initial aspiration to establish the cause rather than surgery has been recommended as a rational approach (Cheetham 1985). Treatment by marsupialisation is widely practised (Davies 1948; Johnson 1961; Jacobson 1966; Mathews 1966). Excision of the cyst using the CO_2 laser has been advocated by some workers (Lashgari and Keene 1986).

4.1.2 Bartholin's Gland Adenoma and Cystadenoma

The two tubo-alveolar glands located on either side of the vulva are common sites of inflammation and cyst formation. Swelling of these glands is most often due to cyst and infrequently carcinoma. The literature is factually silent about the existence of benign neoplastic lesions of these glands. Willis (1948) pointed out that such lesions could indeed occur and described a case of papillary cystadenoma in one

(1987) supports this view. The patient was a 32-year-old woman who presented with a non-tender, 0.3-cm vulval mass composed of multiple branching, focally dilated, mucous-secreting glands set in dense connective tissue stroma. Foushee et al. (1968) reported five instances which were thought to be hyperplastic rather than neoplastic lesions although two of them they considered could be classified as adenomas. All were well-circumscribed but unencapsulated and composed of an increased number of ducts and acini. Thrombosis of the blood vessel was noticed in one and cyst formation in two. Three further cases of adenomas were reported (Honore and O'Hara 1978), and these, too, were composed of hyperplastic secretory alveoli with expansile behaviour, compressing the surrounding tissue.

Grossly, these lesions are unencapsulated, firm in consistency and have a grey-tan cut surface.

4.1.2.1 Microscopical Appearance

The mass consists of closely packed, hyperplastic, secretory alveoli lined by a single layer of mucin-secreting, tall columnar epithelium with minimal atypia or pleomorphism. The ductal components may be increased or fewer in number. A variable amount of fibrous stroma containing chronic inflammatory cells may be present. There may be occasional small cysts lined by low columnar, cuboidal or squamous epithelium representing dilated ducts.

4.1.2.2 Treatment

The malignant potential of these lesions is at present not known. It has been suggested that they should be excised rather than marsupialised in patients over 40 years of age (Dodson et al. 1970; Friedrich 1976).

4.1.3 Mixed Tumours – Benign and Malignant (Pleomorphic Adenoma and Adenocarcinoma)

On rare occasions, a Bartholin's gland may be the site of a pleomorphic adenoma similar to the one occurring in the salivary glands. A similar tumour occurs also in the skin appendages of the vulva. When it is located near the introitus, findings of the Bartholin's gland tissue at the periphery of the tumour provide evidence of the origin in the Bartholin's gland.

The patients are usually elderly.

4.1.3.1 Gross Appearance

These tumours are tan to grey coloured, firm masses of 1–2 cm in size, located at the lower lateral wall of the vagina.

4.1.3.2 Microscopical Appearance

The tumour is composed of both epithelial and mesenchymal cells, the latter forming abundant stromal tissue containing mucin and cartilage. The epithelial cells are cuboidal and form cords and tubules.

Malignant changes with extension to the surrounding structures and perineural infiltration can occur in these tumours. Ordonez et al. (1984) reported a malignant tumour consisting predominantly of adenocystic and anaplastic components in a 69-year-old woman who had to be treated by pelvic exenteration. According to some authors, the mixed tumours of Bartholin's gland should be treated as malignant (Janovski and Douglas 1972).

4.1.4 Bartholin's Gland Carcinoma

Bartholin's gland carcinoma comprises 2% (Crossen 1948) to 7% (Barclay et al. 1964) of vulval malignancies. According to Masterson and Goss (1955), one case of Bartholin's gland carcinoma can be found per thousand female genital cancers. Since the original description by Klob (1864, cited in Dennis et al. 1955), more than 200 cases have been reported in the literature (Dennefors and Bergman 1980).

4.1.4.1 Clinical Features

The average age of the patient is 52 years (Trelford and Deos 1976). The youngest patient reported was 14 (Addison 1977) and the oldest, 91 years old (Pape 1907, cited in Dennis et al. 1955). Rarely, Bartholin's gland carcinoma has been reported in a pregnant woman.

The most common symptoms are unilateral vulval mass, pain or irritations and, less frequently, vaginal discharge and bleeding. The symptoms may be mistaken for inflammation (Dennis et al. 1955; Trelford and Deos 1976) or a benign cyst (Dodson et al. 1970; Trelford and Deos 1976). In almost 50% of cases (Chamlian and Taylor 1972), these two are the initial diagnoses. Occasionally, the patient may present with a fistula draining purulent material (Payan and Kish 1965). Some patients present with the complaint of dyspareunia.

Honan (1897, cited in Dennis et al. 1955) laid down several criteria for the diagnosis of Bartholin's gland carcinoma. These include: correct anatomical location of the tumour should be deep in the labium, connection of the tumour with the gland duct should be established, and intact gland tissue should be present. In the advanced lesion these criteria are difficult to fulfill, particularly when the whole gland is infiltrated and destroyed.

The aetiology of Bartholin's gland carcinoma is not known. Obstetrical trauma, chronic inflammation in the neighbouring and ischio-rectal tissues and involutional and cystic changes in the lobules of Bartholin's glands have been suggested (Sackett 1958). The role of inflammation in the development of malignancy in this gland has not been established, and if there is any, it is probably very minor (Wharton and Everette 1951). It has been argued that if inflammation played any significant role, a higher incidence of malignancy would be expected (Wharton and Everette 1951). In fact, it is in only about 7%–8% of these patients that a past history of Bartholin's gland adenitis (Leuchter et al. 1982) can be obtained.

Mossler et al. (1980) demonstrated low levels of oestrogen and progesterone receptor protein in the tumour tissue and suggested that the tumours could be hormonally responsive.

4.1.4.2 Pathological Features

Grossly Bartholin's gland carcinoma is mostly unilateral; bilateral carcinomas are exceedingly rare (Purola and Widholm 1966; Schweepe and Schlake 1980). The tumour varies in size from 2 to 10 cm with an average of 4 cm. Tumours of the size of a hen's egg (Purola and Widholm 1966) and weighing 160 g (Lulenski and Naji 1964) have been reported. Bartholin's gland carcinoma is an irregular, firm to hard, unencapsulated mass with a reddish-grey to pale grey cut surface which displays areas of haemorrhage, necrosis and cystic changes.

4.1.4.3 Microscopical Appearance

Squamous cell carcinoma and adenocarcinoma are the most common malignant tumours of Bartholin's gland. Although there are some reported variations in the frequencies (Wharton and Everette 1951; Dennis et al. 1955; Leuchter et al. 1982), the incidence of both squamous cell carcinoma and adenocarcinoma appear to be approximately equal (Masterson and Goss 1955; Barclay et al. 1964; Dodson et al. 1970; Chamlian and Taylor 1972; Trelford and Deos 1976), and both types together constitute 85% of the Bartholin's gland carcinomas (Leuchter et al. 1982). The remainder comprise adenocystic, adenosquamous, transitional cell and undifferentiated carcinomas. The histological appearances of squamous cell carcinoma are not different from the squamous cell carcinomas occurring at other sites (Fig. 4.3). The tumour can arise both in the ducts and acini; a transition from the normal acini and ductal epithelium to the tumour can sometimes be identified (Cochran 1956; Chamlian and Taylor 1972; Copeland et al. 1986). The metaplastic squamous epithelium of the proximal duct and the terminal portion of the duct which is normally lined by squamous cells are the likely sites of origin. It is probable that the metaplastic changes occur also in the acini, and squamous carcinoma arises from these metaplastic foci. Adenocarcinomas may occur in typical form or as a papillary (Fig. 4.4), mucoepidermoid (Fig. 4.5) and mucinous variant (Pund and Cole 1942; Payan and Kish 1965; Chamlian and Taylor 1972). Mucin secretion, which is pronounced in some tumours (Lulenski and Naji 1964), may be diffuse or limited

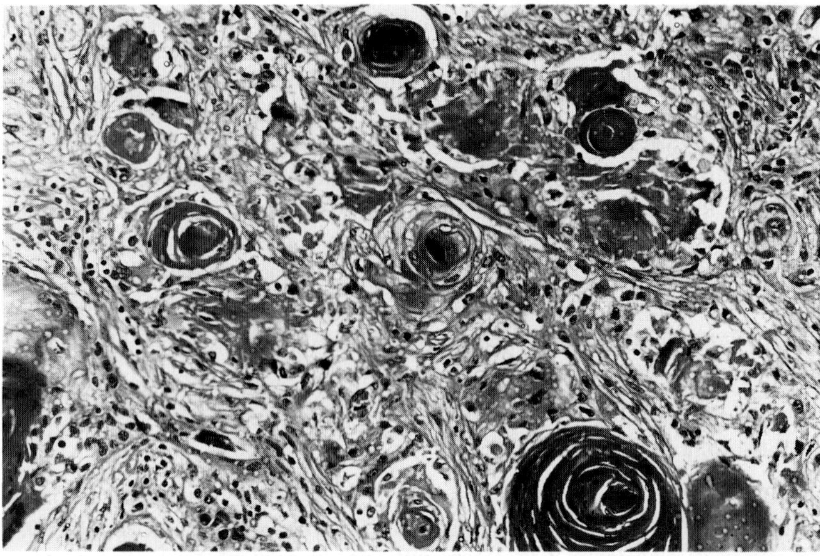

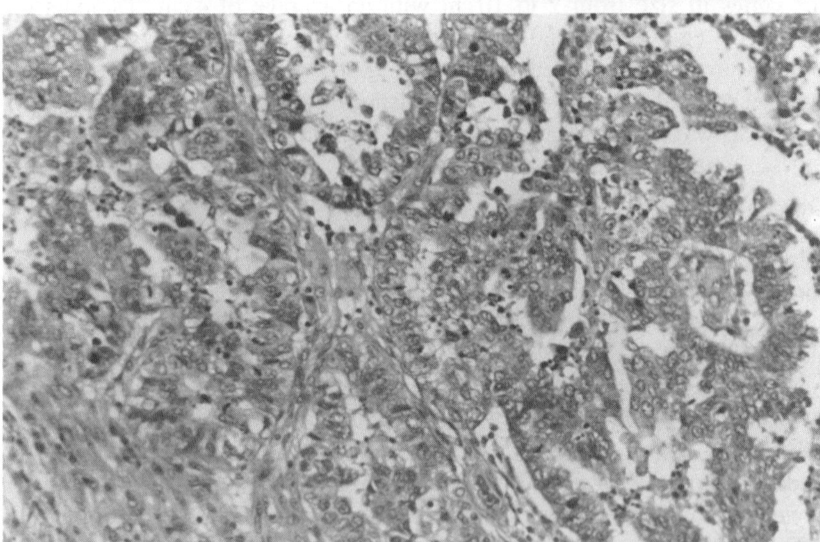

Fig. 4.3. Bartholin's gland carcinoma: a well-differentiated squamous cell carcinoma with epithelial pearls

Fig. 4.4. Bartholin's gland adenocarcinoma

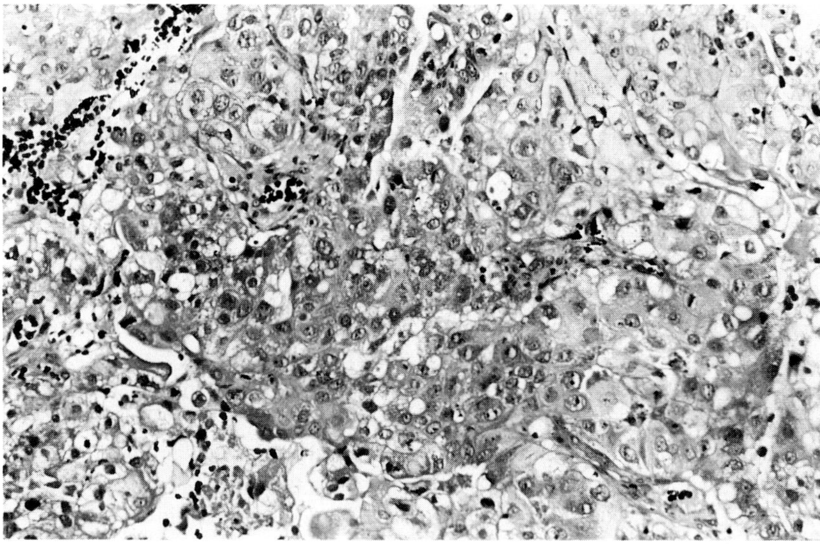

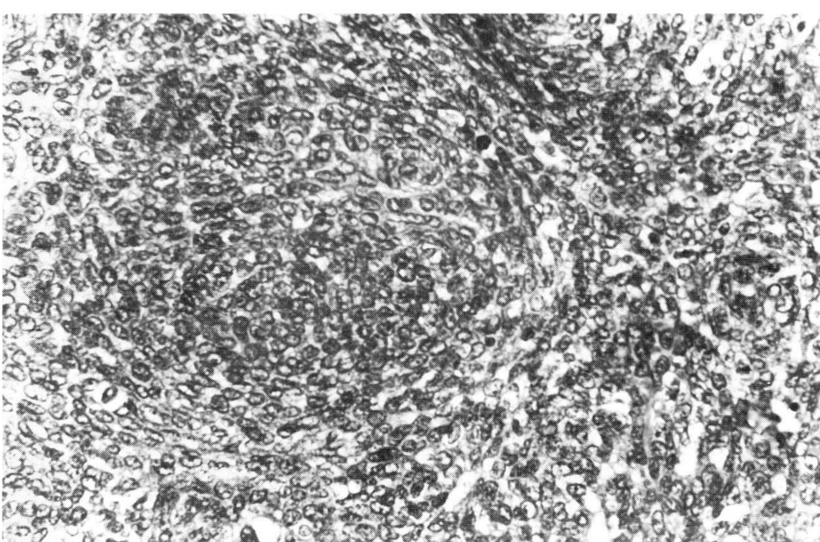

Fig. 4.5. Bartholin's gland carcinoma mucoepidermoid type: composed of sheets of large, mucin-positive cells

Fig. 4.6. Bartholin's gland carcinoma basaloid type: composed of basaloid-type cells

to some portion of the tumour or some acini only. Rarely, signet carcinoma can also occur (Pattison and Schute 1951). The Bartholin's glands are mucin-secreting, racemose-type glands, and some amount of mucin contents can be expected in the adenocarcinomas arising in these glands. An undifferentiated carcinoma may display areas of bizarre nuclei with numerous mitoses and giant cells (Boughton 1943). The rare transitional cell carcinoma (Wahlstrom et al. 1978), probably arising in the ducts, may resemble cloacogenic basaloid carcinoma of the anal ducts (Fig. 4.6).

Squamous differentiation either as benign or malignant foci which occurs not uncommonly in the adenocarcinomas (adenoacanthoma, adenosquamous carcinoma) of the endometrium, endocervix, etc. can also occur in the adenocarcinoma of Bartholin's gland (Van Nagell et al. 1969; Dennefors and Bergman 1980; Wheelock et al. 1984). Such differentiation, however, does not seem to bear any prognostic significance as at the other sites.

Direct extension of the carcinomas from vulval skin and vagina and metastases from cervical and fundal primaries can occur to the Bartholin's glands (Wahrton and Everette 1951). Such possibilities should be excluded when examining a Bartholin's gland carcinoma.

The vulval carcinoma displays a high incidence of association with a second gynaecological primary. This association has also been observed with Bartholin's gland carcinoma. The other notable primaries are those of the cervix and other neoplastic conditions of the vulva (Chamlian and Taylor 1972; Tchang et al. 1973; Webb et al. 1984; Wheelock et al. 1984). Ultrastructurally, three cell types with different sorts of secretory granules have been demonstrated in the adenocarcinoma of Bartholin's gland (Kuzuya et al. 1981): (a) principal cells, the most predominant component with numerous, electron-dense, round, secretory granules like those seen in the ductal cells; (b) cells like goblet cells with low density, large, secretory granules which are also seen in normal Bartholin's glands; and (c) eccrine sweat gland-like cells with moderately dense, large, irregular, secretory granules, tight intercellular junctions, desmosomes, abundant rough endoplasmic reticulum, Golgi complex and secretory vacuoles, as well as acinar structures (Mossler et al. 1980). In an undifferentiated carcinoma these secretory vacuoles may be absent (Advani et al. 1978).

4.1.4.4 Prognosis

The main prognostic determinant of Bartholin's gland carcinoma is the inguino-femoral nodal status. With multiple nodal metastases, the 5-year survival rate is only 18%. When a single node is involved, the outlook is much better, with the 5-year survival rate approaching 71% or more (Leuchter et al. 1982). Although the incidence of inguino-femoral node metastasis has varied in different series from 37.3% (Leuchter et al. 1982) to 55% (Wheelock et al. 1984), it is nevertheless very high. This highlights the high risk associated with this malignancy as well as the importance of early diagnosis. Delay in the diagnosis adversely influence the prognosis.

4.1.4.5 Treatment

Although modalities of treatment have varied in different centres, radical vulvectomy with inguino-femoral lymphadenectomy has been the optimum treatment (Wharton and Everette 1951; Materson and Goss 1955; Leuchter et al. 1982; Wheelock et al. 1984). Whether the pelvic nodes should also be removed is unresolved. When the patients have positive inguino-femoral nodes, 18% of them will also have the risk of deep node involvement (Leuchter et al. 1982). Some workers have advocated routine deep node dissection in addition to the vulverectomy and bilateral inguino-femoral node dissection (Barclay et al. 1964). The Bartholin's glands are situated between the bulbocavernosus muscles and deep perineal compartments. The risk of extension of the tumour to the ischiorectal fossae, beneath the vaginal wall or into the rectum (Leuchter et al. 1982) and directly draining into the deep nodes (Barclay et al. 1964) is high. Some authors therefore emphasise the tumour-free surgical excision margins, which may necessitate resections of portions of levator ani muscles, vagina and/or rectum (Wheelock et al. 1984). When the groin nodes and surgical excision margins are involved, risk of late recurrence is high (Lichtinger et al. 1986). Exploratory laparotomy in addition to the radical vulvectomy has been advocated to exclude extension beyond the pelvis (Cavanagh et al. 1985). To obtain adequate resections some patients may need exenterative surgery (Abrams et al. 1952; Wheelock et al. 1984). Others have achieved satisfactory results with hemivulvectomy or wide local excison (Wharton and Everette 1951; von Lurmann 1974; Copeland et al. 1986).

Reports on the role of radiation as an adjuvant in the management of recurrence (Dodson et al. 1970; Trelford and Deos 1976), residual disease (Wheelock et al. 1984) or primary tumour (Wharton and Everette 1951) are not at present available for a large number of patients. Favourable results with adjuvant radiotherapy have been claimed at some centres (Copeland et al. 1986).

Chemotherapy has been used in the treatment of recurrent disease (Copeland et al. 1986). Its effectiveness has not yet been evaluated in a sufficient number of cases.

4.1.5 Adenoid Cystic Carcinoma

Adenocystic carcinoma of Bartholin's gland, according to some authors (Murphy et al. 1962; Leuchter et al. 1982), is a variant of adenocarcinoma and comprises 1% of all carcinomas of the vulva and 10% of all Bartholin's gland carcinomas (Copeland et al. 1986). Others (Abell 1963; Eichner 1963; Addison and Parker 1977) consider it a distinct histological and clinical entity which pursues an indolent course, tends to recur and spreads by the bloodstream as well as by the perineural lymphatic system (Ortner et al. 1980; Bernstein et al. 1983). This tumour occurs commonly in the salivary glands and breasts and uncommonly in the tracheo-bronchial tree, uterine cervix and maxillary sinuses.

The histogenesis of these tumours is unknown. Ultrastructural and immunochemical studies of tumours from different sites have not resolved the problem. Origin from the glandular and ductal epithelium (Murphy et al. 1962) and from myoepithelial cells of the vascular and lymphatic bed (Eichner 1963) have been suggested.

4.1.5.1 Clinical Features

The age of the patients varies from 25 to 80 years, with bimodal peak incidence about 40 and 70 years (Abrao et al. 1985). The patients present with a vulval nodule or gradually increasing mass, sometimes of a very short duration. Pain is not generally a presenting symptom. A higher frequency of other genital primaries has also been noticed in association with this tumour (Trelford and Deos 1976).

4.1.5.2 Pathological Features

The tumour does not have distinctive gross features which can differentiate it from other carcinomas of Bartholin's gland. It is generally described as an irregular, unencapsulated or partly capsulated mass with a grey and greyish-tan cut surface.

4.1.5.3 Microscopical Appearance

Adenoid cystic carcinoma is composed of irregular nests, anastomosing cords and groups of cells with variable stroma. The component cells closely resemble basal cells which are oval or slightly elongated in shape, possessing scanty cytoplasm with an indistinct cell outline and hyperchromatic oval or slightly elongated nuclei (Fig. 4.7). Under low power view, some areas of the tumour may mimic an adenocystic basal cell carcinoma of the skin (Fig. 4.8). The anastomosing cords are made of one to two layers of cells and surround numerous cystic spaces, creating a sieve-like cribriform pattern which is a characteristic feature (Fig. 4.9). These spaces contain eosinophilic amorphous material which reacts positively with PAS after digestion by diastase. Small duct-like structures lined by a single layer of cuboidal cells are also frequently noticed in different parts of the tumour. In some areas, the neoplastic cells may be arranged in compact sheet and solid masses or cords without containing any cystic spaces. Mitoses are usually very few. The stroma consists of fibrovascular connective tissue often separating the tumour mass into nodules or lobules.

There may be an occasional collision tumour involving squamous cell carcinoma of the excretory duct and adenocystic carcinoma of the gland (Webb et al. 1984).

Histochemical investigations (Mazur and Battifora 1982) reveal both epithelial (stained intensely with mucicarcmine, PAS following diastase digestion and alcian blue following hyaluronidase digestion) and connective tissue mucin (stained by alcian blue prior to digestion by hyaluronidase). It has been inferred that the cysts contain acid mucopolysaccharides (Anthony and James 1975) and the small duct-like structures, neutral mucopolysaccharides (Anthony and James 1975). It

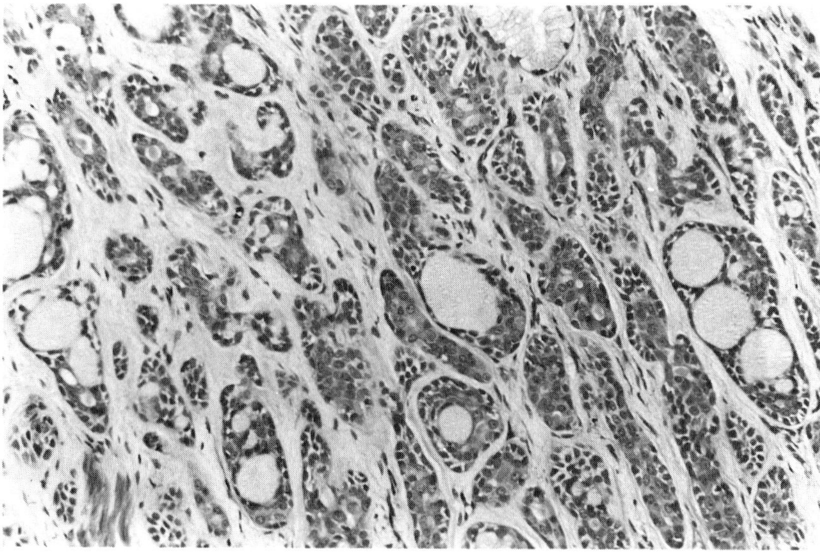

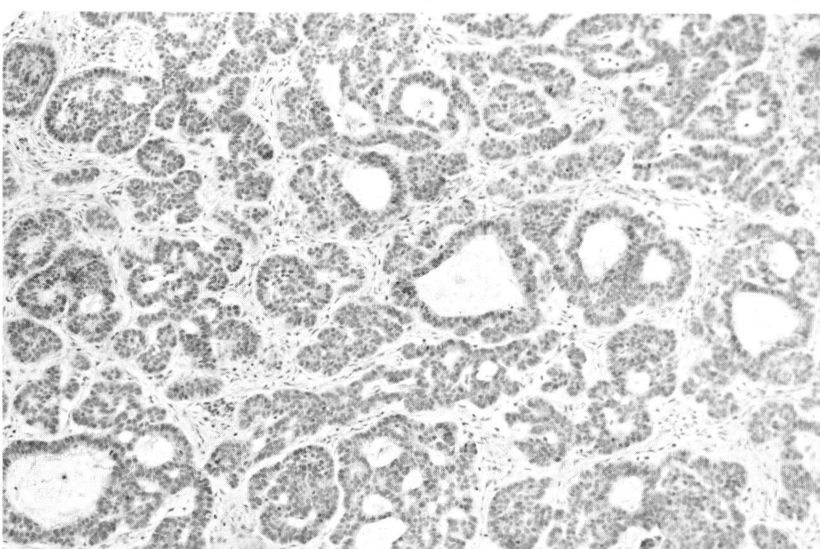

Fig. 4.7. Bartholin's gland carcinoma adenocystic variant: composed of oval cells with oval to elongate nuclei

Fig. 4.8. Bartholin's gland carcinoma adenocystic type: cystic space and basaloid-type cells are reminiscent of adenocystic basal cell carcinoma of the skin

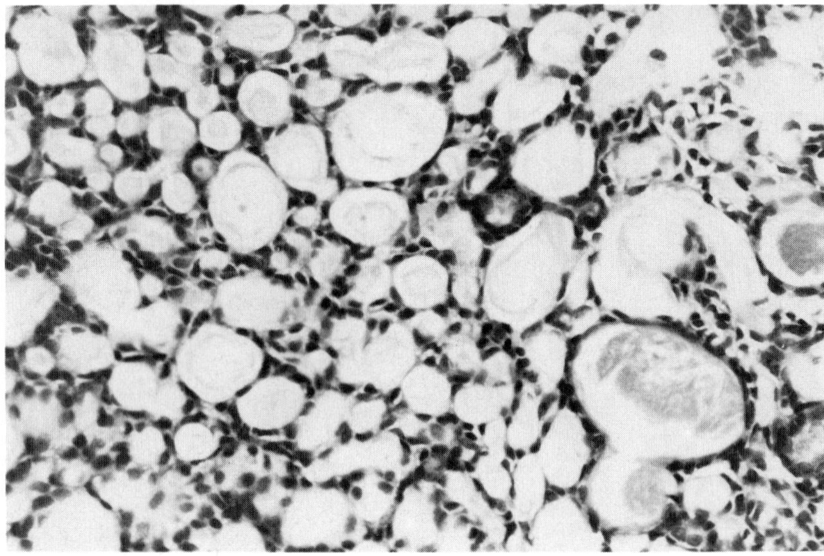

Fig. 4.9. Bartholin's gland carcinoma: sieve-like pattern

has been suggested that the myoepithelial cells which are capable of secreting acid mucopolysaccharides and fibrillary connective tissue constitute the main tumour mass, and the duct-like structures secreting neutral mucin are an attempt at ductal epithelial differentiation. Amichetti and Aldovini (1988) noticed on immunohistochemical examination positive reaction for epithelial membrane antigen at the apex of the duct cells and cup-like positivity with vimentin antibody in the basal cytoplasm. In the adenoid cystic carcinoma of the uterine cervix, the neoplastic cells contain actin and keratin filaments and produce epithelial membrane antigen (Mazur and Battifora 1982).

Ultrastructure studies of these tumours arising in the Bartholin's gland are very few (Bernstein et al. 1983). The presence of desmosomes and occasional microvilli indicates the epithelial nature of the cells. The cystic spaces are lined by the filamentous deposit of basal lamina rather than by microvilli. Similar observations have also been made in the adenoid cystic carcinoma of the salivary gland (Tandler 1971). While the cystic spaces or "pseudocysts" represent extracellular compartments of the tumour, the true lumina lined by microvilli are also scattered in the cellular areas (Tandler 1971). Two cell types have been recognised in the tumour – one elongated and flattened with cytoplasmic filaments, thought to be myoepithelial, and the other plump and polyhedral in shape, possessing desmosomes and epithelial in nature (Gordon et al. 1972).

Although adenoid cystic carcinoma of the Bartholin's gland is said to be less aggressive than squamous cell and adenocarcinoma (Addison and Parker 1977), its biological behaviour does not seem to be different from those developing at other locations. Local recurrences are common before the tumour spreads to the regional nodes and distant sites. After repeated local recurrences over a long period of 27 years, a tumour was reported to develop ultimately widespread lymphatic and haematogenous metastases (Sayre 1949).

4.1.5.4 Treatment

Radical surgery in an attempt to achieve tumour-free margins should be undertaken, if necessary extending to the levator ani muscles in order to remove the deep fascial plane of the urogenital diaphragm (Addison and Parker 1977). Presence of the tumour in the surgical excision margins heralds a poor outlook. All patients with residual malignancies at the surgical margins ultimately succumbed due to distant metastases (Bernstein et al. 1983). The efficacy of inguino-femoral and deep lymphadenectomy has been questioned (Addison and Parker 1977; Wahlstrom et al. 1978; Bernstein et al. 1983). It has been argued that unless there are clinical suspicions of nodal metastases, lymphadenectomy can be omitted (Bernstein et al. 1983). The role of radiotherapy in the treatment of adenoid cystic carcinoma has been disappointing (Sayre 1949; Eichner 1963; Dodson et al. 1978). Copeland et al. (1986) have recommended adunctive radiotherapy in those patients with positive surgical margins. A chemotherapeutic regimen has shown some encouraging results (Skibba et al. 1981; Budd and Groppe 1983) in metastatic salivary gland adenocystic carcinoma, but its efficacy in the treatment of vulval adenoid cystic carcinoma is yet to be sufficiently evaluated (Copeland et al. 1986).

4.1.6 Transitional Cell Carcinoma

The transitional cell carcinoma of Bartholin's gland arises in the duct (Wheelock et al. 1984). The occurrence of this tumour in Bartholin's gland is surprisingly a rare phenomenon, considering the entire length except near the external orifice of the duct is lined by transitional cells. Morphologically, these tumours are composed of groups, sheets and nests of neoplastic transitional cells with a tendency to squamous and acinar differentiation (Wahlstrom et al. 1978; Sackett 1958). This may sometimes structurally resemble cloacogenic carcinoma arising in the anal ducts. Because of their rarity, the behaviour of these tumours is not exactly known. Metastases to the inguinal nodes have been noticed (Dodson et al. 1978).

4.1.7 Undifferentiated Carcinoma

Occasional carcinomas of Bartholin's gland are undifferentiated (Dennis et al. 1955; Chamlian and Taylor 1972; Trelford and Deos 1976) and associated with a poor prognosis (Mossler et al. 1980). The small, round, polygonal and spindle-shaped neoplastic cells with scanty cytoplasm and pleomorphic, hyperchromatic and occasionally bizarre-shaped nuclei are arranged in diffuse sheets and groups separated by incomplete fibrous stroma. Mitoses may be numerous. The cases reported in the past as spindle cell sarcomas are very much more likely to be undifferentiated carcinomas.

4.1.8 Other Rare Malignant Tumours

4.1.8.1 Haemangioendothelioma

The single instance of haemangioendothelioma occurring at this site in a 57-year-old woman was treated by surgery and radiotherapy with no recurrence at 1-year follow-up (Rosenzweig 1960).

4.1.8.2 Melanoma

Reports of melanomas arising at this site are not elaborate. These lesions are probably secondaries from vaginal or vulval primaries.

4.1.8.3 Lymphoma

Involvement of Bartholin's gland in generalised lymphoma is infrequent. The exact incidence of involvement is not known. Unless the lesion causes symptoms, the female genital tract is rarely examined. At routine autopsy the Bartholin's glands seldom draw the attention of the prosector. Nonetheless, lymphomas can infiltrate these glands and produce symptoms. Plouffe et al. (1984) reported a 64-year-old patient with generalised, large cell, immunoblastic lymphoma involving the right Bartholin's gland. These lymphomas belong to the poor prognostic group, and outlook is generally disappointing even with a multiagent chemotherapeutic regimen.

4.2 Minor Vestibular Glands

4.2.1 Adenoma

Of the vestibular glands, the Bartholin's glands appear to be more commonly affected by inflammatory and neoplastic processes than the minor vestibular glands. While inflammatory process may also involve the minor glands (Marinoff and Turner 1986), benign adenomatous masses are distinctly uncommon in both the major and minor vestibular glands. Although Willis (1948) and others (Foushee et al. 1968; Honore and O'Hara 1978) reported cystadenoma and adenoma of the major vestibular glands, it is only recently that adenomas of the minor vestibular glands have been recognised (Axe et al. 1986). The patients have a wide age range and present for surgery after the initial failure of medicinal or ablative treatment of symptoms of localised pain, itchiness, discharge, burning sensation and dyspareunia. The surgical specimens contain nodules of 1–2 cm in diameter which are histologically composed of nests of hyperplastic, mucous-secreting glands traversed and surrounded by irregular bands of the fibrous tissue (Axe et al. 1986).

4.3 Tumour-like Conditions: Malakoplakia of Bartholin's Glands

Malakoplakia is an unusual chronic granulomatous lesion consisting of chronic inflammatory cells, of which histiocytes containing Michaelis-Gutmann bodies are characteristic (see also vulval and vaginal malakoplakia). The two patients reported by Paquin et al. (1986) were 49 and 61 years old. One of them presented with an asymptomatic Bartholin's cyst which was about 4 cm in diameter and contained purulent exudate; the other presented with a rapidly growing, tender swelling which was excised and found to be a cyst 3 cm in size with a haemorrhagic lining. Microscopical examination of the tissue from both patients shows characteristic histological features and remnants of Bartholin's glands.

References

Bartholin Duct Cyst

Aborjaily AN, McSweeny DJ (1958) Bartholin cyst of extraordinary size. Report of a case. Obstet Gynecol 11:350–351

Cheetham DR (1985) Bartholin's cyst: marsupialisation or aspiration? Am J Obstet Gynecol 152:569–570

Davies JW (1948) Bartholin cyst, a simple method for its restoration to function. Surg Gynecol Obstet 86:329–331

Freedman SR, Goldman RL (1978) Mucocele-like changes in the Bartholin's gland. Hum Pathol 9:111–114

Jacobson P (1960) Marsupialisation of vulvovaginal (Bartholin) cysts. Am J Obstet Gynecol 79:73–78

Johnson WD (1961) Vulvovaginal (bartholi) cyst marsupialisation under pudendal anesthesia. Obstet Gynecol 18:277–280

Lashgari M, Keene M (1986) Excision of Bartholin duct cysts using the CO_2 laser. Obstet Gynecol 67:735–737

Mathews D (1966) Marsupialisation in the treatment of Bartholin's cysts and abscesses. J Obstet Gynaecol Br Commonw 73:1010–1012

Rorat E, Ferenczy A, Richart RM (1975) Human Bartholin gland, duct and duct cysts. Arch Pathol 99:367–374

Tancer ML (1965) Bartholin's cyst and paraurethral lesions. Clin Obstet Gynecol 8:982–996

Bartholin Gland Adenoma and Cystadenoma

Chapman GW Jr, Hassan N, Page D et al. (1987) Mucinous cystadenoma of Bartholin's gland: a case report. J Reprod Med 32:939–941

Dodson MG, O'Leary JA, Averette HE (1970) Primary carcinoma of Bartholin's gland. Obstet Gynecol 35:578–584

Foushee JHS, Reeves WJU, McCool JA (1968) Benign masses of Bartholin's gland: solid adenomas, adenomas with cyst and Bartholin's gland with varices or thrombosis or cavernous haemangioma. Obstet Gynecol 31:695–701

Friedrich EG (1976) Vulvar disease. In: Major problems of obstetrics and gynecology, vol 9. Saunders, Philadelphia, pp 51–55

Honore LH, O'Hara KE (1978) Adenoma of the Bartholin's gland: report of three cases. Eur J Obstet Gynaecol Reprod Biol 8:335–340

Willis RA (1948) Epithelial tumours of the vagina and vulva. In: Pathology of tumours. Butterworth, London, pp 547–553

Mixed Tumours of Bartholin Gland

Janovski JA, Douglas CP (1972) Disease of the vulva. Harper and Row, Maryland, p 78

Ordonez NG, Manning JT, Luna MA (1984) Mixed tumour of the vulva: a report of two cases probably arising in Bartholin's gland. Cancer 48:181–186

Bartholin Gland Carcinoma

Abrams BS, Bauer J, Bricker EM (1952) Primary carcinoma of the Bartholin's gland treated by radical surgery. Arch Surg 65:790–794

Addison A (1977) Adenocarcinoma of Bartholin gland a 14 year old girl. Am J Obstet Gynecol 127:214–215

Advani H, Waldo ED, McCarty KS (1978) Bartholin's gland carcinoma: an ultrastructural study. Am J Obstet Gynecol 130:362–364

Barclay DL, Collins CG, Macey HB Jr (1964) Cancer of the Bartholin gland: a review and report of 8 cases. Obstet Gynecol 24:329–336

Boughton TG (1943) Carcinoma of Bartholin's gland. Am J Surg 59:585–591

Cavanagh D, Ruffulo EH, Marsden DE (1985) Adenocarcinoma of the vulva: a clinico-pathologic approach. In Gynecologic cancer. Appleton-Century Crofts, East Norwalk, pp 30–31

Chamlian DL, Taylor HB (1972) Primary carcinoma of Bartholin's gland: a report of 24 patients. Obstet Gynecol 39:489–494

Cochran RB (1956) A very early case of carcinoma of Bartholin's gland. Am J Obstet Gynecol 71:1138–1140

Copeland LJ, Sneige N, Gershenson DM et al. (1986) Bartholin gland carcinoma. Obstet Gynecol 67:794–801

Crossen RJ (1948) Primary carcinoma of Bartholin's gland. Am J Surg 75:597–601

Dennefors B, Bergman B (1980) Primary carcinoma of the Bartholin's gland. Acta Obstet Gynecol Scand 59:95–96

Dennis EJ III, Hester LL Jr, Wilson LA (1955) Primary carcinoma of Bartholin's gland. Obstet Gynecol 6:291–296

Dodson MG, O'Leary JA, Averette HE (1970) Primary carcinoma of Bartholin's gland. Obstet Gynecol 35:578–584

Honan J (1897) Über die Carcinome der Glandulae Bartholini. Inaugural Dissertation. University of Berlin

Klob JM (1864) Carcinoma of Bartholin's gland. In: Pathologische Anatomie der weiblichen Sexualorgane. Braunmüller, Vienna

Kuzuya K, Matsuyama M, Nishi Y et al. (1981) Ulstrastructure of adenocarcinoma of Bartholin's gland. Cancer 48:1392–1398

Leuchter RS, Hacker NF, Voet RL et al. (1982) Primary carcinoma of Bartholin's gland: a report of 14 cases and review of the literature. Obstet Gynecol 60:361–368

Lichtinger M, Girtanner R, Averette H et al. (1986) Primary malignant Bartholin's gland tumors. J Reprod Med 31:981

Lulenski CR, Naji AF (1964) Mucin secreting adenocarcinoma of Bartholin gland. Obstet Gynecol 24:542–544

Masterson JG, Goss AS (1955) Carcinoma of Bartholin gland. Review of the literature and report of a new case in an elderly patient treated by radical operation. Am J Obstet Gynecol 69:1323–1332

Mossler JA, Woodard BH, Addison A et al. (1980) Adenocarcinoma of Bartholin's gland. Arch Pathol Lab Med 104:523–526

Pape W (1907) Carcinom der Bartholinschen Drüse von einer jährigen Frau. Dtsch Med Wochenschr 33:1620

Pattison DS, Schute D (1951) Carcinoma of Bartholin's gland. Can Med Assoc J 64:249–250

Payan H, Kish M (1965) Carcinoma of Bartholin gland. Obstet Gynecol 25:268–269

Pund ER, Cole WC (1942) Carcinoma of Bartholin's gland. Am J Obstet Gynecol 43:887–890

Purola E, Widholm O (1966) Primary carcinoma of Bartholin's gland. Acta Obstet Gynecol Scand 45:205–210

Sackett NB (1958) Carcinoma primary in Bartholin's gland. Am J Obstet Gynecol 75:183–188

Schweppe KW, Schlake W (1980) Adenocarzinom der Bartholinschen Drüse. Geburtshilfe Frauenheilkd 40:437–443

Tchang F, Okagaki T, Richart RM (1973) Adenocarcinoma of Bartholin's gland associated with Paget's disease of vulvar area. Cancer 31:221–225

Trelford JD, Deos PH (1976) Bartholin's gland carcinomas: five cases. Gynecol Oncol 4:212–221

Van Nagell JR Jr, Tweeddale DN, Roddick JW Jr(1969) Primary adenoacanthoma of the Bartholin gland. Obstet Gynecol 34:87–90

Von Lurmann K (1974) Das primäre Karzinom der Bartholinschen Drüse. Zentralbl Gynäkol 96:1044–1047

Wahlstrom TM, Vesterinen MDE, Saksela E (1978) Primary carcinoma of Bartholin's glands: a morphological and clinical study of six cases including a transitional cell carcinoma. Gynecol Oncol 6:354–362

Webb JB, O'Sullivan JC, Azzopardi JG (1984) Combined adenoid cystic and squamous carcinoma of Bartholin's gland. Case report. Br J Obstet Gynaecol 91:291–295

Wharton LR Jr, Everette HS (1951) Primary malignant bartholin gland tumors. Obstet Gynecol Surv 6:1–8

Wheelock JB, Goplerud DR, Dunn LJ et al. (1984) Primary carcinoma of the Bartholin gland: a report of ten cases. Obstet Gynecol 63:820–824

References of Adenocystic, Transitional, Undifferentiated Carcinomas and Other Rare Malignancies

Abell MR (1963) Adenocystic (pseudoadenocarcinomatous) basal cell carcinoma of vestibular glands of vulva. Am J Obstet Gynecol 86:470–482

Abrao FS, Marques AF, Marziona F et al. (1985) Adenoid cystic carcinoma of Bartholin's gland: review of the literature and report of two cases. J Surg Oncol 30:132–137

Addison A, Parker RT (1977) Adenoid cystic carcinoma of the Bartholin's gland: a review of the literature and report of a patient. Gynecol Oncol 5:196–201

Amichetti M, Aldovini D (1988) Primary adenoic cystic carcinoma of the Bartholin's gland: a clinical, histological and immunocytochemical study of a case. Eur J Surg Oncol 14:335–339

Anthony PP, James PD (1975) Adenoid cystic carcinoma of the breast: prevalance, diagnostic criteria and histogenesis. J Clin Pathol 28:647–655

Bernstein SG, Voet RL, Lifshig S et al. (1983) Adenoid cystic carcinoma of Bartholin's gland. Case report and review of the literature. Am J Obstet Gynecol 147:385–390

Budd GT, Groppe CW (1983) Adenoid cystic carcinoma of the salivary gland. Cancer 51:589–590

Chamlian DK, Taylor HB (1972) Primary carcinoma of bartholin gland. Obstet Gynecol 39:489–494

Copeland LJ, Sneige N, Gershenson DM et al. (1986) Adenoid cystic carcinoma of Bartholin gland. Obstet Gynecol 39:489–494

Dennis ES III, Esther LL, Wilson LA (1955) Primary carcinoma of Bartholin's gland: review. Obstet Gynecol 6:291–296

Dodson MG, O'Leary JA, Orfei E (1978) Adenoid cystic carcinoma of the vulva. Malignant Cylindroma. Obstet Gynecol 51 [Suppl]:26–29

Eichner E (1963) Adenoid cystic carcinoma of Bartholin gland: review of the literature and report of a case. Obstet Gynecol 21:608–613

Gordon HW, McMahon NJ, Agliozzo CM et al. (1972) Adenoid cystic (cylindromatous) carcinoma of the uterine cervix: report of two cases. Am J Clin Pathol 58:51–57

Leuchter RS, Hackder NF, Voet RL et al. (1982) Primary carcinoma of bartholin's gland: a report of 14 cases and review of the literature. Obstet Gynecol 60:361–368

Mazur MT, Battifora HA (1982) Adenoid cystic carcinoma of the uterine cervix: ultrastructure, immunofluorescence and criteria for diagnosis. Am J Clin Pathol 77:494–500

Mossler JA, Woodard BH, Addison A et al. (1980) Adenocarcinoma of Bartholin's gland. Arch Pathol Lab Med 104:523–526

Murphy J, Wilson JM, Bickel DA (1962) Adenoid cystic carcinoma of the Bartholin gland and pregnancy. Am J Obstet Gynecol 83:612–614

Ortner VA, Barbee W, Mikuz A et al. (1980) Adenoidzystisches Karzinom (Zylindrom) der Bartholinschen Drüse. Zentralbl Gynakol 102:59–63

Plouffe L Jr, Tulandi T, Rosenberg A et al. (1984) Non-Hodgkins's lymphoma in Bartholin's gland: case report and review of literature. Am J Obstet Gynecol 148:608–609

Rosenzweig E (1960) Un cas rare de sarcome vulvaire dans la region de la glande de Bartholin (sa hemangioendothelial). Gynaecologia 149:608–609

Sackett NB (1958) Carcinoma primary in Bartholin's gland. Am J Obstet Gynecol 75:183–188

Sayre GP (1949) Cylindroma of the vulva: adenocarcinoma, cylindroma type of the vulva, report of a case of twenty seven years duration. Mayo Clin Proc 24:224–233

Skibba JL, Hurtley JD, Ravelo HC (1981) Complete response of a metastaic adenoid cystic carcinoma of the parotid gland to chemotherapy. Cancer 47:2543–2548

Tandler B (1971) Ultrastructure of adenoid cystic carcinoma of salivary gland origin. Lab Invest 24:504–512

Trelford JD, Deos PH (1976) Bartholin's gland carcinoma: five cases. Gynecol Oncol 4:212–221

Webb JB, Lott M, O'Sullivan JC et al. (1984) Combined adenoid cystic and squamous carcinoma of Bartholin's gland. Br J Obstet Gynecol 91:291–295

Whalstrom TM, Vesterinen MDE, Saksela E (1978) Primary carcinoma of bartholin's glands: a morphological and clinical study of six cases including a transitional cell carcinoma. Gynecol Oncol 6:354–362

Wheelock JB, Gopelerud DR, Dunn LJ et al. (1984) Primary carcinoma of the Bartholin gland: a report of ten cases. Obstet Gynecol 63:820–824

Adenoma of Minor Vestibular Glands

Axe S, Parmley T, Woodruff JD et al. (1986) Adenomas in minor vestibular glands. Obstet Gynecol 68:16–18

Foushee JHS, Reeves WJ, McCool JA (1968) Benign masses of Bartholin gland: solid, adnomas, adenomas with cyst, and Bartholin's gland with varices or thrombosis or cavernous hemangioma. Obstet Gynecol 31:695–701

Honore LH, O'Hara KE (1978) Adenoma of Bartholin's gland: report of three cases. Eur J Obstet Gynaecol Reprod Biol 8:335–340

Marinoff SC, Turner MLC (1986) Hypersensitivity to vaginal candidiasis or treatment vehicles in the pathogenesis of minor vestibular gland syndrome. J Reprod Med 31:796–799

Willis RA (1948) Epithelial tumours of the vagina and vulva. In: Pathology of tumours. Butterworth, London, pp 547–553

Malakoplakia of Bartholin's Gland

Paquin ML, Davis JR, Weiner S (1986) Malakoplakia of Bartholin's gland. Arch Pathol Lab Med 110:757–758

5 Tumours and Tumour-like Conditions of Ectopic Tissue in the Vulva

5.1 Ectopic Breasts, Cysts and Breast Tumours

5.1.1 Normal Breast Tissue

5.1.1.1 Ectopic Breast Tissue in the Vulva

The mammary ridges appear as an ectodermal thickening along the ventrolateral surface of the embryo, extending from the axilla to the upper medial surface of the thigh. The mammary buds appear in these ridges, and only those in the pectoral region persist. Subsequently, the caudal two-thirds of the ridges disappears. Ectopic breasts develop when the mammary ridges of the caudal part of the embryo fail to atrophy.

An aberrant breast may be suspected when a painful vulval swelling (Reeves and Kaufman 1980) or a vulval mass is first noticed during pregnancy (Levin and Diener 1968) and the postnatal period (Woodruff and Seeds 1962). In the non-pregnant and non-lactating woman (Tow and Shanmugaratnam 1962), it may be present as an asymptomatic vulval lump, commonly a semicystic mass of the size of a plumstone in one of the labia majora, often misdiagnosed as a lipoma or fibroma (McFarland 1931). Infrequently, the breast tissues are found in the labia minora (Mengert 1935). The majority of the affected women are multiparous.

The lesions are usually unilateral. Bilateral lesions are discovered more often during pregnancy and puerperium (Garcia et al. 1978). On rare occasions, ectopic breasts develop concamitant with vulval breasts at other sites such as in the axillae (Looney et al. 1959). A nipple and areola are not usually seen on ectopic breasts. Like normal pectoral breasts, the aberrant breast tissues may show hyperplasia, secretory activities and even undergo neoplastic changes.

5.1.1.1.1 Microscopical Appearance

The mass is made up of breast lobules consisting of ductules which are lined by two layers of cells (Fig. 5.1). On the luminal side, the cells are cuboidal, and on the outer side they are flattened myoepithelial. The intralobular connective tissue is loose and generally contains a few lymphocytes and plasma cells. The lobules are separated by dense bands of collagen containing interlobular ducts lined by two layers of cuboidal cells.

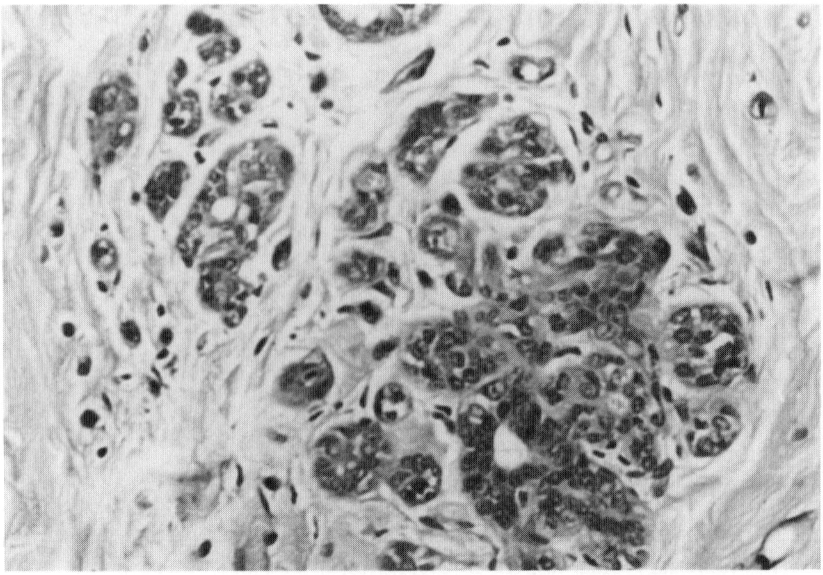

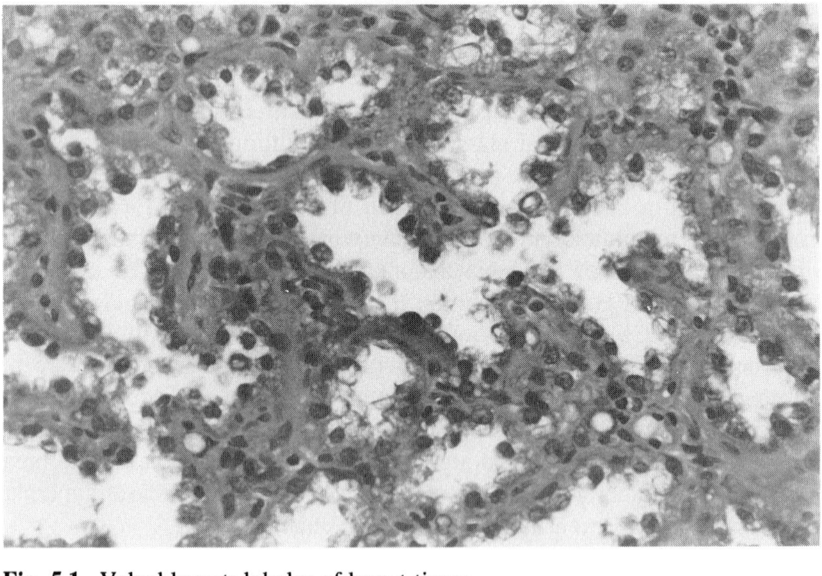

Fig. 5.1. Vulval breast: lobules of breast tissue

Fig. 5.2. Vulval breast lactation changes: secretory vacuoles within the cells

Abscess formation, galactocele and neoplastic changes may complicate the lesion. According to Hassim (1969), the common pathological change in the ectopic breast is the occurrence of fibroadenoma. There are also reports indicating that the vulval breast tissues have the same malignant potential as the pectoral breast and that adenocarcinoma can develop in them (Greene 1936; Hendrix and Behrman 1956). See 8.5.1.

5.1.1.1.2 Treatment
Simple excision is adequate.

5.1.1.2 Vulval Lactating Breast

In almost half of all patients, supernumerary breast tissue is first discovered during pregnancy due to gradual swelling or appearance of a mass on one or both labia majora. Like the pectoral breasts, supernumerary vulval breasts may undergo similar pregnancy changes such as hyperplasia and secretory activities and at times even exude milk fluid. Some patients may notice a sudden increase in the size of an otherwise indolent nodule in the labium majus during late pregnancy or the lactating period.

5.1.1.2.1 Gross Appearance
The nodules are usually small, well-demarcated and soft. They may occasionally be large, weighing up to 40 g (Gugliotta et al. 1983).

5.1.1.2.2 Microscopical Appearance
The breast nodules are composed of crowded acini lined by one to two layers of cells. The basal layer is formed by elongated myoepithelial cells containing a moderate amount of pale eosinophilic cytoplasm and small, round nuclei. The luminal layer is made up of cuoidal or low columnar cells with round or oval nuclei. The cytoplasm of these cells display apical vacuoles and snouts of active secretion (Fig. 5.2). The hyperplastic acini with ducts may be grouped in a lobular fashion. Eosinophilic secretory products may be present in the lumen of both acini and ducts.

5.1.1.2.3 Treatment
Treatment is by excision.

5.1.2 Breast Cyst

5.1.2.1 Milk Cyst

An excessive collection of milky fluid within the lactating breast may occasionally cause cystic distension as large as a fist or an orange (Bergner 1934). The patient complains of a rapidly growing lump in a labium majus, causing difficulty in walking. Aspiration of the cyst reveals milky fluid.

To avoid repeated collection of fluid and risk of rupture and infection, the cyst needs to be excised.

5.1.3 Breast Tumours

5.1.3.1 Fibroadenoma and Giant Fibroadenoma (Cystosarcoma Phyllodes)

5.1.3.1.1 Clinical Features

Fibroadenomata are the most common pathological change which occurs in vulval breasts. The patients are usually between 14 and 48 years of age (Smith-Foushee and Pruitt 1967), but the women in 5th and 6th decades can also develop these lesions. Generally, the patient presents with a slowly growing lump in the vulva. Most often the tumour is discovered incidentally. Infrequently, the tumour appears during the lactation period, pregnancy and menses, when it increases in size and becomes tender (Smith-Foushee and Pruitt 1967). Of the vulval breast lesions diagnosed in non-gravid women, 78% are likely to be neoplastic (Garcia et al. 1978). Rarely the tumour appears as a perineal lump (Fisher 1947).

5.1.3.1.2 Gross Appearance

The lesion is most frequently unilateral; bilateral tumours are indeed rare (Hassim 1969). The tumour is an unencapsulated, well-circumscribed and slightly lobulated mass of 1–3 cm in size and of firm and rubbery consistency. The cut surfaces are bulging, solid and grey-white to grey-tan in colour. Occasionally, it may be cystic, containing papillary fronds and gelatinous material (Siegler and Gordon 1951).

5.1.3.1.3 Microscopical Appearance

The tumour consists of ducts and ductules lined by cuboidal to columnar and a few myoepithelial cells arranged haphazardly or in an orderly fashion in loose myxoid or oedematous connective tissue (Fig. 5.3). The exuberant stroma may elongate, bend and distort the tubular configurations of the ducts and ductules to various degrees. Branching or budding may lead to the formation of new tubules.

Cystosarcoma phyllodes, also known as giant fibroadenoma, can occur in ectopic breasts (Singh et al. 1980). Although the tumour may attain an enormous size, it can be very small. According to Treves and Sunderland (1951), increased cellularity and a marked growth pattern are more important distinguishing characteristics. This fibroepithelial tumour displays sinusoidal clefts, blunt papillae, slit-like spaces lined by cuboidal cells and densely cellular, exuberant, oedematous and myxoid connective tissue stroma. The disproportionate stromal proliferation sometimes converts blunt papillae into leaf-like structures. These tumours are essentially benign, but a small minority of them are malignant and metastasise. They may be locally aggressive and recur. There are no satisfactory histological criteria to differentiate the benign from malignant tumours. Because of this, clinical correlation with the histological features has remained a difficult problem (Blichert-Toft et al. 1975).

Vulval fibroadenomas have been suggested to be of local apocrine gland origin (Burger and Marcuse 1954). The majority opinion at present favours an ectopic breast origin.

5.1.3.1.4 Treatment

Treatment is simple excision. Recurrence has not been reported after surgical removal. Adenocarcinoma complicating ectopic breast is obviously rare and should be treated similarly to other vulval malignant lesions.

5.1.3.2 Intraduct Papilloma

Intraduct papilloma consisting of papillary projections with a double layer of cells supported on a connective tissue core (Fig. 5.4) with occasional foci of apocrine metaplasia, a not uncommon condition of the pectoral breast, has also been reported in the vulval ectopic breast (Rickert 1980).

Intraduct epithelial proliferation (epitheliosis) is more frequent than intraduct papilloma in the pectoral breast. In vulval breasts fibroadenoma is thought to be the msot common of pathological changes (Hassim 1969). The papillary lesions in the vulval breast are mostly hidradenomas which most likely arise in the apocrine sweat glands. Although the intraduct papillomas can occur in genital breasts (Meeker et al. 1962; Rickert 1980), they are, indeed, rare lesions and according to some authors are analogous to hidradenoma papilliferum (Cunningham and Hardy 1947). While it is difficult to differentiate these two lesions, some differences are thought to exist. The intraduct papillomas are larger and tend to be multiple (Meeker et al. 1962). The presence of breast tissue or fibroadenomatous changes with the papillary lesions are helpful points for the diagnosis of intraduct papilloma. Nevertheless, the breasts are modified sweat glands, and the two lesions in question arising in the breast can display some degree of structural similarity. From the mangement point of view, the distinction appears arbitrary as both lesions have very low malignant potential (Gugliotta et al. 1983).

5.1.4 Tumour-like Conditions

5.1.4.1 Endometriotic Cysts, Endometriosis

Endometriosis of the vulva is uncommon. The patients are usually in their 30s and present with a painful nodule which may enlarge during menstruation (Healy 1956). The lesion is usually located on the labium majus (Henry 1927; Kirk 1950) as subcutaneous nodules or in the vestibule and fourchette as submucosal, sharply localised tumours (Williams 1965). It can develop in an episiotomy scar (Brougher 1947; Nussbaum and Motyloff 1957) and in the groin with preference for the right side, often in association with inguinal hernia (Catherwood and Cohen 1951; Clausen and Nielsen 1987). The patient may complain of gradually increasing

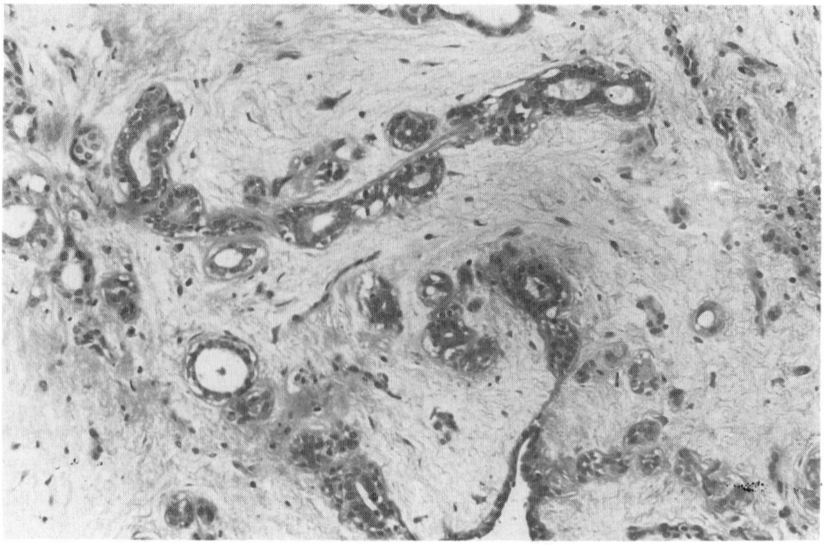

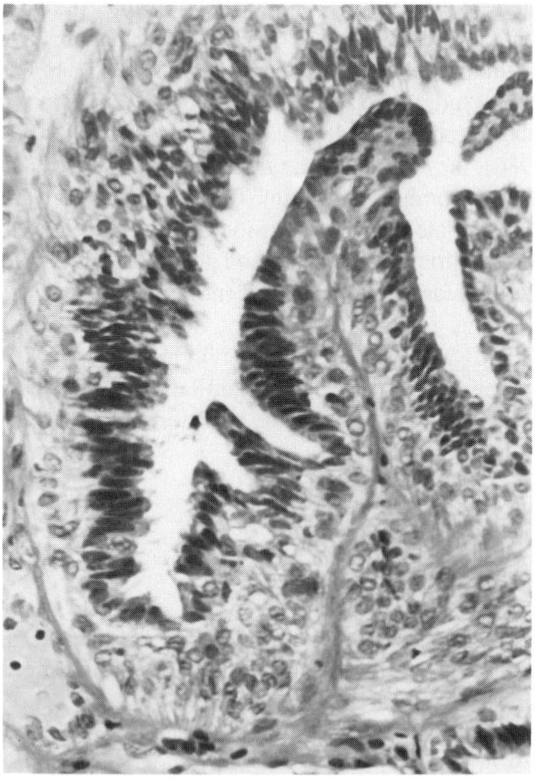

Fig. 5.3. Vulval breast: fibroadenoma showing irregularly arranged acini in mucoid stroma

Fig. 5.4. Vulval breast: papillae lined by two layers of cells and supported on a fibrovascular core

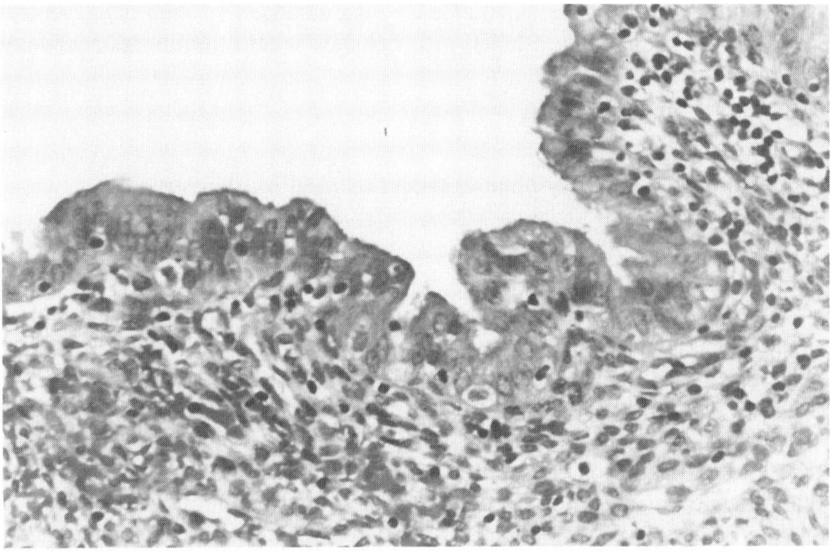

Fig. 5.5. Endometriotic cyst: gland lined by columnar cells and surrounded by stromal cells

painful nodules, dyspareunia and irritation. The nodules are 1.5 cm in average diameter, round or oval in shape, bluish in colour and firm in consistency.

5.1.4.1.1 Microscopical Appearance

The lesion consists of endometrial glands and stroma with variable fibroblastic stroma (Fig. 5.5) which may display marked myxoid changes and inflammatory cell reaction. Macrophages laden with haemosiderin pigments may be arranged in sheets around the glands. Recent haemorrhages may be seen in some lesions (Steck and Helwig 1966).

The histogenesis of these lesions was linked by von Recklinghausen to the embryological association of Wolffian body and round ligament. These structures were thought to harbour the cell rests which could give rise to endometriosis (Rothman 1949). Both implantation and metaplasia could be possible mode of genesis.

5.1.4.1.2 Treatment

Treatment is surgical excision.

5.1.4.2 Deciduoma

Small nodules of decidualised endometriosis can on rare occasions be seen in the episiotomy scar of the vulva (Catherwood and Cohen 1951) and may resemble hidradenoma, hypertrophic scar or a fibroepithelial polyp. They may appear initially as reddish granulation tissue with an elevated surface (Nussbaum and Motyloff 1957) but later become firm, fibrous and tan coloured. The microscopic features consist of endometrial glands surrounded by decidualised stromal cells. At a later stage only a few haemosiderin-laden macrophages within the fibrous scar may be seen.

5.1.4.2.1 Treatment

The lesions are most often symptomless and excised for diagnosis.

5.1.4.3 Choriostoma

Choriostoma is the presence of a mass of normal tissue in an abnormal site. This uncommon phenomenon has been reported to occur at several locations. A frequent example is the Meckel's diverticulum harbouring pancreatic and gastric tissue. Willis (1968) reported gastrointestinal and respiratory epithelium in a cystic mass on the face. In the female genital tract, choriostoma is rare. The presence of thyroid and parathyroid tissues in the vagina (Kurman and Chandra Prabha 1973) and pancreatic tissue on the fallopian tube (Mason and Quagliarello 1976) have been previously noticed. Whether some of these unusual lesions represent a benign teratoma is not clear. Marwah and Bergman (1980) reported a 4-cm gelatinous mass on the left labium majur of a 38-year-old woman, which on microscopic examination was found to be salivary gland composed of lobules of normal serous and mucinous acini set in a myxoid stroma, an island of cartilage and respiratory epithelium. Yeoh et al. (1987) noticed an ulcerated lesion on a labium majus which consisted of colonic mucosa.

Several theories have been proposed: abnormal migration of progenitor cells, misplaced blastema which has differentiated in an abnormal location, teratoma and abnormal transformation from the urogenital sinus (Marwah and Bergman 1980). The last phenomenon is known as heteroplasia in contrast to metaplasia, which occurs in an already differentiated tissue.

5.1.4.3.1 Treatment

All these lesions are benign and are excised.

References

Ectopic Breasts

Garcia JJ, Verkauf BS, Hockberg CJ et al. (1978) Aberrant breast tissue of the vulva. Obstet Gynecol 52:225–228

Greene HJ (1936) Adenocarcinoma of supernumerary breasts of the labia majora in a case of epidermoid carcinoma of the vulva. Am J Obstet Gynecol 31:660–663

Hassim AM (1969) Bilateral fibroadenoma in supernumerary breasts of the vulva. J Obstet Gynaecol Br Commonw 76:275–277

Hendrix RC, Behrman SJ (1956) Adenocarcinoma arising in a supernumerary mammary gland in the vulva. Obstet Gynecol 8:238–241

Levin N, Diener RL (1968) Bilateral ectopic breast of the vulva. Obstet Gynecol 32:274–276

Looney CM, Reichman SC, Noel OF (1959) Ectopic breast tissue: report of unusual case. Am Surg 25:219–222

McFarland J (1931) Mammary gland situated on the labium majus. Arch Pathol 11:236–240

Mengert WF (1935) Supernumerary mammary gland on labia minora. Am J Obstet Gynecol 29:891–892

Reeves KO, Kaufman RH (1980) Vulvar ectopic breast tissue mimicking periclitoral abscess. Am J Obstet Gynaecol 137:509–511

Tow SH, Shanmugaratnam K (1962) Supernumerary mammary gland in the vulva. Br Med J II:1234–1236

Woodruff JD, Seeds AE Jr (1962) Benign and malignant adenomatous lesions of the vulva: summaries of six cases. Obstet Gynecol 20:690–695

Lactating Breasts

Gugliotta P, Fibbi ML, Fessia L et al. (1983) Lactating supernumerary mammary gland tissue in the vulva. Appl Pathol 1:61–65

Milk Cyst

Bergner EA (1934) A case of milk cyst in the labium majus. Acta Obstet Gynecol Scand 14:205–206

Fibroadenoma

Blichert-Toft M, Hansen JPH, Hansen OH et al. (1975) Clinical course of cystosarcoma phyllodes related to histologic appearance. Surg Gynecol Obstet 140:929–932

Burger RA, Marcuse PM (1954) Fibroadenoma of vulva. Am J Clin Pathol 24:965–968

Fisher JH (1947) Fibroadenoma of supernumerary mammary gland tissue in vulva. Am J Obstet Gynecol 53:335–337

Garcia JJ, Verkauf BS, Hockberg CJ et al. (1978) Aberrant breast tissue of the vulva. Obstet Gynecol 52:225–228

Hassim AM (1969) Bilateral fibroadenoma in supernumerary breasts of the vulva. J Obstet Gynaecol Br Commonw 76:275–277

Siegler AM, Gordon R (1951) Fibroadenoma in a supernumerary breast in the vulva. Am J Obstet Gynecol 62:1367–1369

Singh J, Singh B, Chander J (1980) Extramammary cystosarcoma phyllodes with bilateral breast involvement. Aust NZ J Surg 50:56–58

Smith-Foushee JH, Pruitt AB Jr (1967) Vulvar fibroadenoma from aberrant breast tissue: report of 2 cases. Obstet Gynecol 29:819–823

Treves N, Sunderland DA (1951) Cystosarcoma phyllodes of the breast: a malignant and a benign tumour; a clinicopathologic study of seventy seven cases. Cancer 4:1286–1332

Intraduct Papilloma

Cunningham JA, Hardy J (1947) Hidradenoma of the vulva: report of four cases with an evaluation of them in the light of analogous breast lesions. South Surg 13:831–838

Gugliotta P, Fibbi ML, Fessia L et al. (1983) Lactating supernumerary mammary gland tissue in the vulva. Appl Pathol 1:61–65

Hassim AM (1969) Bilateral fibroadenoma in supernumerary breasts of the vulva. J Obstet Gynaecol Br Commonw 76:275–277

Meeker JH, Neubecker RD, Helweg EB (1962) Hidradenoma papilliferum. Am J Clin Pathol 37:182–195

Rickert RR (1980)Intraductal papilloma arising in supernumerary breast tissue. Obstet Gynecol 55 [Suppl]:84–87

Endometriosis

Brougher JC (1947) Endometrial cyst in an episiotomy scar. Am J Obstet Gynecol 54:127–128

Catherwood AE, Cohen ES (1951) Endometriosis with decidual reaction in episiotomy scar. Am J Obstet Gynecol 62:1364–1366
Clausen I, Nielsen KT (1987) Endometriosis in the groin. Int J Gynecol Obstet 25:469–471
Healy JJ (1956) Bilateral endometriosis of the vulva. Am J Obstet Gynecol 72:1361–1363
Henry JS (1927) An endometrial growth in right labium majus. Surg Gynecol Obstet 44:637–645
Kirk EW (1950) Endometrioma in the posterior half of the labium majus. J Obstet Gynaecol Br Emp 57:237–238
Nussbaum W, Motyloff L (1957) Endometriosis of the vulva during pregnancy. Am J Obstet Gynecol 73:215–216
Rothman ED (1949) Endometriosis of the vulva. West J Surg Obstet Gynecol 57:297–300
Steck ED, Helwig EB (1966) Cutaneous endometriosis. Clin Obstet Gynecol 9:373–383
Williams GA (1965) Post surgical and post traumatic tumors. Clin Obstet Gynecol 8:1020–1034

Deciduoma

Catherwood AE, Cohen ES (1951) Endometriosis with decidual reaction in episiotomy scar. Am J Obstet Gynecol 62:1364–1366
Nussbaum W, Motyloff L (1957) Endometriosis of the vulva during pregnancy. Am J Obstet Gynecol 73:215–216

Choristoma

Kurman RJ, Chandra Prabha A (1973) Thyroid and parathyroid glands in the vaginal wall: report of a case. Am J Clin Pathol 59:503–507
Marwah S, Berman ML (1980) Ectopic salivary gland in the vulva (choriostoma): report of a case and review of the literature. Obstet Gynecol 50:389–391
Mason TE, Quagliarello JR (1976) Ectopic pancreas in the fallopian tube; a case report. Obstet Gynecol 48 [Suppl]:70–73
Willis RA (1968) Some unusual developmental heterotopias. Br Med J III:267–272
Yeoh G, Bannatyne P, Kossard S et al. (1987) Intestinal heterotopia: an unusual cause of vulval ulceration; case report. Br J Obstet Gynaecol 94:600–602

6 Intra-epithelial and Invasive Carcinomas of Squamous Cell Origin

6.1 Vulval Intra-epithelial Neoplasia

The three types of lesions – Bowen's disease, Queyrat's erythroplasia, and squamous cell carcinoma-in-situ – once recognised as distinct entities have been regrouped into a single category by the International Society for the Study of Vulvar Disease (1976). The terms Bowen's disease and Queyrat's erythroplasia have been abolished, and these two together with intra-epithelial carcinoma simplex have been put into a single category as carcinoma-in-situ. As there are only subtle histopathological differences (Kaufman and Gardner 1965), many overlapping similarities among them and occasionally wide variations of appearances in the same lesion, the pathologists are not often unanimous in their diagnoses (Woodruff and Hildebrandt 1958) of these conditions. Most importantly, the biological behaviour of these lesions are similar and often necessitate a similar mode of management. The Society has defined carcinoma-in-situ as disorientation of epithelial architecture which extends throughout the full thickness of the epithelium, not including surface layers above the granular zone, and put dysplasia under vulval atypia which may exist with or without dystrophy (International Society for the Study of Vulvar Disease 1976). In a small percentage of lesions, the epithelium may not be involved in its full thickness, and there may be squamous "pearls" at the tips of rete pegs with loss of the normal basal cell layer. The present trend is to encompass all intra-epidermal atypias as intra-epithelial neoplasia (VIN) in accordance with the criteria used for defining cervical intra-epithelial neoplasia.

Paget's disease of the vulva and melanoma in situ have been put under a separate category as non-squamous type of intra-epithelial neoplasia by the ISSVD.

A consistent body of evidence has over the past 2 decades accumulated to indicate that most of the vulval, vaginal and cervical intra-epithelial neoplasias are sexually transmitted viral diseases, implicating initially herpes simplex virus (HSV) type 2 and subsequently human papillomaviruses (HPV) as the related agents. A high incidence of association between the vulval, vaginal and cervical carcinomas amply supports the theory that a common agent or agents are responsible for multifocal origin (Franklin and Rutledge 1972) of some of the carcinomas of the female genital tract. Both herpes and papillomaviruses have been fairly extensively investigated recently with regard to their causative role. Initially, the viruses could be demonstrated only occasionally in intra-epithelial neoplasms (Kimura et al. 1978;

Korhonen et al. 1982), but by employing the in situ hybridisation technique with tritium-labelled, single-stranded, viral DNA, Crum et al. (1981) detected HSV-2 messenger RNA in the tissue from 6% of grade 3 intra-epithelial neoplasms of the vulva and vagina. It was suggested that in the process of neoplastic transformation, only a small portion of the viral genome was incorporated. This was followed by the transcription of mRNA and production of viral proteins. The protein produced during the early part of infection has been identified as the non-structural DNA binding protein (Dressman et al. 1980).

Using the immunocytochemical method, Kaufman et al. (1981) were able to localise the proteins VP143 and 34/35 in the biopsy specimens from carcinoma-in-situ or severe dysplasia of the vulva in 9 of 10 women. Positive results were also noticed by Cabral et al. (1982), who by using hyperimmune sera demonstrated non-structural glycoprotein VP143 and envelope glycoprotein VP119 in biopsies exhibiting severe dysplasia, carcinoma-in-situ and invasive carcinoma. Although these and other epidemiological studies suggest a link between HSV-2 and squamous intra-epithelial neoplasia of the female genital tract, the morphological and more elaborate in situ hybridisation techniques have tilted the balance largely in favour of HPV (Meisels et al. 1977; zur Hausen 1976). The increase in the incidence of these lesions in recent years (Boutselis 1972; Wolcott and Gallup 1984) and shift in the median age of occurrence from the mid-50s 30 years ago (Woodruff and Hildebrandt 1958) to the mid-30s (Buscema et al. 1980b; Friedrich et al. 1980) in the 1980s have paralleled the increase in the incidence of genital infections with HPV among women of reproductive age. It is now apparent that there is a high association between condylomata acuminata and VIN. The koilocytic atypia which are seen in the condylomatous lesions of cervix (Meisels et al. 1977) are also seen in a high percentage of VIN (Crum et al. 1984). The problem of understanding the mechanism linking condylomata, a proliferative lesion with virus infection as the aetiological agent, to the development of intraepithelial neoplasia as well as invasive carcinoma is yet to be solved. Although immunoperoxidase (Woodruff et al. 1980; Ferenczy et al. 1981; Rueda-Leverone et al. 1987) and in situ hybridisation techniques have been able to demonstrate several types of HPV in many atypical epidermal lesions including condyloma acuminatum, intra-epithelial neoplasia and invasive squamous cell carcinoma of the lower female genital tract, the causative role of these viruses in the genesis of genital cancer has not been conclusively established. It has been suggested that both HPV and HSV may act synergistically (zur Hausen 1982) or that HPV is a co-carcinogen acting with other carcinogenic agent or agents; one such agent may be HSV-2. Recently, Kaufman et al. (1988) have found HPV DNA in the tissue and HSV-2 antigen in the sera of 91% of patients with VIN. The most common HPV in early vulval neoplasia has been the type 16 (Gupta et al. 1987).

6.1.1 Clinical Features

The age of the patients ranges from 19 to 72 years, with a mean age of 38 years. Some 38% (Caglar et al. 1982) to 48% (Bernstein et al. 1983) of the patients are under 41 years of age.

The lesions are symptomatic in 75% of patients (DiPaola et al. 1982). This is in contrast to CIN which is mostly asymptomatic (Iversen et al. 1981). Pruritus is by far the most common complaint. The patient may sometimes notice changes in the vulval architecture due to white patch, ulcer, 'bumps' or other palpable abnormalities such as warty elevations. Some patients may complain of bleeding, pain and vaginal discharge. Up to 25% of the patients may not be aware of their disease. In 25%–60% of patients, a second, primary, malignant lesion in other genital areas, particularly in the cervix and vagina, has been noticed (Collins et al. 1970; Boutselis 1972; Forney et al. 1977; Friedrich et al. 1980). Seski et al. (1978) noticed abnormalities of lymphocyte transformation in response to mitogen in some of these patients and suggested that immunosuppression could probably explain the occurrence of neoplasia at multiple sites.

6.1.2 Gross Appearance

The lesion may be small, circumscribed or diffuse, affecting the whole vulva. The warty lesions are seen in 20% of cases (Buscema et al. 1980a), and 90% of them exhibits a raised surface (Friedrich et al. 1980). The colour varies from white to grey to shades of brown. In 34% of the patients the lesion is hyperpigmented and darker than the surrounding skin (Friedrich et al. 1980). The lesions are multifocal, and multicentricity is particularly common in young women, who tend to have discrete unifocal lesions (Benedet et al. 1982). Friedrich Jr. (1981) summarised the clinical features with "p" factors – papular, parakeratotic and pigmented.

6.1.3 Microscopical Appearance

The basic histological changes in VIN are distortion and disorganisation of the epidermal layer, which is thickened irregularly, with the rete pegs often elongated and expanded (Fig. 6.1). In VIN III, the whole thickness of the epidermis is composed of crowded abnormal cells displaying abnormal maturation, mitosis and nuclear aberrations (Fig. 6.2). Although there is considerable overlapping, the morphological changes in VIN III are expressed in two basic patterns (Buckley et al. 1984). In some, the cells are basal or parabasal cell type which extend to the upper strata of the epidermis and involve the whole thickness (Fig. 6.3). These cells are smaller than mature squamous cells, possess a scanty amount of cytoplasm around the hyperchromatic and pleomorphic nuclei and display a high nucleo-cytoplasmic ratio. In other lesions, the cells bear an apparent similarity to normal squamous cells but with reduced cytoplasm, larger hyperchromatic nuclei, prominent nucleoli

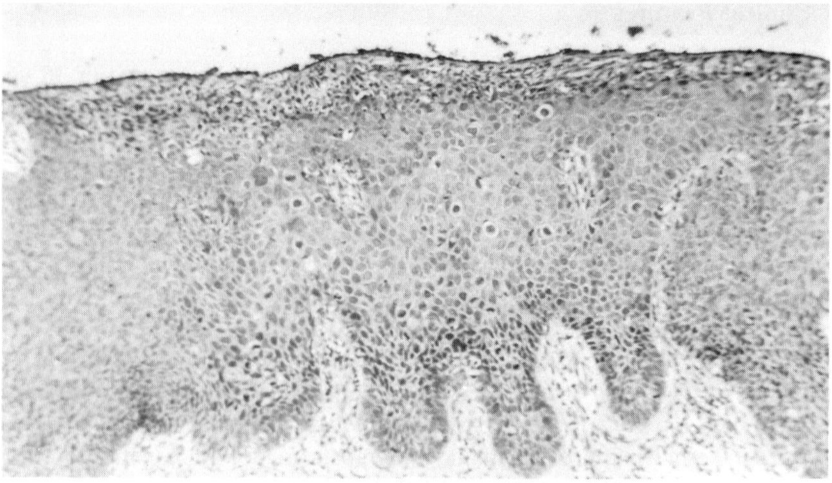

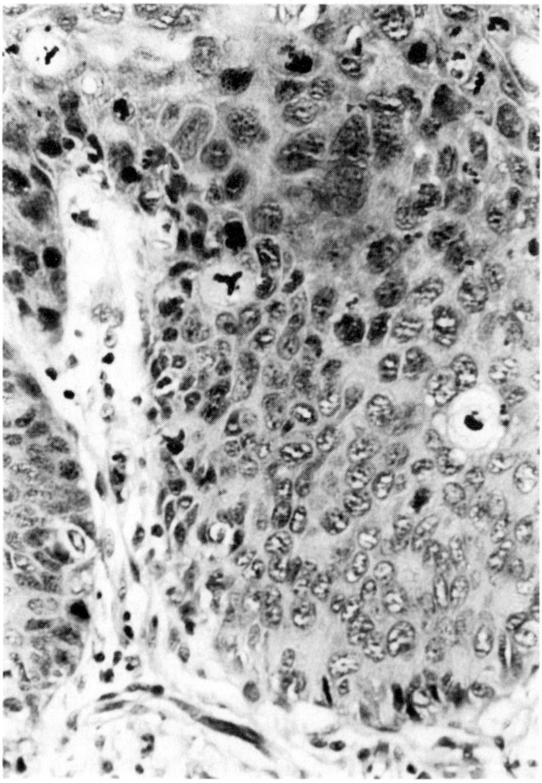

Fig. 6.1. Vulval intra-epithelial neoplasia: thickened epidermis with irregular rete peg

Fig. 6.2. Vulval intra-epithelial neoplasia III: abnormal cells showing pleomorphic nuclei and mitoses

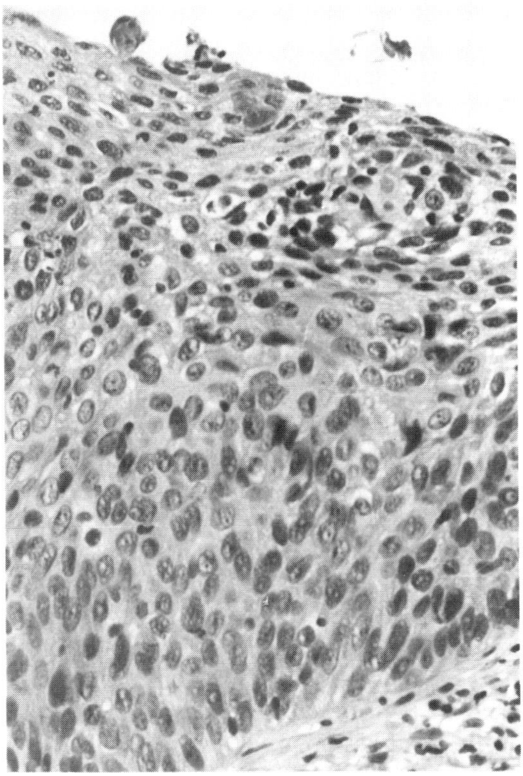

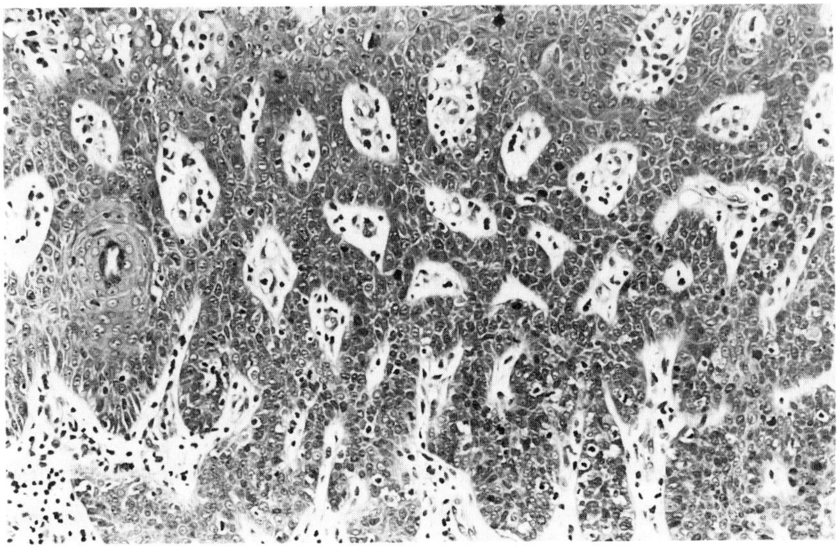

Fig. 6.3. Vulval intra-epithelial neoplasia III: basal and parabasal type cells extending to upper strata of epidermis

Fig. 6.4. Vulval intra-epithelial neoplasia III: cribriform pattern with intercommunicating rete ridges

and altered nucleo-cytoplasmic ratio. In this type the cellular atypia in general is not very marked. The rete ridges which are frequently elongated may be replaced by neoplastic cells. Mitotic figures are always present and may be quite frequent. In some lesions, there are occasional bizarre and monstrous nuclei in the suprabasal zone, corps ronds characterised by pyknotic nuclei surrounded by clear halos of pale or vacuolated cytoplasm and individual keratinised cells with dense eosinophilic cytoplasm. Focal areas containing koilocytes can be seen in the upper strata of the lesion. Surperficially, the lesions are covered by a layer of hyperkeratotic plugs and parakeratotic cells. These features were previously recognised as those of intra-epithelial carcinoma simplex type. In others, the lesions are composed of hyperplastic epidermis with markedly thickened and broader rete pegs containing numerous isolated keratinised cells scattered in all strata of abnormal epidermis, multinucleate cells, corps ronds, monstrous forms of nuclei and pronounced hyperkeratosis and parakeratosis. Occasionally, a cribriform pattern with interconnecting rate ridges can be seen in these lesions (Fig. 6.4). Koilocytes are also more frequent in these lesions. There are always variable, inflammatory, cellular infiltrations comprising lymphocytes, plasma cells and macrophages at the dermo-epidermal junctions. These correspond to what has been coined as the bowenoid type of intra-epithelial neoplasia. These lesions tend to occur in younger patients (Abell 1965), are multicentric and may regress (Berger and Horu 1978; Friedrich et al. 1980; Bernstein et al. 1983). In some, abundant melanin pigments and increased melanocytes can be demonstrated. Such lesions have been labelled as multicentric, pigmented Bowen's disease (Lloyd 1970; Kimura et al. 1978). Except for pigmentation, there are not histologically distinctive features to delineate them as an entity. Some authors (Wade et al. 1979; Ulbright et al. 1982) have advocated separation of Bowen's dysplasia from carcinoma-in-situ on clinical grounds and on the basis of histological features; the latter include the presence of dyskeratotic cells, multinucleate keratinocytes, nuclear uniformity and absence of pilosebaceous involvement, although these authors admit that overlapping does exist in both conditions. Ultrastructural studies of Nordquist et al. (1970) demonstrated virus-like particles in 6 or the 7 lesions, which could not be confirmed by others (Lupulesen et al. 1977; Faber and Hagedorn 1981).

An unusual histological feature characterised by atypical cellular maturation (Fig. 6.5) with pearl formation in the rete pegs in the setting of normal-looking superficial epidermis is occasionally noticed in VIN (Buscema et al. 1980b; Zacur et al. 1980). Such a feature, labelled by some workers as differentiated VIN III, should warrant a thorough search for areas of early invasion. Occasionally, the changes from normal epithelium to in situ neoplasia are very abrupt (Buscema et al. 1980a).

Suggestions have been made for grading VIN in accordance with the grading system used in CIN (Buckley et al. 1984): grade I signifying mild, grade II moderate and grade III severe atypia and carcinoma-in-situ. In a later modification (Kaufman and Gordon 1986), the International Society for the Study of Vulval Diseases has classified VIN into (a) squamous type with or without HPV changes and (b) non-squamous type which includes Paget's disease and melanoma-in-situ.

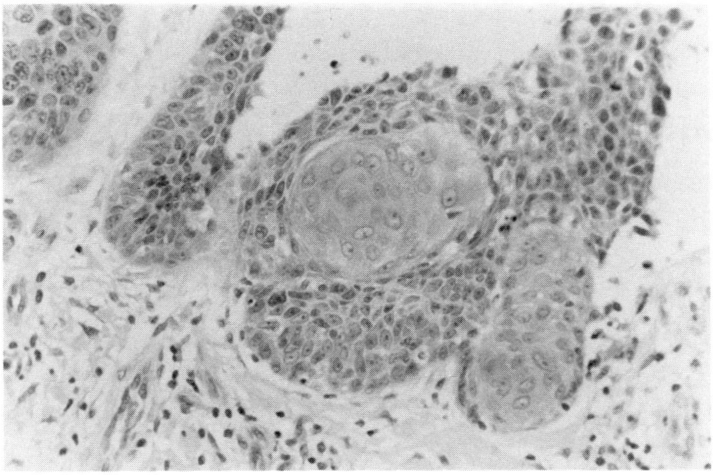

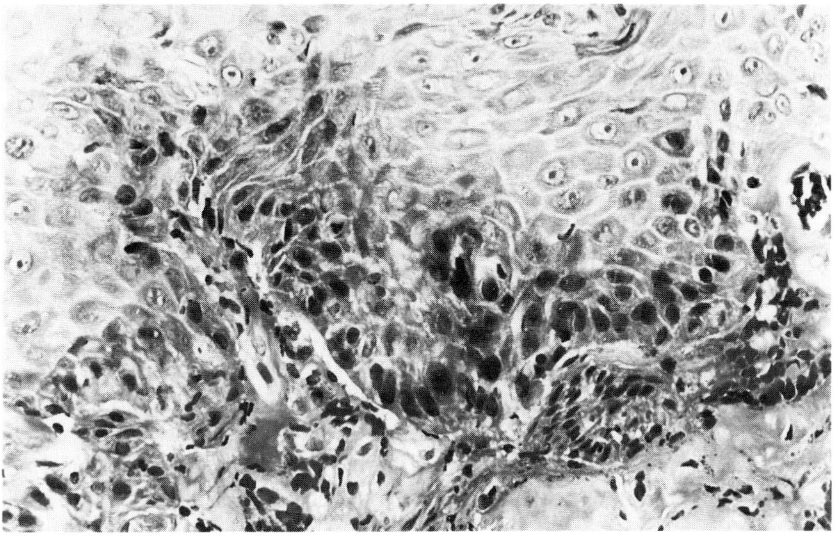

Fig. 6.5. Vulval intra-epithelial neoplasia III: atypical cellular maturation at the tip of rete ridge

Fig. 6.6. Vulval intra-epithelial neoplasia I: cellular pleomorphism limited to lower one-third of epidermis

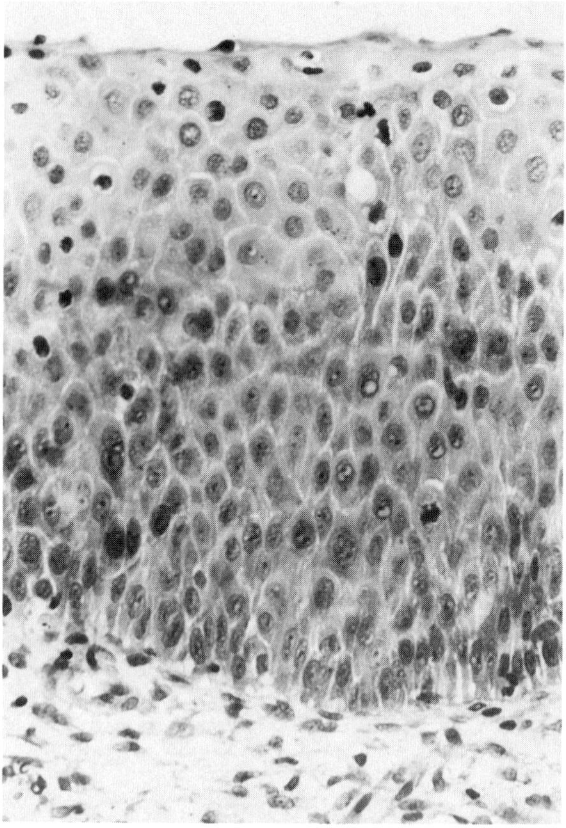

Fig. 6.7. Vulval intra-epithelial neoplasia II: cellular atypia limited to lower two-thirds of epidermis

The squamous type has been classified as mild dysplasia (VIN I), in which cellular atypia with loss of maturation and nuclear hyperchromasia, pleomorphism, mitosis and cellular crowding is limited to the lower one-third of the epidermis (Fig. 6.6). Dyskeratosis, corps ronds, hyperkeratosis and parakeratosis may be present. In moderate dysplasia (VIN II) the above-mentioned changes are limited to the lower two-thirds of the epidermis (Fig. 6.7). In severe dysplasia (VIN III) the cellular atypia involves more than the lower two-thirds and in carcinoma-in-situ (VIN III), nearly or full thickness of the epidermis. The differentiated VIN III lesions, as mentioned earlier, are those in which the constituent cells possess prominent eosinophilic cytoplasm and display keratin or pearl within the involved epidermis or at its rete tips. Bowenoid papulosis has not been accepted by the Society as an entity (Wilkinson et al. 1986). The inclusion of Paget's disease and melanoma-in-situ in the category of intra-epithelial neoplasia may not be universally acceptable, as the histogenesis and biological behaviour of both conditions are yet to be conclusively elucidated.

6.1.3.1 Ultrastructural Studies

Faber and Hagedorn (1981) noticed enlarged nucleoli, fewer desmosomes, aggregation of tonofilaments, intra-cytoplasmic inclusions containing parts of dyskeratotic cells, and intra-cytoplasmic vacuoles. The basal cells display cytoplasmic projections which extend into the dermis through the basement membrane (Olson et al. 1985). Individual cell keratinisation was reflected ultrastructurally in condensed cytoplasm, few cytoplasmic organelles and an increased number of tonofilaments (Korhonen et al. 1982). Abnormalities of the basement membrane and tonofilaments have also been noticed by others (Stegner 1986). There are several studies which demonstrated virus particles within the nuclei (Skinner et al. 1973; Rastkar et al. 1982) or cytoplasm (Nordquist et al. 1970).

6.1.4 Diagnosis

Cytological technique is not a popular method of diagnosis of VIN. The nuclear stain toludine blue is useful in detecting parakeratotic cells, which retain the dye even after application of 1% acetic acid for decolourisation. Although its value is controversial (Collins et al. 1966), it can be used during colposcopy to delineate the lesion (Broen and Ostergard 1971). In experienced hands, colposcopy is a very reliable tool for screening the macroscopically unrecognisable lesions (Caglar et al. 1982). Biopsy, however, has remained the most important of all diagnostic methods, and all chronic vulval lesions should be subjected to biopsy diagnosis.

6.1.5 Natural History

The progression rate of VIN to invasive carcinoma is very low. Buscema et al. (1980b) observed that only 4 patients (4%) in a series of 102 with carcinoma-in-situ developed invasive carcinoma during the follow-up period of up to 15 years, although the recurrence rate was much higher. In another series of 9 patients, only one who was immunosuppressed (Friedrich et al. 1980) developed an invasive lesion. The recurrence rate of VIN has been estimated to be about 25% and rate of invasion between 2% (Andreasson and Bock 1985) and 8% (Powell et al. 1986). While regression occurs mostly in younger patients, old age and immunosuppression are high risk factors for invasion. The area around the anal orifice, which is subjected to many irritants and trauma, is a high risk area particularly in older patients (Buscema and Woodruff 1980). Untreated, multifocal lesions in middle and late adult life also entail a much higher potential for progression (Jones and McLean 1986). The histological appearance of intra-epithelial carcinoma with characteristic epithelial pearls in the rete pegs in older patients is significant (Buscema and Woodruff 1980) and may portend impending invasion. By Feulgen microspectrophotometric nuclear study, Fu et al. (1981) observed that all carcinoma-in-situ had an aneuploid pattern and postulated that low ploidy stem cell lines (less than

3N) among these aneuploid lesions had a greater risk of progression to invasive carcinoma. With immunoperoxidase techniques, only 2.8% of the aneuploid lesions stained positive for HPV (Crum et al. 1982), and it was postulated that VIN was formed of immature cells which were not permissive for viral replication. However, the predictive values of both histopathological appearances and DNA analysis for the biological behaviour of the lesion are at present considered limited (Bernstein et al. 1983).

6.1.6 Treatment

Several factors, namely age of the patient, extent and multiplicity of the lesion and other associated conditions, are taken into consideration in the management of VIN. Several modalities like local excision, skinning vulvectomy followed by graft (Rettenmaier et al. 1987), vulvectomy, cryosurgery, laser and application of 5-fluorouracil are practised. However, in view of the likelihood of regression and low risk of invasion, particularly in young patients, the general tendency nowadays is to treat VIN conservatively. Local excision with shallow circular removal of individual lesions taking 0.5 cm margin of grossly and colposcopically normal skin was used in 16 patients without any recurrence in 14 for a period ranging from 1 to 8 years. The 2 patients with recurrences had positive margins (Bernstein et al. 1983). With wide local excision in 13 patients, recurrences followed in 2 patients, and with re-excision of the lesion, the patients remained disease free for 4 and 5 years (Caglar et al. 1982). A clear excision margin has been emphasised as an important factor in the reduction of recurrence rates. Wolcott and Gallup (1984) did not see any recurrence within 5 years in patients treated by wide local excision with clear margins. Rare recurrences can occur several years later even in skin grafts, indicating the importance of follow-up of these patients (Cox et al. 1986). Post-operative skin grafting has been advocated for cosmetic and functional reasons in sexually active women (Rutledge and Sinclair 1968), particularly with multifocal lesions (Underwood and Hester 1971; DiSaia and Rich 1981). Some workers (Dean et al. 1974; Wolcott and Gallup 1984) have recommended simple vulvectomy which lowers the recurrence risk and can be considered for older patients with minor medical problems. It is imperative, however, that a thorough histological examination of the specimen should be done to exclude the presence of any invasive focus. Recently, several authors (Baggish and Dorsey 1981; Townsend et al. 1982; Leuchter et al. 1984; Reid 1985; Wright and Davies 1987) also indicated that provided adequate biopsies had ruled out invasive carcinoma, the benefits of ablative treatment by CO_2 laser can be comparable with that of other surgical treatment, and the procedure can be used in unifocal, multifocal and recurrent vulval intra-epithelial lesions with maximum preservation of vulval integrity and sexual functions. Eradication of tissue to a depth of 5 mm has been advocated by Mene and Buckley (1985) as the appendages up to the depth of 4.6 mm from the surface of the epidermis are involved in more than 50% of patients with VIN. Successful results have also been reported with cryosurgical treatment in smaller lesions (Forney et al. 1977). Topical chemotherapy with 5-fluorouracil has been tried by many (Carson et al. 1976; Forney et al. 1977; Krupp and Bohm 1978; Lifshitz and Roberts 1980) with a very high failure rate. Many patients abandon the treatment due to pain and discomfort caused by this agent. Local immunotherapy with dinitrochlorbenzene (DNCB) has been used with some response (Foster and Woodruff 1981), but the number of cases studied are very few.

6.2 Superficially Invasive Carcinoma, Stage 1a (Microinvasive) Carcinoma

At present, there is no accepted definition of microinvasive carcinoma of the vulva. The variations in criteria of invasion with regard to depth, points at which depth measurement is made and discrepancies in the results of similar treatment in different series are so wide that the issue of microinvasive carcinoma as an entity is very much clouded with confusion.

Attempts at defining microinvasive carcinoma either of the cervix or vulva has mainly centred around the characterisation of an invasive lesion which is still microscopic and does not show metastatic potential to the regional lymph nodes or distant sites. Wharton et al. (1974) took an arbitrary depth of 5 mm invasion beneath the surface and found no lymphatic invasion in 25 patients. With a similar criterion of 5 mm limit, Parker et al. (1975) on the other hand noticed lymph node metastasis in 3 of 58 patients. There is general agreement that the incidence of lymph node metastases at vulvectomy is about 10%, when the depth of invasion is 5 mm or less (Wilkinson et al. 1982). When 3 mm is taken as the cut-off point, the incidence of nodal metastases is substantially lower; nonetheless, metastasis still occurs (Nakao et al. 1974; Magrina et al. 1979; Hoffman et al. 1983). There are still some lesions (Jafari and Cartnic 1976b; Yzigi et al. 1978) in which the depth of invasion is less than 2 mm, yet the patients develop nodal metastases. One patient died of metastatic disease with a lesion of less than 1 mm invasion (Jafari and Cartnic 1976a) and another patient had lymph node recurrence following local excision of microinvasive carcinoma with a depth of invasion of only 0.76 mm (Atamdede and Hoogerland 1989). Woodruff (1982) concluded that an invasion to a depth of more than 0.8 mm from the top of the deepest rate peg must be considered at risk. There is also wide variability in the method of measurement of invasion, which has hindered comparison of results in different series. Some researchers (Woodruff 1982) measured invasion from the base of the deepest rete pegs, others from the surface (Iverson et al. 1981) and granular cell layer (Husseinzadeh et al. 1983). Kurzl et al. (1988) compared methods of measurement with regard to their prognostic value and found that measurement of tumour thickness from the surface to the deepest point of invasion was a better indicator if 0.5 cm was taken as an endpoint; the median survival of the patients with a tumour thickness over 0.5 cm was 1.1 years, while it was 5.3 years with a thickness up to 0.5 cm.

Although Donaldson et al. (1981) found a lower incidence of nodal metastases in lesions less than 3 cm in size and a considerably higher incidence (72.4%) with larger lesions, nodal metastases occurred with lesions 2 cm or less in diameter (DiPaola et al. 1975; Parker et al. 1975; Magrina et al. 1979). Even lesions 1 cm or smaller are no guarantee against the possible risk of metastases (Nakao et al. 1974; Barnes et al. 1980).

Confluent or spray patterns of invasion by small cords of cells were also associated with lymph node metastases (Barnes et al. 1980), although such a correlation could not be confirmed in all studies (Magrina et al. 1979; Buscema et al. 1981). Parker et al. (1975) concluded that confluency as an isolated parameter was of no significance. It is evident that the definition of confluency has not been uniform. Magrina et al. (1979) defined it "as a group of tumour cells filling an area of 2 mm or more", whereas according to Hoffman et al. (1983) it was "a mass of invasive carcinoma which filled a 1 mm or greater field". While lymphatic permeation was also not considered to be an important variable by many (Magrina et al. 1979; Buscema et al. 1981; Boice et al. 1984), Donaldson et al. (1981) stressed that a lesion with neoplastic cells in the lymphatic space and only 1.1-mm stromal invasion could metastasise to the inguinal nodes. A correlation between lymphatic permeation and lymph nodal metastases as well as survival was, on the other hand, claimed in other studies (Iversen et al. 1981; Kolstad et al. 1982).

In an attempt to characterise the natural history on the basis of cellular differentiation, these lesions have been classified into large cell keratinising, large cell non-keratinising and small cell non-keratinising types (Parker et al. 1975; Kolstad et al. 1982); well, moderately and poorly differentiated types (Hoffman et al. 1983); or well differentiated, moderately differentiated and mixed differentiated types (Buscema et al. 1981; Woodruff 1982). Grading into 1 to 4 according to Broder's classification has also been tried (Magrina et al. 1979). The predictive value of cellular differentiation in relation to the biological behaviour has not, however, been found very accurate. It has been thought to be important by some workers (Parker et al. 1975; DiSaia et al. 1979; Buscema et al. 1981; Chu et al. 1981; Crissman and Azoury 1981) and of no great value by others (Iversen et al. 1981; Woodruff 1982; Hoffman et al. 1983). Husseinzadeh et al. (1983) concluded that the degree of tumour differentiation taken with depth of invasion was a more reliable predictor of nodal metastasis than either parameter alone. Franklin and Rudledge (1971) were of the opinion that size, extent and histologic differentiation of the lesion should all be considered together. According to others (Dvoretsky et al. 1984) the neoplastic thickness was a significant parameter and was defined as the maximal vertical dimension from the tip of the adjacent non-neoplastic rete ridge to the point of deepest stromal infiltration. The estimation of tumour volume (*V*) is now considered to be significantly more important. This can be done by measuring the radius of the surface of the lesion (*r*1), depth of invasion (*D*) and radius at deepest point of invasion (*r*2) and plotting the value according to the formula:

$$V = \frac{\pi D}{3} (r_1^2 + r_1 r_2 + r_2^2)$$

(Wilkinson et al. 1982). The tumour with volume not exceeding 1000 m^3 and depth of invasion not beyond 5 mm has the least risk of nodal metastases. Pickel and Haas

(1986) applying the mathematical formula calculated the 3-dimensional parameters of the lesion and came to the conclusion that a poorly differentiated microcarcinoma should not exceed a volume of $300\,mm^3$ and a well-differentiated one, $500\,mm^3$. Some have attempted to characterise the lesion by the pattern of invasion. It has been suggested that the spray, pseudoglandular and small cell superficially invasive carcinomas might be particularly aggressive (Hacker et al. 1983). Others held that the microinvasive carcinoma which progressed from an intra-epithelial carcinoma was at little risk of nodal metastases (Barnes et al. 1980; Chu et al. 1981).

This wide range of observations and inference reflect a gap in understanding the so-called microinvasive carcinoma of the vulva, and many have cast doubt on the existence of this entity. The task force and subcommittee of ISSVD on microinvasive cancer of the vulva has recently stated that "the term microinvasive cancer of the vulva is misleading and dangerous when taken with its current definition" and recommended that the term be discontinued and the designation "stage 1a cancer of vulva" be used for a small group of lesions; for the purposes of study, these lesions should be solitary and confined to a maximum of 2 cm diameter and 1 mm depth of stromal invasion. The depth of invasion is measured as the distance from the epithelial stromal junction of the most superficial, adjacent, dermal papillae to the deepest point of invasion of the tumour (Wilkinson et al. 1986).

6.2.1 Clinical Features

The overwhelming majority of patients are over 50 years old with ages ranging from 25 to 86 years (Boice et al. 1984). 60% being under 60 years old (Wharton et al. 1974). The presenting symptoms are pruritus, lump, ulceration, pain and bleeding. Some patients may be asymptomatic.

6.2.2 Pathological Features

The lesions may appear erythematous, grey, pink, brown or pigmented and may be flattened, raised, papular, warty or ulcerated. They may be multifocal in 30% of cases (Kunschner et al. 1978). In 65% of cases, the lesions are unilateral (Buscema et al. 1981), affecting the labia majora more frequently (Kunschner et al. (1978). Clitoris, fourchette and perineum may be involved in as many as 35% of cases (Buscema et al. 1981). Some 80% of patients may have associated other vulval lesions such as vulval dystrophy, intra-epithelial carcinoma and chronic vulvovaginitis (Magrina et al. 1979). Intra-epithelial carcinoma has been noticed in 18% (Gosling et al. 1961) to 70% of patients (Barnes et al. 1980).

The incidence of sexually transmitted granulomatous lesions like syphilis and lymphogranuloma venereum in association with microinvasive carcinoma is low. Condylomata acuminata are also not seen as frequently with the vulval microinvasive lesion as with intra-epithelial carcinoma (Buscema et al. 1981). Other malignancies which may be associated in as many as 20% of cases include those of the cervix, uterus, vagina, ovary, breast, oesophagus, tongue and rectum (Magrina et al. 1979; Japaze et al. 1977).

6.2.3 Diagnosis

To delineate the biopsy sites, colposcopy and toludine blue are useful (Broen et al. 1971; Forney et al. 1977), although with both false positive and false negative results are known to occur (Hughes 1971).

6.2.4 Microscopical Appearance

The histological appearances vary widely. Barnes et al. (1980) observed two types of microscopical appearance. One was associated with the overlying intra-epithelial carcinoma which consisted of (a) classic bowenoid type to intermediary form of

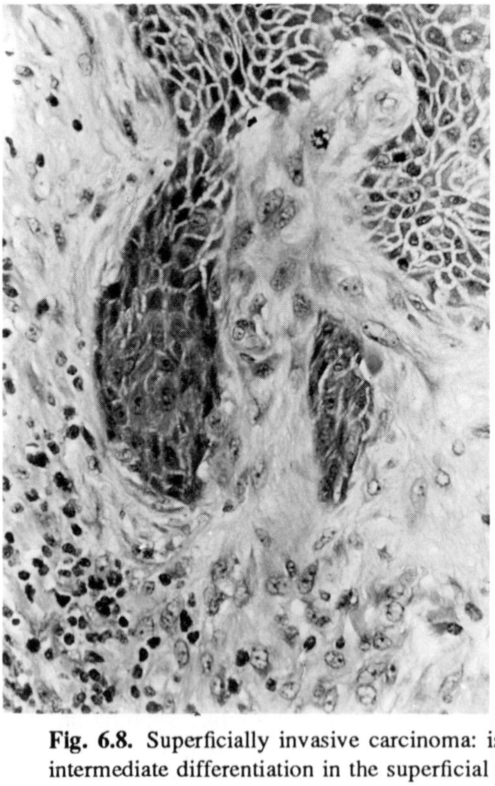

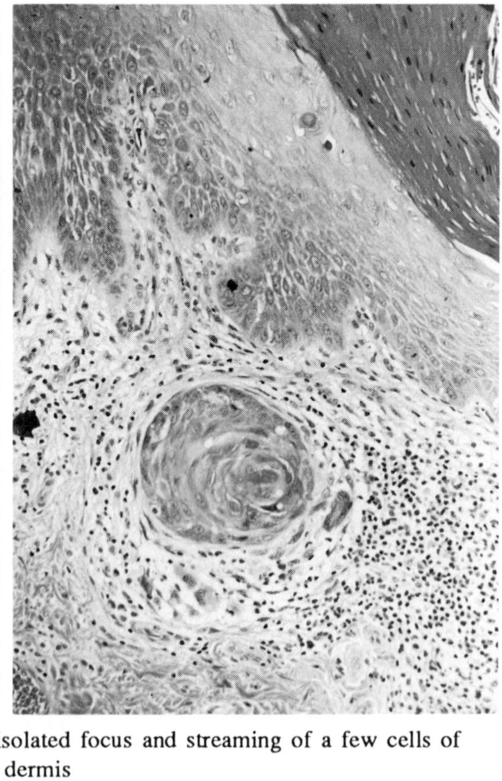

Fig. 6.8. Superficially invasive carcinoma: isolated focus and streaming of a few cells of intermediate differentiation in the superficial dermis

Fig. 6.9. Superficially invasive carcinoma: cells of the epidermis and invading cells are well-differentiated

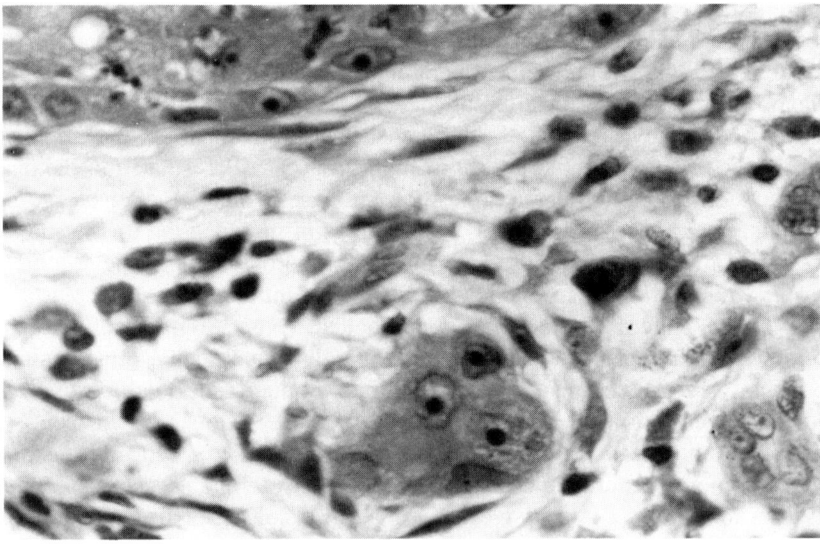

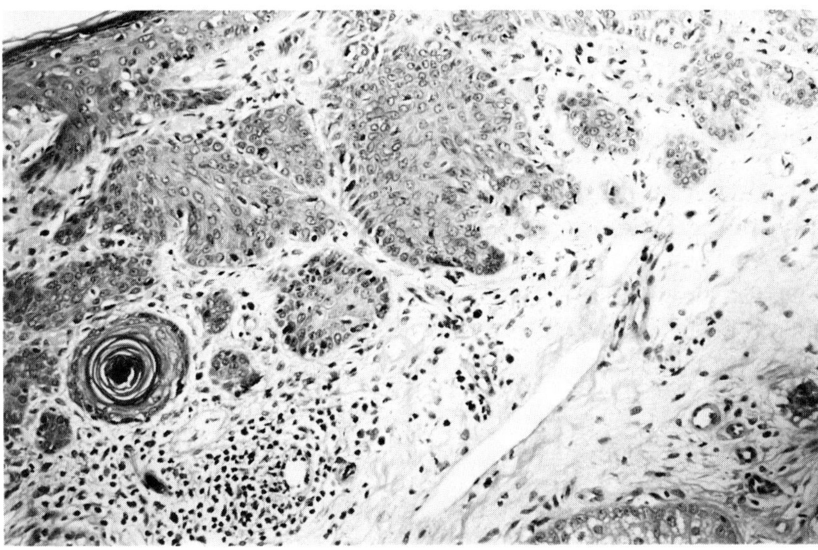

Fig. 6.10. Superficially invasive carcinoma: isolated focus of invasion with surrounding oedema, fibroblastic and inflammatory cell reactions

Fig. 6.11. Superficially invasive carcinoma: spray pattern of invasion with multiple foci of invasion over a wide area

undifferentiated cells, with the invasive component made up of one or more isolated foci of single cords or groups of cells infiltrating the stroma (Fig. 6.8) and (b) diffuse epithelial atypia with prominent keratinisation and focal areas of microinvasive carcinoma composed of well-differentiated cells (Fig. 6.9). In an occasional lesion, assessment of the invasion may be difficult because of broad and pushing deeper margins. Serial sectioning may reveal a small group of cells isolated in the dermis and surrounded by a mild degree of desmoplastic and cellular reactions (Fig. 6.10). Such a pattern used to be labelled as verrucoid form in which the invasion did not exceed 2 mm measuring from the base of the normal epithelium. The second type of lesion, which is not associated with significant intra-epithelial neoplasia, displays a 'spray' pattern of the invasive component (Fig. 6.11). In this, the single or multiple foci of well-differentiated cells expand symmetrically, often containing a prominent area of keratinisation, and infiltrate by numerous small cords, groups or individual cells from the expanding focus. In some lesions, the adjacent squamous epithelium is acanthotic with minimal atypia, and then a sudden transition to infasive carcinoma occurs which may be very well-differentiated or even anaplastic (Chu et al. 1981). The invasive focus may also consist of irregular groups of dyskeratotic epithelial cells beneath the basement membrane (Rastkar et al. 1982). The invading cells may be arranged as nests in the stroma beyond the level of the rete pegs or as groups in the papillae (Jafari and Cartnic 1976). Kunschner et al. (1978) designated a lesion as "questionable microinvasion" when isolated epithelial cells are present in the underlying stroma. Ross and Ehrmann (1987) have identified three patterns of invasion, namely (a) carcinoma-in-situ with early stromal invasion (one or more isolated foci of single cords or narrow tongue of cells, without regard to length, arising from the carcinoma-in-situ and infiltrating the stroma without coalescence), (b) pushing pattern with broad smooth front of invasion and (c) infiltrative, which includes all other types of invasion. Ehrmann et al. (1988) observed defective laminin around the nests of invading carcinoma by immunoperoxidase techniques and concluded that defective laminin beneath the carcinoma-in-situ might indicate early stromal invasion.

6.2.5 Treatment

Because of uncertainty of the definition of the condition, the treatment has varied widely from local excision to radical vulvectomy with or without lymphadenectomy. Due to the high risk of nodal metastases in vulval microinvasive carcinoma in contrast to cervical microinvasive carcinoma, which has a much lower incidence, radical surgery has been the choice of treatment. Hemivulvectomy with removal of the inguinal and femoral lymph nodes for the unilateral lesion and radical vulvectomy with bilateral inguino-femoral lymphadenectomy for a central lesion were advocated by Iversen et al. (1981). Parker et al. (1975) selected radical vulvectomy with lymphadenectomy for the lesions with invasion more than 5 mm in depth, vascular invasion and cellular anaplasia. Patients with an invasion less than 5 mm deep, no vascular involvement and anaplasia underwent radical vulvectomy without lymphadenectomy. When the vulvectomy specimen revealed residual disease, vascular involvement and anaplasia, staged lymphadenectomy was performed. It has also been advocated that midline lesions with more than 1 mm of stromal invasion should be treated by radical vulvectomy with bilateral inguino-femoral lymphadenectomy and a lateralised lesion by radical vulvectomy with ipsilateral inguino-femoral and contralateral superficial inguinal lymphadenectomy (Hacker et al. 1983). Figge and Gaudnez (1974) considered radical vulvectomy and inguino-femoral lymph node dissection as minimal treatment for invasive carcinoma. As nodal metastases were noticed in the lesion with any depth of invasion, the value of a pathological examination of the lymph nodes was particularly emphasised. Dean et al. (1974) advocated wide excision only in selected cases of microinvasive carcinoma. DiSaia et al. (1979) recommended immediate frozen section examination of the bilateral superficial inguinal nodes for a lesion 1 cm or less in diameter and 5 mm or less depth of invasion, and if the nodes were negative, wide local excision with a 3-cm margin of normal skin. Wide local excision has also been advocated by other workers (Zucker and Berkowitz 1985; Ross and Ehrmann 1987); Ross and Ehrmann (1987) observed a lower recurrence rate with wide local excision and concluded that the incomplete surgical margins rather than the omission of radical vulvectomy were related to recurrence. An almost similar view has been expressed by Rowley et al. (1988), who consider that ipsilateral superficial inguinal node dissection in addition to wide local excision is an effective treatment for the superficially invasive carcinoma of the vulva. It is apparent now that with proper evaluation of the lesions, drastic surgery which may be mutilating at times could be avoided.

6.3 Invasive Carcinoma

Carcinoma of the vulva constitutes 3.4% (Rutledge et al. 1970) of all female genital cancers and less than 1%–2% (Charles 1972) of all cancers in women (Kelly 1972).

6.3.1 Clinical Features

Although the lesion has been reported in a girl of 14 (Lister and Akinla 1972), vulval carcinoma is usually a disease of postmenopausal women. Some 7% of the patients are above the age of 60 years old (Green 1978) and approximately 27% of the patients are between 20 and 50 years (Rutledge 1965). Carcinoma complicating the granulomatous disease tends to occur in younger patients. Rare cases have been reported in association with pregnancy (Rahman 1982; Managhan and Lindeque 1986).

Pruritus is by far the most common symptom, followed by mass, dysuria, pain, discharge and bleeding. Paraneoplastic hypercalcaemia is occasionally noticed in a patient with vulval carcinoma (Buchsbaum 1969; Nichols and Bonney 1973;

Niebyl et al. 1975), particularly bulky tumour. This causes mental confusion which improves dramatically after removal of the tumour (Niebyl et al. 1975).

Several risk factors, namely obesity, hypertension, heart disease and diabetes, thought to be associated with vulval cancers are probably age-related. In some series, nulliparous women constituted about 16%–20% of the total (Garcia and Bornow 1972; Figge and Gaudenz 1974). In the earlier literature, granulomatous and non-granulomatous venereal disease were linked to the aetiology (Alexender and Shields 1953; Saltztein et al. 1956; Green et al. 1958; Mickal et al. 1966; Hay and Cole 1969; Rutledge et al. 1970). Of the patients from Jamaica 51% have been shown to have co-existing or pre-existing granulomatous disease (Sengupta 1981). Condylomata acuminata have been found in association with 5%–10% (Franklin and Rutledge 1972) and squamous carcinoma-in-situ of the lower female genital tract with an increasing frequency. There is at present a strong belief that HPV are oncogenic and related to some neoplasias of the female genital tract. HPV-6 and 11 have been demonstrated in 78% of squamous carcinoma of the vulva in one study (Sutton et al. 1987) and HPV-6 and 16 in three of the five patients in another study (Carson et al. 1988). HSV-2-related antigens have also been demonstrated in squamous carcinoma-in-situ of the vulva (Kauffman et al. 1981). Although the aetiological significance of these findings is not clear, a synergistic oncogenic effect of these viruses has been suggested (zur Hausen et al. 1984).

The risk of invasion of vulval carcinoma-in-situ is known to be much less than that of CIN; although in only less than 20% can an in situ component be seen in the adjacent epithelium (Buscema et al. 1980a), just 4% of the patients progress to invasive cancer over a period of 15 years (Buscema et al. 1980b). It has been suggested that, in contrast to CIN which progresses to invasive cancer, VIN and invasive carcinoma are not related diseases (Evans et al. 1987). The occurrence of a unifocal invasive carcinoma from a multifocal carcinoma-in-situ and a wide time lag between the intra-epithelial phase and invasion and response to local excision suggest, according to Evans et al. (1987), that these two are separate entities.

The most frequently associated lesions with vulval squamous cell carcinoma are the vulval dystrophies reported under various terms as leukoplakia, kraurosis and dystrophy (Bibby 1957). The noted incidence has been as high as 60%. These lesions have been considered both as aetiological factors (Taussig 1940) and as coincidental vulval disease (Figge and Gaudenz 1974). Taussig (1940) held strong views that the leukoplakic vulvitis was a pre-malignant condition, and 50% of women with this condition would develop invasive carcinoma. This conclusion could not be confirmed by the subsequent studies of Jeffcoate (1966) and Kauffman and Gardner (1978). These later researchers estimated that approximately 1%–5% of cases of vulval dystrophies could in the course of time progress to invasive carcinoma.

The incidence of second primary malignant tumours in association with invasive vulval carcinoma has baried from 6% (Boutselis et al. 1963) to 27% (Podratz et al. 1983), and cervical carcinoma has been the most frequently associated genital malignancy (Marcus 1960; Jimmerson and Merrill 1970). Vulval carcinoma may often be a part of a regional multicentric disease involving the cervix, vagina, perineum and anus (Choo and Morley 1980). Apart from cervical cancer, cancers of other genital organs and breast account for nearly 60% of the second primaries (Podratz et al. 1983).

Immunosuppression is an important predisposing factor for lower genital tract malignancy even in young patients (Lindeque et al. 1987).

6.3.1.1 Sites of Lesion

The frequency of distribution of lesion has varied in different series. The anterior part of the vulva involving the labia is the most common site. The clitoris and prepuce may be primarily affected (Sawyer et al. 1949). Primary clitoral origin has been noted in 12% (Boutselis et al. 1963) to 26% cases (Andreasson et al. 1982). The vestibule, perineum and posterior commissure can also be primarily affected.

6.3.1.2 Clinical Staging

The International Federation of Gynaecology and Obstetrics (FIGO) formulated a TNM staging system which was based on tumour assessment by size and location (T), lymph node status (N) as determined by palpation and distant metastases (M):

Stage 1 – All lesions confined to the vulva with maximum diameter of 2 cm or less and no suspected groin nodes.
Stage 2 – All lesions confined to the vulva with diameter greater than 2 cm and no suspicious groin nodes.
Stage 3 – Lesions extending beyond the vulva to adjacent areas.
Stage 4 – Lesions extending to rectal and bladder mucosa.
(Nodes: N1, palpable but not suspicious; N2, nodes suspicious; N3, clinically malignant)
Metastases: M1A, palpable deep pelvic nodes; M1B, distant metastases)

This classification is complex and has not gained wide acceptance (Krupp et al. 1975).

6.3.2 Pathological Features

The vulval carcinoma can present as indurated ulcers with irregular margins, an irregular hard nodule with subsequent ulceration, an irregular polypoidal or fungating, cauliflower-like mass (Fig. 6.12) and less commonly an infiltrating growth with ill-defined margins. Carcinomas developing in the granulomatous lesions tend to be larger lesions and present with ulceration and bleeding which are late manifestations in the usual type of carcinoma (Saltzstein et al. 1956). Hay and Cole (1969) noticed a higher incidence of lymph node involvement (32%) and associated carcinoma-in-situ (54%). Carcinoma developing in condylomata acuminata is larger and cauliflower-like in appearance, ulcerates and bleeds. The lesion is similar to the giant condylomata of Buschke and Löwenstein.

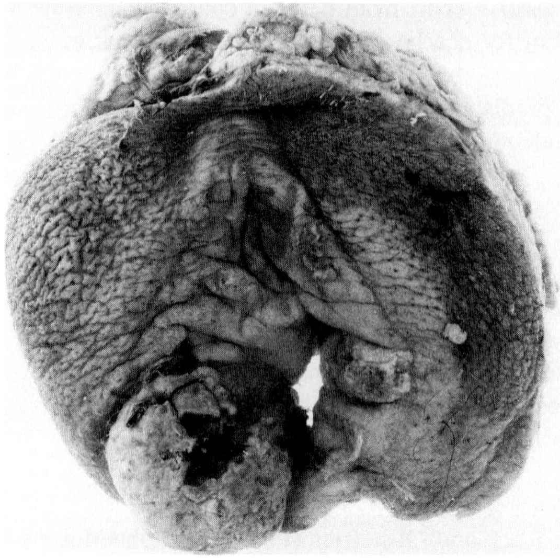

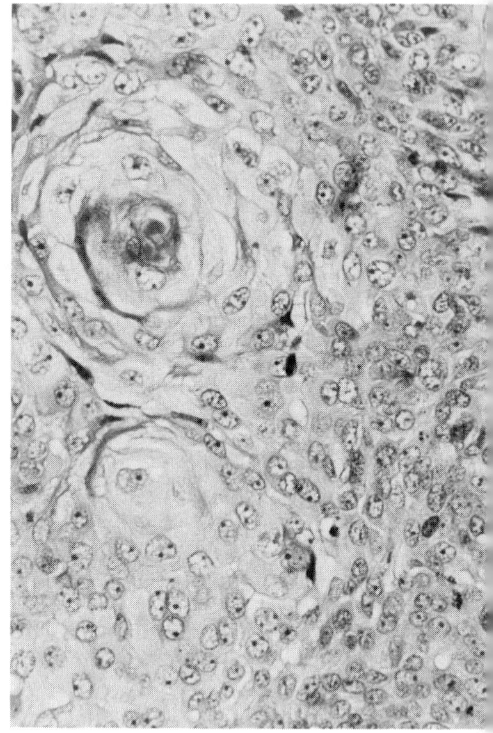

Fig. 6.12. Vulval carcinoma: ulcerated polypoid mass at posterior end of labia

Fig. 6.13. Vulval carcinoma: well-differentiated squamous cells displaying neoplastic characters of pleomorphism, epithelial pearls

6.3.2.1 Microscopical Appearance

Squamous cell carcinomas are the most common invasive tumours of the vulva, constituting about 95% of all vulval malignancies (Palmer et al. 1949; Andreasson et al. 1982). In contrast to squamous cell carcinoma of the cervix, the majority of carcinomas of the vulva are well or moderately differentiated (Way 1960; Gosling et al. 1961; Merrill and Ross 1961; Woodcock 1976; Wright 1976) in approximately 90%–95% of cases. In the well-differentiated type, the atypical squamous cells forming broad masses and sheets of invading neoplastic tissue show prominent inter-cellular bridges and cytoplasmic keratin. Keratin whorls and keratin masses are conspicuous features of this type (Fig. 6.13). Nuclear atypia are not outstanding, but mitotic figures are at times frequent. The moderately differentiated carcinoma shows more cellular pleomorphism, less keratinisation and a few mitoses (Fig. 6.14). In the poorly differentiated type, which constitutes about 4% of this group (Lundwell 1961), cells are very pleomorphic with scanty cytoplasm containing little or no keratin and have a very high mitotic rate (Fig. 6.15).

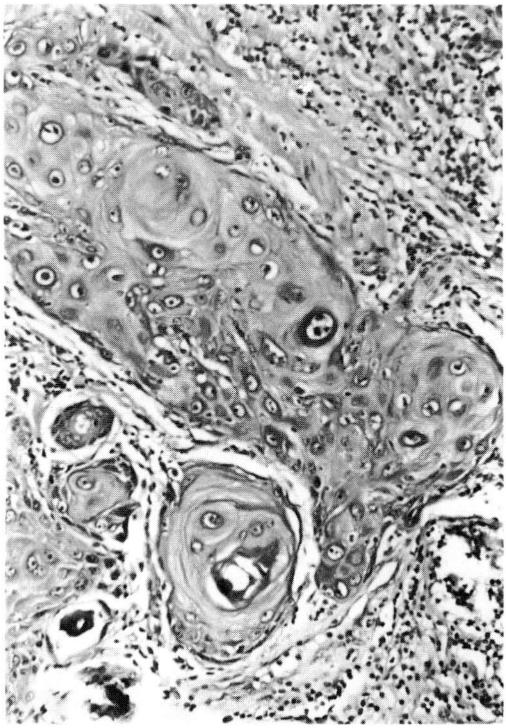

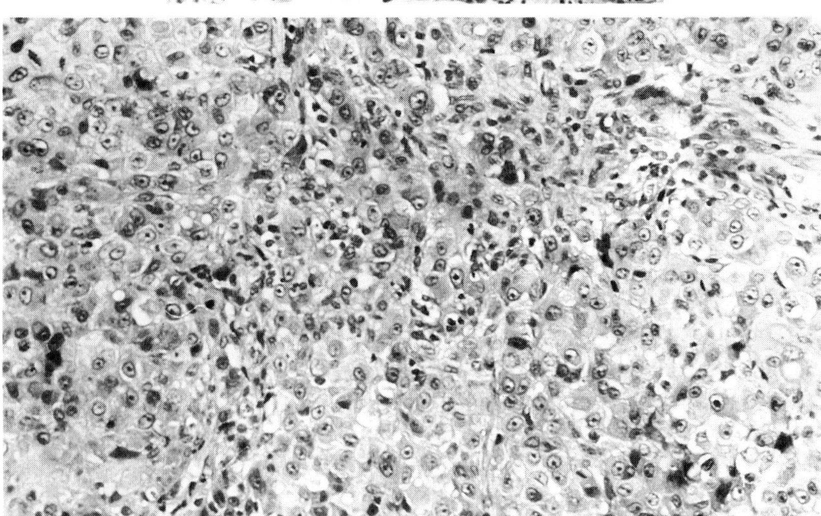

Fig. 6.14. Vulval carcinoma: cells are moderately differentiated with an attempt at formation of whorls which are also not well keratinised

Fig. 6.15. Vulval carcinoma: small, poorly differentiated cells containing scanty cytoplasm and no keratin

The arrangement of the infiltrating cells may vary from solid mass, anastomosing columns, cords, scattered islands or interrupted rows. Lasser et al. (1974) noticed a pseudoglandular arrangement of the neoplastic cells with gland-like spaces lined by keratinised cells (Fig. 6.16). If looked for carefully, these features can be seen in approximately 5% of well and moderately differentiated squamous cell carcinomas. Varying degrees of desmoplastic reaction and lymphocyte and plasma cell infiltration are almost always noticeable around the area. In an occasional moderately differentiated carcinoma, eosinophils may outnumber other cellular infiltrates (Fig. 6.17) and form eosinophilic micro-abscesses within and around the tumour (Lowe and Fletcher 1984). The blood eosinophilia associated with tumour eosinophilia was seen particularly in patients who had metastatic disease and a poor prognosis (Lowe and Fletcher 1984). Dysplasia and squamous carcinoma-in-situ are seen in one-fourth to one-fifth of patients at the adjacent area on the superficial skin surface which often contains a mass of keratin debris. Dystrophic changes – atrophic, hypertrophic or mixed types – are noticed in more than 50% of squamous cell carcinoma (Gosling et al. 1961; Buscema et al. 1980a). Frankman and Kabulski (1983), using a pattern of tumour growth – superficial papillomatous, inverted papillomatous and non-papillomatous – together with mitosis, nuclear pleomorphism and tumour-host relationship, found a histological correlation with lymph node metastases and prognosis. The low-scoring tumours, which were predominantly verruciform and well-differentiated, had little nuclear pleomorphism, low mitoses, well-defined tumour borders and a good cellular response, showed a predictably better prognosis.

In the majority of the carcinomas, the component cells are polyhedral, but in the occasional poorly differentiated tumours, the cells are predominantly spindle-shaped (Gosling et al. 1961; Copas et al. 1982), and such lesions may at times be misdiagnosed as sarcomas (Fig. 6.18). The ultrastructural demonstration of desmosomes and tonofilaments and immunohistochemical techniques are helpful in establishing the diagnosis.

Way (1960) observed tumours consisting of giant cells which were undoubtedly variants of a very poorly differentiated carcinoma. These lesions were very aggressive, had a short growth period and metastased with a fatal outcome. Wilkinson et al. (1988) identified two groups of giant cell tumours of similar histological appearance and studied them by immunoperoxidase techniques. One group was amelanotic melanoma and the other, squamous cell carcinoma.

The invasive features of postgranulomatous carcinoma may be masked by florid granulomatous reactions. Pseudo-epitheliomatous hyperplasia is also common in these lesions and should be differentiated from true invasive carcinoma (Saltzstein et al. 1956). The post-granulomatous carcinomas tend to be poorly differentiated. The recognition of squamous carcinoma arising in condylomata acuminata may be difficult both macroscopically and microscopically. However, multiple biopsies from long-standing condylomata may reveal infiltrating columns of atypical squamous cells with formation of keratin masses or pearls in the underlying connective tissue. Clinically, a history of a recent rapid increase in size, induration and ulcer-

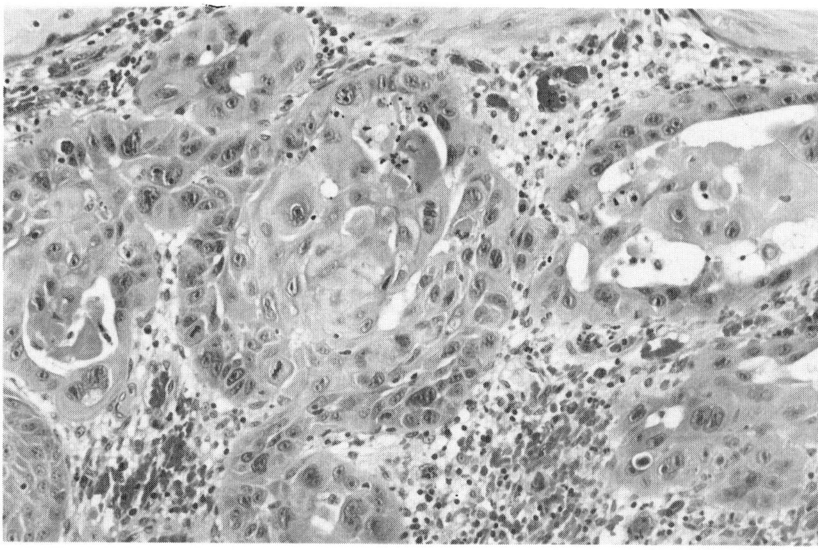

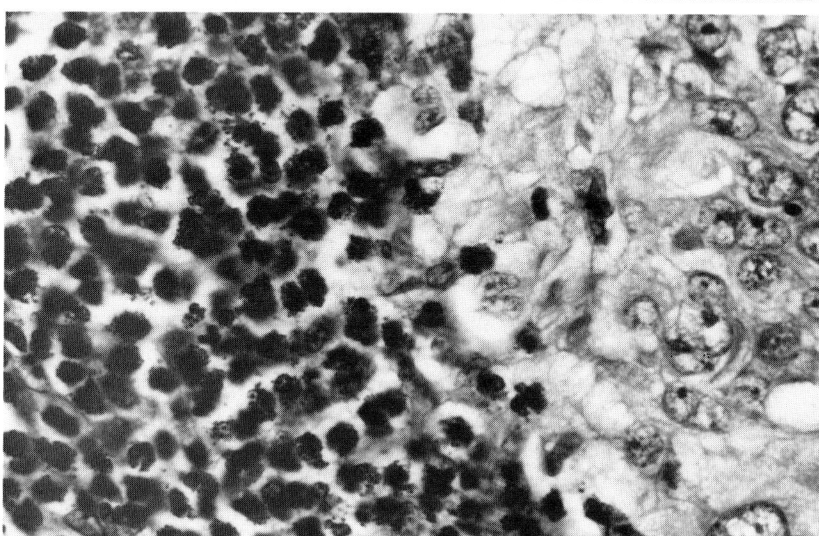

Fig. 6.16. Vulval carcinoma pseudo-glandular arrangement: keratinised squamous cells around pseudo-acini

Fig. 6.17. Vulval carcinomas: diffuse sheets of heavily granulated eosinophils bordering the tumour cells

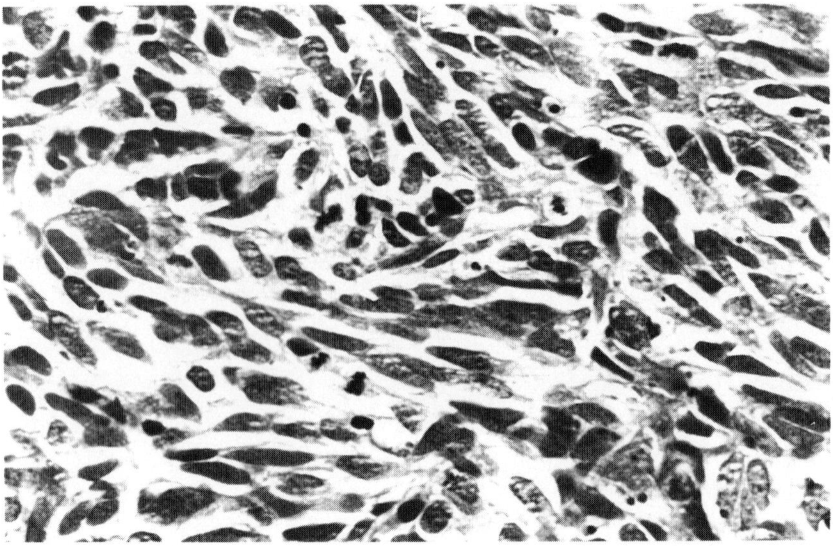

Fig. 6.18. Vulval carcinoma: spindle-shaped malignant squamous cells may be mistaken for sarcoma

ation should prompt biopsies. These patients are younger than those with classic vulval carcinoma (Embrey 1961; Shafeek et al. 1979).

6.3.2.2 Special Studies

Several authors (Clark et al. 1960; Thomas 1965; Punnonen et al. 1977) noticed an increased uptake of radioactive phosphorous by the vulval malignant and premalignant lesions and advocated its use as a diagnostic tool. Feulgen microspectrophotometric analysis of the DNA content of pre-invasive and invasive squamous cell carcinoma of the vulva revealed low ploidy stem cells (less than 3N) in 70% of invasive lesions (Fu et al. 1981) and in 82% of the intra-epithelial neoplasms in the vicinity of an invasive carcinoma. It has been suggested by Fu et al. (1981) that the intra-epithelial neoplasms with low ploidy stem cells have a greater potential to be invasive, and low ploidy invasive carcinoma shows a higher rate of lymph node metastases. Katayama et al. (1972) observed marked chromosomal aneuploidy with some peritriploid components in the well-differentiated (mature) carcinoma, which had a greater frequency of lymph node metastases, whereas the immature (poorly differentiated) tumours had chromosomes in the diploid range and no nodal metastases. Immunohistochemically, the invasive carcinomas react positively for pre-keratin, which is helpful in differentiating the spindle cell variant of squamous cell carcinoma from amelanotic spindle cell melanoma and many mesenchymal tumours composed of spindle cells. Nadji et al. (1984) found a weaker immunochemical reaction for carcinoembryonic antigens (CEA) in the invasive than in intra-epithelial carcinoma, but radioimmunoassay of CEA with plasma of a small number of patients showed a raised value which dropped to anormal level after complete removal of the lesion (DiSaia et al. 1976).

6.3.2.3 Spread

Squamous carcinoma of the vulva grows slowly and spreads mainly by direct extension and the lymphatic system (Way 1948; Parry-Jones 1960; Krupp and Bohm 1978). Extension to neighbouring structures occurs with an increase in the size of the lesion. The vagina, urethra, urinary bladder, perineum, anus and rectum may be infiltrated in advanced cases with a worsening prognosis.

6.3.2.4 Lymph Node Metastases

The incidence of nodal metastases has varied widely in different series, from 20% (Figge et al. 1985) to 58% (Taussig 1938; Green et al. 1958). In a collective review of 466 patients, Boutselis (1972) noted an incidence of positive nodes in 46%. The incidence of positive inguinal nodes among these was 60%.

The vulva has a rich lymphatic supply, being covered by a multilayered, anastomotic, fine meshwork of lymphatic vessels. Way (1948) divided the draining system into six groups: (a) superficial inguinal nodes lying along the inguinal ligament and slightly below it; (b) the sub-inguinal or superficial femoral nodes grouped round the great saphenous vein just before its passes through the fossa ovalis to join the femoral vein; (c) deep femoral nodes passing along the femoral vessels, the uppermost and constant node being known as the lymph node of Cloquet or Rosenmüller; (d) the external iliac nodes consisting of three groups, the medial group lying infero-medial to the external iliac vein. These receive afferents from the node of Cloquet and pass their own efferents to the common iliac nodes; (e) deep inguinal nodes which are inconstant and lie in the inguinal canal along the course of the round ligament; (f) pre-symphyseal lymph nodes, which are inconstant and lie in the fat in the lower part of mons veneris, usually around the root of the clitoris.

The vulva, being a bilateral organ, displays free anastomoses of the lymphatics from both sides. In general, the lymphatics from the anterior part of the vulva run upward to the mons veneris then laterally to drain to the superficial inguinal node, and those from the psoterior part run transversely and also to the superficial inguinal nodes.

Saltzstein et al. (1956) observed a very low incidence of nodal metastases in the carcinomas arising in association with granulomatous diseases and thought to be due to the blockage of lymphatic channels by the granulomatous process. Metastases to the pelvic lymph nodes occurred when the perirectal tissue was infiltrated by carcinoma (Hay and Cole 1969). While some perineal lymphatics close to the anus may drain to the anal and pelvic nodes at the posterior part, some lymphatics drain anteriorly from the clitoris, directly to Cloquet's nodes and the pelvic nodes accompanying the dorsal vein of the clitoris.

Free anastomoses of the lymphatic vessels from both sides permit contralateral nodal metastases (Shingleton et al. 1970; Iversen 1983) even in the absence of ipsilateral positive nodes (Green et al. 1958; Merrill and Ross 1961; Macafee 1962). In one series, this occurred in 15.3% of patients (Krupp 1978). However, the overall incidence of such occurrences does not appear to be very high. The deep nodes are also known to be involved in the absence of superficial positive nodes (Cassidy et al. 1957; Way 1960; Merrill and Ross 1961; Collins et al. 1963; Krupp and Bohm 1978), particularly from midline clitoral lesions. The incidence of deep node involvement in the absence of superficial positive nodes is low and has been estimated to be about 2% (Franklin and Rutledge 1972). In recent years, early diagnosis of the lesion is being made increasingly frequently, resulting in a declining trend of lymph node metastases (Green 1978).

6.3.3 Treatment

Up to 1940, the 5-year survival rate with this lesion was of the order of 20%–30%. Taussig (1940) and Way (1948, 1954), using radical resection of the vulva and removal of regional lymphatics, improved the prognosis of the condition substantially from its overall bleak prognosis to a most optimistic level. Surgery is now accepted as the principle mode of treatment. This includes complete removal of the vulva and bilateral inguinal and pelvic lymphadenectomy in stages I, II and III (Way 1960; Collins et al. 1963; Rutledge 1965; Krupp 1978). The value of routine inclusion of the pelvic lymph nodes has remained somewhat controversial. Some researchers (Morley 1976; Benedet et al. 1979) do not recommend routine resection of the pelvic nodes unless the superficial nodes are positive. The usefulness of routine dissection of the pelvic nodes has been seriously questioned (Boyce and Mehram 1974; Curry et al. 1980; Hacker et al. 1983), considering the fact that the incidence of deep node metastases in the absence of superficial nodal involvement is low (Morris 1977), the survival rate with deep nodal metastases is poor, and the post-operative morbidity associated with extension of the surgical procedure is high. According to Monaghan and Hammond (1984), the decision to perform dissection of pelvic nodes should be influenced by tumour size and degree of differentiation and reserved for tumours more than 4 cm in diameter. The necessity for a greater selectivity of the patients and individualisatiaon of the treatments has been amply stressed in this disease. Metastases in the pelvic nodes are usually suspected when the primary lesion is extensive, and there are metastases in the inguinal and Cloquet's nodes. In such circumstances, pelvic lymphadenectomy has been advocated (Rutledge et al. 1970). Benedet et al. (1979) performed pelvic lymphadenectomy for the clitoral lesion and when the inguino-femoral nodes were positive. Piver and Xynos (1977) also observed that even in the clitoral lesion routine dissection of the pelvic nodes in the absenceof histologically proven positive inguinal nodes is not of much benefit. In one series (Morley 1976), patients with stage I and II disease treated by radical vulvectomy and groin node dissection had a corrected 5-year survival rate of 90% and 95%, respectively. Also in this series, of the 65 patients in stage III, 48 were treated by radical vulvectomy and groin node dissections and 17 by radical vulvectomy and both groin and pelvic node dissections, resulting in survival rates of 45.2% and 40.0%, respectively (Morley 1976). These indicated that routine dissection of the pelvic nodes did not improve the survival rates significantly. Similar observations were made by several other researchers (Boyce and Mehream 1974; Hacker et al. 1983). Homesley et al. (1986) advocated adjunctive groin and pelvic irradiation after radical vulvectomy and inguinal lymphadenectomy when the groin nodes were found to be positive. Unilateral node dissection has also been advocated in patients with small and one-sided lesions (Figge and Gaudenz 1974). Morris (1977) achieved 81% 5-year survival in 21 patients by unilateral dissections of the negative inguinal nodes.Melfetano et al. (1985) recommended wide local excision with ipsilateral node dissection to treat a lesion 1 cm or less in diameter and with a depth of invasion 1 mm or less. Treatment of the central lesion of this size and depth should include bilateral inguinal lymphadenectomy. All other stage I and II lesions should be treated by radical vulvectomy and bilateral inguinal node dissection (Melfetano et al. 1985). In advanced carcinoma involving the urethra or rectum, pelvic exenterative surgery has been used (Thornton and Flanagan 1973; Kaplan and Kaufmann 1975; Phillips et al. 1981; Cavanagh and Shepherd 1982). In selected cases, an overall salvage rate can be expected up to 75% (Krupp et al. 1975).

Earlier, the results of radiotherapy in vulval cancer were disappointing (Taussig 1940; Smith and Pollack 1947; Lunin 1949). Because of the poor results, about 20% salvage rate and severe local reactions, radiation treatment has long been considered unsuitable (Collins et al. 1963; Ballon and Lamb 1975). In recent years, however, there is a renewed interest in its use either as an adjunct to surgery or as primary treatment for palliation and cure (Frischbier and Thomson 1971; Nobler 1972; Daly and Million 1974; Helgason et al. 1977; Acosta et al. 1978; Iversen 1982; Fairey et al. 1985; Homesley et al. 1986). By using radiation alone or in combination with surgery, encouraging results of up to 92% survival rate have been reported in two small series (Jafari and Magalotti 1981; Fairey et al. 1985). Kucera and Weghaupt (1988) employing an electrosurgical operation coupled with post-operative irradiation of the inguinal lymph nodes achieved an absolute cure rate of 60% for 5 years. The uncorrected 5-year survival rate in their series of 607 patients was 78% in FIGO stage I, 70.5% in stage II, 56.5% in stage III and 11.7% in stage IV. Levin et al. (1986) used radiotherapy and chemotherapy to reduce the size of an advanced tumour prior to surgery with positive results. The efficacy of cryosurgery (Wallach 1975; Renziehausen 1974) or immunotherapy (Freedman et al. 1983; Morley 1976) is uncertain, as only a very small number of patients have been treated with these modalities. Chemotherapeutic treatment in recurrent and metastatic disease (Deppe et al. 1979; Kalra et al. 1981) has been claimed to be of some success, but support with some larger series is yet to be published.

6.3.4 Recurrences

The incidence of recurrences in vulvar carcinoma varies from 9% (Bartholdson et al. 1982) to about 35% (Iversen et al. 1980; Rutledge et al. 1970). From 75% (Podratz et al. 1983) to 92% (Franklin and Rutledge 1971) of the recurrences appear within the first 2 years after surgery. The vulval area is the site of recurrences in 60% and inguinal area in 40% (Morley 1976). In one report (Buchler et al. 1979), 60% of the recurrences involved the perineum. About 20% of the patients with clinically positive groin nodes risk skin recurrences in the groin region after surgery (Daly and Million 1974). The high rate of recurrences is due to microscopic permeation or embolisation of paravaginal, pararectal or paraurethral lymphatics (Podratz et al. 1983). The size of the tumour is an important factor in recurrences. The tumours 1 cm in diameter or above have a 10% probability of recurrence, which increases to 35% for tumours 6 cm in diameter (Melfetano et al. 1985).

6.3.5 Prognosis and Survival

The size of the primary lesions and existence of lymph node metastases are important prognostic parameters (Hoffman et al. 1985) which greatly influence the survival rate. Shimm et al. (1986) concluded that survival was heavily dependent upon tumour size, nodal state, stage of the disease, age of the patient and presence or absence of lymphatic permeation. Dissociated tumour growth, tumour thickness, and ulceration have also been observed to influence the prognosis (Kurzl and Messerer 1989). The incidence of nodal metastasis correlates fairly well with the size and extent of the disease. The risk of nodal metastasis is about 30% when the disease is confined to the vulva but increases to 50% when the lesion involves the anus, urethra and vagina (Franklin and Rutledge 1971). Several researchers noted that histological differentiatiaon of the tumour was also an important prognostic parameter (Garcia and Bornow 1972; Kabulski and Frankman 1978; Donalson et al. 1981; Bartholdson et al. 1982; Zaino et al. 1982; Husseinzadeh et al. 1983; Podratz et al. 1983), a better survival rate being associated with the well differentiated tumours.

Table 1. The 5-year survival rate (in %) according to the stage of disease in some recent series

	Stage I	Stage II	Stage III	Stage IV
Benedet et al. (1979)	85	58	24	–
Iversen et al. (1980)	93	75	50	–
Podratz et al. (1983)	90	81	68	20
Kucera and Weghaupt (1988)	78	70.5	56.5	11.7

There is at present general agreement that a good 5-year surfival rate can be achieved with adequate treatment. Although the approach and statistical analysis have varied in different series, the overall results are encouraging (Table 1).

6.4 Verrucous Carcinoma

Verrucous carcinoma was first described by Ackerman (1948). It is a locally infiltrative, non-metastasising lesion which occurs in the oral cavity, larynx and anogenital region. In recent years, these lesions are being recognised with increasing frequency in the female lower genital tract.

6.4.1 Aetiology

Because of similarities of the lesions with condylomata acuminata which is now known to be caused by papovavirus (HPV), the probability of verrucous carcinoma being associated with these viruses is very strong (Partridge et al. 1980). HPV DNA has, in fact, been detected in both conditions (Ubben et al. 1979). Type 6 has been found in the majority of genital warts (Gissmann et al. 1982, 1983) and also in verrucous carcinoma (Rando et al. 1986). Type 11 has also been demonstrated in some verrucous lesions (Crowther et al. 1988). Rando et al. characterised a subtype 6b which, according to these workers, undergoes genetic changes and becomes tumorigenic, causing a benign condylomatous lesion to transform into a more aggressive verrucous carcinoma. The condyloma of Buschke and Löwenstein is considered to be the same or a similar lesion to verrucous carcinoma, both grossly and hstilogically. It is highly probable that condylomata acuminata, giant condylomata of Buschke and Löwenstein and verrucous carcinoma are but variants of the same pathological process (Judge 1969).

6.4.2 Clinical Features

The age of the patients ranges from 29 to 86 years old, with an average of 54 years (Japaze et al. 1982). The patients present with vulval growth, pruritus, discharge and pain.

6.4.3 Gross Appearance

The appearances vary from warty nodules to cauliflower-like masses of 0.5–10 cm in size, which may be ulcerated and covered with necrotic material emitting a putrid smell. The growth is usually pink or grey-white in colour and on cut section presents grey and buffy appearances with well-demarcated deeper margins. The most common site is one of the labia, but the confluent area involving both labia, mons and perineum may be affected.

6.4.4 Microscopical Appearance

The tumour consists of large and bulky papillary fronds which are composed of well-differentiated squamous cells with abundant eosinophilic cytoplasm and regular, oval to round, vesicular nuclei and covered by layers of parakeratotic cells and heaps of keratin. Nuclear vacuolations may be noticed in some cells and are pronounced in some areas. The epidermis is markedly thickened and displays well-demarcated, pushing deeper margins and bulbous rete pegs (Fig. 6.19). Epithelial pearls or abnormal cellular maturations are not seen, and evidence of invasion of the underlying connective tissue is absent. The cells are regular and uniform with no nuclear anaplasia. Mitoses are usually absent. Variable numbers of lymphocytes, plasma cells and histocytes are always seen in the stroma along the deeper margins. Distinction from the well-differentiated squamous cell carcinoma and pseudoepitheliomatous hyperplasia is always a problem. Pseudoepitheliomatous hyperplasia, which also consists of well-differentiated squamous cells, is usually seen at the edge of an ulcer and has sharp, tapering deeper margins. The irregular infiltrating margins, irregular cords and isolated groups of invading cells with features of malignancy help characterisation of squamous cell carcinoma. Condylomata acuminata contain a fibrovascular stalk and irregular and slender rete pegs. Autoradiographic study with tritiated thymidine demonstrated a thick layer of non-proliferating, non-keratinised cells between the surface and basal layers similar to the non-reactive malpighian layer of the normal epidermis (Prioleau et al. 1980). Ultrastructurally, focal collections of hemidesmosomes in these cells have been correlated with the non-invasive tendency (Prioleau et al. 1980).

6.4.5 Clinical Course

The lesion is considered to be a low grade, slowly evolving and relentlessly expanding tumour not eager to metastasise (Kraus and Perez-Mesa 1966). Although regional nodes may be enlarged due to associated infections, metastasis occurs very rarely, if ever (Foye et al. 1969; Jennings and Barclay 1972; Lucas et al. 1974).

6.4.6 Treatment

Surgery is the best treatment for this condition. Because of its low malignant potential, local excision with wide margins is considered adequate by several researchers (Judge 1969; Zaaijman and Slabber 1978; Stehman et al. 1980); others advocate radical surgery as a preventive measure against recurrence, and for recurrent and anaplastic growths (Vayrynen et al. 1981; Gallousis 1972; Isaacs 1976; Powell et

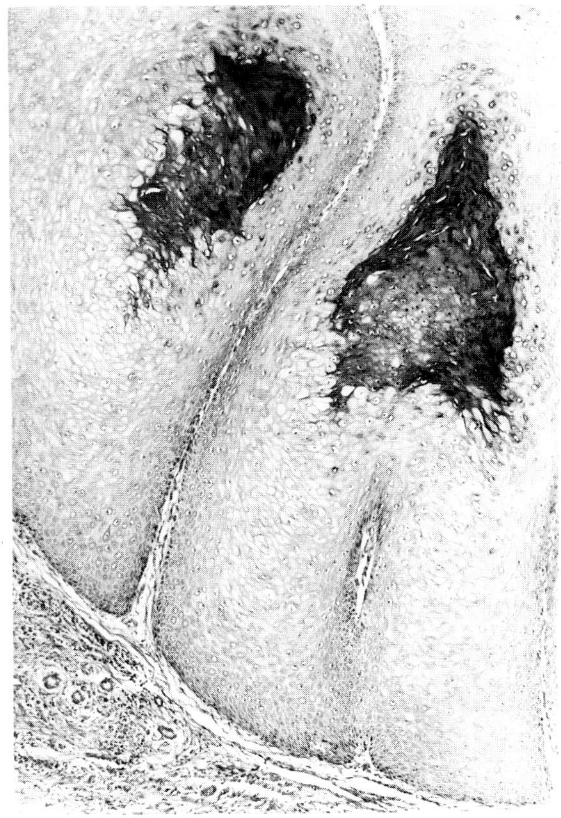

Fig. 6.19. Verrucous carcinoma: bulbous rete pegs with pushing deeper margin

al. 1978). When there is histological evidence of invasion, radical surgery with regional lymphadenectomy should be considered (Selim and Lankerani 1979). The growth is radio-resistant; the tumour recurs after initial regression after irradiation (Vayrynen et al. 1981). It can even be dangerous as anaplastic changes (Foye et al. 1969; Gallousis 1972) and invasion (Demian et al. 1973) are known to occur following radiation therapy. Treatment with bleomycin was reported to be unsuccessful (De Graaff and van der Harten 1975).

References

Intraepithelial Neoplasia

Abell MR (1965) Intraepithelial carcinomas of epidermis and squamous mucosa of vulva and perineum. Surg Clin North Am 45:1179–1198

Andreasson B, Bock J (1985) Intraepithelial neoplasia in the vulvar region. Gynecol Oncol 21:300–305

Baggish MS, Dorsey JH (1981) CO_2 laser for the treatment of vulvar carcinoma in situ. Obstet Gynecol 57:371–375

Benedet JL, Murphy KJ (1982) Squamous carcinoma in situ of the vulva. Gynecol Oncol 14:213–219

Berger BW, Horu Y (1978) Multicentric Bowen's disease of the genitalia. Arch Dermatol 114:1698–1699

Bernstein SG, Kovacs BR, Townsend DE et al. (1983) Vulvar carcinoma in situ. Obstet Gynecol 61:304–307

Boutselis JG (1972) Intraepithelial carcinoma vulva. Am J Obstet Gynecol 113:733–738

Broen EM, Ostergard DR (1971) Toludin blue and colposcopy for screening and delineating vulvar neoplasia. Obstet Gynecol 38:775–778

Buckley CH, Butler EB, Fox H (1984) Vulvar intraepithelial neoplasia and microinvasive carcinoma of the vulva. J Clin Pathol 37:1201–1211

Bucsema J, Woodruff JD (1980) Progressive histologic alterations in the development of vulvar cancer. Report of five cases. Am J Obstet Gynecol 138:146–150

Buscema J, Stern J Woodruff JD (1980a) The significance of the histological alterations adjacent to invasive vulvar carcinoma. Am J Obstet Gynecol 137:902–909

Buscema J, Woodruff JD, Parmley TH et al. (1980b) Carcinoma in situ of the vulva. Obstet Gynecol 55:225–230

Cabral GA, Marciano-Cabral F, Fry D et al. (1982) Expression of herpes simplex virus type 2 antigens in pre-malignant and malignant vulvar cells. Am Obstet Gynecol 143:611–619

Caglar H, Tamer S, Hreschyshyn MM (1982) Vulvar intraepithelial neoplasia. Obstet Gynecol 60:346–349

Carson TE, Hoskins WJ, Wurzel JF (1976) Topical 5-fluorouracil in the treatment of carcinoma in situ of the vulva. Obstet Gynecol 47 [Suppl]:59–62

Collins CG, Hansen LH, Theriot E (1966) A clinical stain for use in selecting biopsy sites in patients with vulvar disease. Obstet Gynecol 28:158–163

Collins CG, Roman-Lopez JJ, Lee FYL (1970) Intraepithelial carcinoma of the vulva. Am J Obstet Gynecol 108:1187–1191

Cox SM, Kaufman RH, Kaplan A (1986) Recurrent carcinoma in situ of the vulva in a skin graft. Am J Obstet Gynecol 155:177–179

Crum CP, Galliway DA, McDougall JK et al. (1981) Intraepithelial neoplasia of the vulva and vagina: an analysis for herpes simplex 2 by in-situ hybridization techniques. Lab Invest 44:13A

Crum E, Braun LA; Shah KV et al. (1982) Vulvar intraepithelial neoplasias: correlation of nuclear DNA content and presence of human papilloma virus structural antigen. Cancer 49:468–471

Crum C, Liskow A, Petras P et al. (1984) Vulvar intraepithelial neoplasia (severe atypia and carcinoma in situ): a clinico-pathologic analysis of 41 cases. Cancer 54:1429–1434

Dean RE, Taylor ES, Weisbrod DM et al. (1974) Treatment of premalignant and malignant lesions of the vulva. Am J Obstet Gynecol 119:59–68

DiPaola GR, Rueda-Leverone NG, Belardi MG et al. (1982) Vulvar carcinoma in situ: a report of 28 cases. Gynecol Oncol 14:236–242

DiSaia PJ, Rich WM (1981) Surgical approach to multifocal carcinoma in situ of the vulva. Am Obstet Gynecol 140:136–145

Dressman GR, Burek J, Adam E et al. (1980) Expression of herpes virus induced antigens in human cervical cancer. Nature 283:591–593

Faber M, Hagedorn M (1981) A light and electron microscopic study of Bowenoid papulosis. Acta Dermatovener (Stockh) 61:397–403

Ferenczy A, Braun L, Shah KV (1981) Human papilloma virus (HPV) in codylomatous lesions of the cervix. Am J Surg Pathol 5:661–670

Forney JP, Morrow CP, Townsend DE et al. (1977) Management of carcinoma in situ of vulva. Am J Obstet Gynecol 127:801–806

Foster DC, Woodruff JD (1981) The use of Dinitrochlorbenzene in the treatment of vulvar carcinoma in situ. Gynecol Oncol 11:330–339

Franklin EW, Rutledge F (1972) Epidemiology of epidermoid carcinoma of the vulva. Obstet Gynecol 39:165–170

Friedrich EG, Wilkinson EJ, Fu Y-S (1980) Carcinoma in situ of the vulva: a continuing challenge. Am J Obstet Gynecol 136:830–843

Friedrich EG Jr (1981) Intraepithelial neoplasia of vulva. In: Coppleson M (ed) Gynecologic oncology, vol 1. Churchill Livingstone, Edinburgh, pp 303–319

Fu Y-S, Reagan JW, Townsend DE et al. (1981) Nuclear DNA study of vulvar intraepithelial and invasive squamous neoplasms. Obstet Gynecol 57:643–652

Gupta J, Pilotti S, Shah KV et al. (1987) Human papilloma virus associated early vulvar neoplasia investigated by in-situ hybridisation. Am J Surg Pathol 11:430–434

International Society for the Study of Vulvar Disease (1976) New nomenclature for vulvar disease I. Obstet Gynecol 47:122–123

Iversen T, Abeler V, Kolstad P (1981) Squamous cell carcinoma in situ of the vulva: a clinical and histopathological study. Gynecol Oncol 11:224–229

Jones RW, McLean MR (1986) Carcinoma in situ of the vulva: a review of 31 cases treated and five untreated cases. Obstet Gynecol 68:499–503

Kaufman RH, Gardner HL (1965) Intra-epithelial carcinoma of the vulva. Clin Obstet Gynecol 8:1035–1050

Kaufman R, Gordon A (1986) Squamous carcinoma in situ of the vulva, pt 1. Br J Sex Med 13:24–27

Kaufman RH, Dressman GR, Burek J et al. (1981) Herpes induced antigens in squamous cell carcinoma in-situ of the sulva. N Engl Med J 305:484–488

Kaufman RH, Bornstein J, Adam E et al. (1988) Human papilloma virus and herpes simplex virus in vulvar squamous carcinoma in situ. Am J Obstet Gynecol 158:862–871

Kimura S, Hirai A, Harada R et al. (1978) So called multicentric pigmented Bowen's disease. Dermatologica 157:229–237

Korhonen MO, Kaufman RH, Roberts D et al. (1982) Carcinoma in-situ of the vulva: the search for viral particles. J Reprod Med 27:746–748

Krupp PJ, Bohm JW (1978) 5-Fluorouracil topical treatment of in-situ vulvar cancer. Obstet Gynecol 51:702–706

Leuchter RS, Townsend DE, Hacker NF et al. (1984) Treatment of vulvar carcinoma in situ with the CO2 laser. Gynecol Oncol 19:314–322

Lifshitz S, Roberts JA (1980) Treatment of carcinoma in-situ of the vulva with topical 5-fluorouracil. Obstet Gynecol 56:242–244

Lloyd KM (1970) Multicentric pigmented Bowen's disease of the groin. Arch Dermatol 101:48–51

Lupulesen A, Mehregan AH, Ranbari H et al. (1977) Venereal warts vs Bowen disease: a histologic and ultrastructural study of five cases. JAMA 237:2520–2522

Meisels A, Fortin R, Roy M (1977) Condylomatous lesions of the cervix II: cytological, colposcopic and histopathologic study. Acta Cytol (Baltimore) 21:379–290

Mene A, Buckley CH (1985) Involvement of vulvar skin appendages by intraepithelial neoplasia. Br J Obstet Gynaecol 92:634–638

Nordquist RE, Olson RL, Everett MA et al. (1970) Virus like particles in Bowen's disease. Cancer Res 30:288–293

Olson RL, Nordquist RE, Everett MA (1985) An ultrastructural study of Bowen's disease. Cancer Res 28:2078–2085

Powell LC Jr, Dinh TV, Rajaraman S et al. (1986) Carcinoma in situ of the vulva: a clinicopathologic study of 50 cases. J Reprod Med 31:808–814

Rastkar G, Okagaki T, Twiggs LB et al. (1982) Early invasive and in-situ warty carcinoma of the vulva: clinical, histologic and electron microscopic study with particular reference to viral association. Am J Obstet Gynecol 143:814–820

Reid R (1985) Superficial vulvectomy. Am J Obstet Gynecol 152:504–509

Rettenmaier MA, Berman ML, DiSaia PJ (1987) Skinning vulvectomy for treatment of multifocal vulvar intraepithelial neoplasia. Obstet Gynecol 69:247–250
Rueda-Leverone NG, DiPaola GR, Meiss RP et al. (1987) Association of human papillomavirus infection and vulvar intraepithelial neoplasia: a Morphological and immunohistochemical study of 30 cases. Gynecol Oncol 26:331–339
Rutledge F, Sinclair M (1968) Treatment of intraepithelial carcinoma of the vulva by skin excision and graft. Am J Obstet Gynecol 102:806–818
Seski JC, Reinholter ER, Silva J Jr (1978) Abnromalities of lymphocyte transformations in women with intraepithelial carcinoma of the vulva. Obstet Gynecol 52:332–336
Skinner MS, Sternberg WH, Ichinose H et al. (1973) Spontaneous regression of Bowenoid atypia of the vulva. Obstet Gynecol 42:40–46
Stegner HE (1986) Ultrastructure of preneoplastic lesion of the vulva. J Reprod Med 31:815–820
Townsend DE (1987) Recurrent carcinoma in situ of vulva in skin graft. Am J Obstet Gynecol 156:1041
Townsend DE, Levin RU, Richart RM et al. (1982) Management of vulvar intraepithelial neoplasia by carbon dioxide laser. Obstet Gynecol 60:49–52
Ulbright TM, Stehman FB, Roth LM et al. (1982) Bowenoid dysplasia of the vulva. Cancer 50:2910–2919
Underwood PB, Hester LL Jr (1971) Diagnosis and treatment of premalignant lesions of the vulva: a review. Am J Obstet Gynecol 110:849–857
Wade TR, Kopf AW, Ackerman B (1979) Bowenoid papulosis of the genitalia. Arch Dermatol 115:306–308
Wilkinson EJ, Kneale B, Lynch PJ (1986) Report of the ISSVD terminology committee. J Reprod Med 31:973–974
Wolcott HD, Gallup DC (1984) Wide local excision in the treatment of vulvar carcinoma in situ: a reappraisal. Am J Obstet Gynecol 150:695–698
Woodruff JD, Hildebrandt EE (1958) Carcinoma in situ of the vulva. Obstet Gynecol 12:414–424
Woodruff JD, Braun L, Cavalieri R et al. (1980) Immunologic identification of papilloma virus antigen in paraffin-processed condyloma tissues from the female genital tract. Obstet Gynecol 56:727–752
Wright VC, Davies E (1987) Laser surgery for vulvar intraepithelial neoplasia: principles and results. Am J Obstet Gynecol 156:374–378
Zacur H, Genadry R, Woodruf JD (1980) The patient at risk for development of vulvar cancer. Gynecol Oncol 9:199–208
zur Hausen H (1976) Condylomata acuminata and human genital cancer. Cancer Res 36:794
zur Hausen H (1982) Human genital cancer: synergism between two viral infections or synergism between a viral infection and initiating event? Lancet II:1370–1372

Superficially Invasive Carcinoma

Atamdede F, Hoogerland D (1989) Regional lymph node recurrence following local excision for microinvasive vulvar carcinoma. Gynecol Oncol 34:125–128
Barnes AE, Crissman JD, Shellhas HF et al. (1980) Microinvasive carcinoma of the vulva: a clinicopathologic evaluation. Obstet Gynecol 56:234–238
Boice CR, Seraj IM, Thrasher T et al. (1984) Microinvasive squamous carcinoma of the vulva: present status and reassessment. Gynecol Oncol 18:71–76
Broen EM, Ostergard DR (1971) Toludine blue and colposcopy for screening and delineating vulvar neoplasia. Obstet Gynecol 38:775–778
Buscema J, Stern JL, Woodruff JD (1981) Early invasive carcinoma of the vulva. Am J Obstet Gynecol 140:563–569
Chu J, Tamini HK, Ek M et al. (1981) Stage I vulvar cancer. Obstet Gynecol 59:716–719
Crissman JD, Azoury RS (1981) Microinvasive carcinoma of the vulva: a report of 2 cases with regional lymph node metastasis. Diagn Gynecol Obstet 3:75–85

Dean RE, Taylor ES, Weisbrod DM et al. (1974) Treatment of premalignant and malignant lesions of the vulva. Am J Obstet Gynecol 119:59–68

DiPaola GR, Gamoze-Rueda N, Arrighi L (1975) Relevance of microinvasive carcinoma of the vulva. Obstet Gynecol 45:647–649

DiSaia PJ, Creasman WT, Rich MM (1979) An alternate approach to the early cancer of the vulva. Am J Obstet Gynecol 133:825–832

Donaldson ES, Powell DE, Hanson MB et al. (1981) Prognostic parameters in invasive vulvar cancer. Gynecol Oncol 11:184–190

Dvoretsky PM, Bonfiglio TA, Helmkamp BF et al. (1984) The pathology of superficially invasive thin vulvar squamous cell carcinoma. Int J Gynecol Pathol 3:331–342

Ehrmann RL, Dwyer IM, Yavner D et al. (1988) An immunoperoxidase study of laminin and type IV collagen distribution in carcinoma of the cervix and vulva. Obstet Gynecol 72:257–262

Figge D, Gaudenz R (1974) Invasive carcinoma of the vulva. Am J Obstet Gynecol 119:382–395

Forney JP, Morrow CP, Townsend DE et al. (1977) Management of carcinoma in-situ of the vulva. Am J Obstet Gynecol 127:801–806

Franklin EW III, Rutledge FD (1971) Prognostic factors in epidermoid carcinoma of the vulva. Obstet Gynecol 37:892–901

Gosling JRG, Abell MR, Drolette BM et al. (1961) Infiltrating squamous cell (epidermoid) carcinoma of vulva. Cancer 13:330–343

Hacker NF, Nieberg RK, Berek JS et al. (1983) Superficially invasive vulvar cancer with nodal metastases. Gynecol Oncol 15:65–77

Hoffman JS, Kumar NB, Morley GW (1983) Microinvasive carcinoma of the vulva: search for a definoition. Obstet Gynecol 16:615–618

Hughes R (1971) Early diagnosis and management of premalignant and early invasive cancers of the vulva. South Med J 64:1490–1492

Husseinzadeh N, Zaino R, Nahhas WA et al. (1983) The significance of histologic findings in predicting nodal metastases in invasive squamous cell carcinoma of the vulva. Gynecol Oncol 16:105–111

Iversen T, Abelar V, Aalders J (1981) Individualized treatment of stage I carcinoma of the vulva. Obstet Gynecol 57:58–59

Jafari K, Cartnick EN (1976a) Microinvasive squamous cell carcinoma of the vulva. Am J Obstet Gynecol 125:274

Jafari K, Cartnick EN (1976b) Microinvasive squamous cell carcinoma of the vulva. Gynecol Oncol 4:158–166

Japaze H, Garcia-Bunnel R, Woodruff JD (1977) Primary vulvar neoplasia: a review of in-situ and invasive carcinoma: 1935–1972. Obstet Gynecol 49:404–411

Kolstad P, Iversen T, Abeler V et al. (1982) Microinvasive carcinoma of the vulva – definition and the treatment problems. Clin Oncol 1:355–362

Kunschner A, Kanbour AJ, David B (1978) Early vulvar carcinoma. Am J Obstet Gynecol 132:599–606

Kurzl R, Messerer D, Baltzer J et al. (1988) Comparative morphometric study on the depth of invasion in vulvar carcinoma. Gynecol Oncol 29:12–25

Magrina JF, Webb MJ, Gaffey TA et al. (1979) Stage I squamous cell carcinoma of the vulva. Am J Obstet Gynecol 134:453–459

Nakao CY, Nolan JF, DiSaia PJ et al. (1974) Microinvasive epidermod carcinoma of the vulva with an unexpected natural history. Am J Obstet Gynecol 120:1122–1123

Parker RT, Duncan I, Rampone J et al. (1975) Operative management of early invasive epidermoid carcinoma of the vulva. Am J Obstet Gynecol 123:349–355

Pickel H, Haas J (1986) Microcarcinoma of the vulva. J Reprod Med 31:831–835

Rastkar C, Okagaki T, Twiggs LB et al. (1982) Early invasive and in-situ warty carcinoma of the vulva: clinical, histologic and electron microcopic study with particular reference to the viral association. Am J Obstet Gynecol 143:814–820

Ross MJ, Ehrmann RL (1987) Histologic prognosticator in stage 1 squamous cell carcinoma of the vulva. Obstet Gynecol 70:774–784

Rowley KC, Gallion HH, Donaldson ES et al. (1988) Prognostic factors of early vulvar cancer. Gynecol Oncol 31:43–49

Wharton JT, Gallagher S, Rutledge FN (1974) Microinvasive carcinoma of the vulva. Am J Obstet Gynecol 118:159–162

Wilkinson EJ, Rico MJ, Pierson EK (1982) Microinvasive carcinoma of the vulva. Int J Gynecol Pathol 1:29–39

Wilkinson EJ, Kneale B, Lynch PJ (1986) Report of the ISSVD Terminology Committee. J Reprod Med 31:973–974

Woodruff JD (1982) Early invasive carcinoma of the vulva. Clin Oncol 1:349–354

Yazigi R, Piver S, Tsukuda Y (1978) Microinvasive carcinoma of the vulva. Obstet Gynecol 51:368–370

Zucker PK, Berkowitz RS (1985) The issue of microinvasive squamous cell carcinoma of the vulva: an evaluation of the criteria of diagnosis and methods of therapy. Obstet Gynecol Surv 40:136–143

Invasive Squamous Cell Carcinoma

Acosta AA, Given FT, Frazier AB et al. (1978) Preoperative radiation therapy in the management of squamous cell carcinoma of the vulva. Am J Obstet Gynecol 132:198–206

Alexender LJ, Shields TL (1953) Squamous cell carcinoma of the vulva secondary granuloma inguinale. Arch Dermatol Syphilol 67:395–402

Andreasson B, Boek JE, Weberg E (1982) Invasive cancer in the vulvar region. Acta Obstet Gynecol Scand 61:113–119

Ballon SC, Lamb EJ (1975) Separate inguinal incisions in the treatment of advanced malignancy of the vulva. Surg Gynecol Obstet 140:81–84

Bartholodson L, Eldh J, Eriksson E et al. (1982) Surgical treatment of carcinoma of the vulva. Surg Gynecol Obstet 155:655–661

Benedet JL, Turko M, Fairey RN et al. (1979) Squamou carcinoma of the vulva: results of treatment 1938 to 1976. Am J Obstet Gynecol 134:201–207

Bibby AVG (1957) Carcinoma of the vulva – a review of 71 cases. J Obstet Gynaecol Br Emp 64:263–266

Boutselis JG (1972) Radical vulvectomy for invasive squamous cell carcinoma of the vulva. Obstet Gynecol 39:827–836

Boutselis JG, Ullery JC, Teteris NJ (1963) Epidermoid carcinoma of the vulva. Obstet Gynecol 22:713–724

Boyce CR, Mehram, AH (1974) Management of vulvar malignancies. Am J Obstet Gynecol 119:48–58

Buchler DA, Kline JC, Tunea JC et al. (1979) Treatment of recurrent carcinoma of the vulva. Gynecol Oncol 8:180–184

Buchsbaum HJ (1969) Hypercalcemia associated with vulvar carcinoma. Gynecologia (Basel) 168:203–208

Buscema J, Stern J, Woodruff JD (1980a) The significance of the histologic alterations adjacent to invasive vulvar carcinoma. Am J Obstet Gynecol 137:902–909

Buscema J, Woodruff JD, Parmley TH et al. (1980b) Carcinoma in situ of the vulva. Obstet Gynecol 55:225–230

Carson LF, Twiggs LB, Okagaki T et al. (1988) Human papillomavirus DNA in adenosquamous carcinoma and squamous cell carcinoma of the vulva. Obstet Gynecol 72:63–67

Cassidy RE, Braden FR, Ceha HT (1957) Factors that might influence prognosis in malignancies of the vulva. Am J Obstet Gynecol 74:361–367

Cavanagh D, Shepherd JH (1982) The place of pelvic exenteration in the primary management of advanced carcinoma of the vulva. Gynecol Oncol 13:318–322

Cavanagh D, Shepherd JH, Praphet H et al. (1982) Invasive carcinoma of the vulva. J Fl Med Assoc 69:447–452

Cavanagh D, Ruffulo EH, Marsden DE (1985) Cancer of the vulva. In: Gynecologic cancer: a clinicopathologic approach. Appleton-Century Crofts, East-Norwalk Ct, pp 1–40 Charles AH (1972) Carcinoma of the vulva. Br Med J 1:397–402

Choo V-C, Morley GW (1980) Multiple primary neoplasms of the anogenital region. Obstet Gynecol 56:365–369

Clark DGC, Zumoff B, Brunschwig A et al. (1960) Preferential uptake of phosphate by premalignant and malignant lesions of the vulva. Cancer 13:775–779

Collins CG, Collins JH, Barclay DL et al. (1963) Cancer involving the vulva. Am J Obstet Gynecol 87:762–772

Copas P, Dyer M, Comas FV et al. (1982) Spindle cell carcinoma of the vulva. Diagn Gynecol Obstet 4:235–241

Curry SL, Whareton JT, Rutledge F (1980) Positive lymphnodes in the vulva squamous cell carcinoma. Gynecol Oncol 9:63–67

Daly JW, Million RR (1974) Radical vulvectomy combined with electrive node irradiation for TXNO squamous carsinoma of the vulva. Cancer 34:161–165

Deppe G, Cohen CJ, Bruckner HW (1979) Chemotherapy of squamous cell carcinoma of the vulva: a review. Gynecol Oncol 7:345–348

DiSaia PJ, Morrow P, Haverback BJ et al. (1976) Carcinoembryonic antigen in cervical and vulvar cancer patients: serum levels and disease progress. Obstet Gynecol 47:95–99

Donaldson ES, Powell DE, Hanson MB et al. (1981) Prognostic parameters in invasive vulvar cancer. Gynecol Oncol 11:184–190

Embrey MP (1961) Vulval carcinoma complicating condylomata acuminata. J Obstet Gynaecol Br Commonw 68:503–504

Evans AS, Monaghan JM, Anderson MC (1987) A nuclear deoxyribonucleic acid analysis of normal and abnormal vulvar epithelium. Obstet Gynecol 69:790–793

Fairey RN, Mackay PA, Benedet JL et al. (1985) Radiation treatment of carcinoma of the vulva: 1950–1980. Am J Obstet Gynecol 151:591–597

Figge DC, Gaudenz R (1974) Invasive carcinoma of the vulva. Am J Obstet Gynecol 119:382–395

Figge DC, Tamini HK, Green BE (1985) Lymphatic spread in carcinoma of the vulva. Am J Obstet Gynecol 152:387–394

Franklin EW, Rutledge F (1971) Prognostic factors in the epidermoid carcinoma of the vulva. Obstet Gynecol 37:892–901

Franklin EW, Rutledge F (1972) Epidemiology of epidermoid carcinoma of the vulva. Obstet Gynecol 39:165–172

Frankman O, Kabulski Z (1983) Malignancy grading and prognosis from a biopsy only in cases of electrocoagulate squamous cell carcinoma of the vulva: stages I and II. Int J Gynecol Obstet 21:119–124

Freedman RS, Bowen JM, Hersen JH et al. (1983) Innunotherapy for vulvar carcinoma with virus-modified homolog extracts. Obstet Gynecol 62:707–714

Frischbier HJ, Thomson K (1971) Treatment of cancer of the vulva with high energy electrons. Am J Obstet Gynecol 111:431–435

Fu Y-S, Reagan JW, Townsend DE et al. (1981) Nuclear DNA study of vulvar intraepithelial and invasive squamous neoplasm. Obstet Gynecol 57:643–652

Garcia CG Jr, Bornow RC (1972) Carcinoma of the vulva. South Med J 65:237–240

Gosling JRG Abell MR, Drolette BM et al. (1961) Infiltrative squamous cell (epidermoid) carcinoma of the vulva. Cancer 14:330–343

Green TH Jr (1978) Carcinoma of the vulva: a reassessment. Obstet Gynecol 52:462–469

Green TH Jr, Ulfelder H, Meigs JV (1958) Epidermoid carcinoma of the vulva: an analysis of 258 cases. Am J Obstet Gynecol 75:848–864

Hacker NF, Berek JS, Lagasse LD et al. (1983) Management of regional lymphnodes and their prognostic influence of vulvar cancer. Obstet Gynecol 61:408–412

Hay DM, Cole FM (1969) Primary invasive carcinoma of the vulva in Jamacia. J Obstet Gynaecol Br Commonw 76:821–830

Helgason NM, Hass AC, Latonrette HB (1977) Radiation therapy in carcinoma of the vulva. Cancer 30:997–1000

Hoffman JS, Kumar NB, Morley GW (1985) Prognostic significance of groin lymph node metastases in squamous carcinoma of the vulva. Obstet Gynecol 66:402–405

Homesley HD, Bundy BN, Sedlis A et al. (1986) Radiation therapy versus pulvic node dissection for carcinoma of the vulva with positive groin node. Obstet Gynecol 68:733–740

Husseinzadeh N, Zaino R, Nahhas WA et al. (1983) The significance of histologic findings in predicting nodal metastases in invasive squamous cell carcinoma of the vulva. Gynecol Oncol 26:112–118

Iversen T (1982) Irradiation and bleomycin in the treatment of inoperable vulvar carcinoma. Acta Obstet Gynecol Scand 61:195–197

Iversen T (1983) Lymph drainage from the vulva. Gynecol Oncol 16:179–189

Iversen T, Alders JG, Christensen A et al. (1980) Squamous carcinoma of the vulva: a review of 424 patients 1956–1974. Gynecol Oncol 9:271–279

Jafari K, Magalotti M (1981) Radiation therapy in carcinoma of the vulva. Cancer 47:686–691

Jeffcoate TNA (1966) Chronic vulval dystrophies. Am J Obstet Gynecol 95:61–74

Jimerson GK, Merrill JA (1970) Multicentric squamous malignancy involving both cervix and vulva. Cancer 26:150–153

Kabulski Z, Frankman O (1978) Histologic malignancy grading in invasive squamous cell carcinoma of the vulva. Int J Gynecol Obstet 16:233–237

Kalra JK, Grossman AM, Krumholz BA et al. (1981) Preoperative chemotherapy for carcinoma of the vulva. Gynecol Oncol 12:256–260

Kaplan AL, Kaufman RH (1975) Management of advanced carcinoma of the vulva. Gynecol Oncol 3:220–232

Katayama KP, Woodruff JD, Jones HW Jr et al. (1972) Chromosomes of condylomata acuminata, Paget's disease, in-situ carcinoma, invasive squamous cell carcinoma and malignant melanoma of the human vulva. Obstet Gynecol 39:346–356

Kauffman RH, Gardner HL (1978) Vulvar dystrophies. Clin Obstet Gynecol 21:1082–1106

Kauffman RH, Dreesman GR, Burek GR et al. (1981) Herpes virus induced antigens in squamous cell carcinoma in-situ of the vulva. N Engl J Med 305:483–488

Kelly J (1972) Malignant disease of the vulva. J Obstet Gynaecol Br Commonw 79:265–272

Krupp PJ (1978) Cancer of the vulva. Surg Clin North Am 58:19–23

Krupp P, Bohm JW (1978) Lymph gland metastases in invasive squamous cell cancer of the vulva. Am J Obstet Gynecol 130:943–952

Krupp PJ, Lee FYL, Bohm JW (1975) Prognostic parameters and clinical staging criteria in epidermoid carcinoma of the vulva. Obstet Gynecol 46:84–88

Kucera H, Weghaupt K (1988) The electrosurgical operation of vulvar carcinoma with post operative irradiation of inguinal lymphnodes. Gynecol Oncol 29:158–167

Kurzl R, Messerer D (1989) Prognostic factors in squamous cell carcinoma of the vulva: a multivariate analysis. Gynecol Oncol 32:143–150

Lasser A, Cornog JL, Morris JM (1974) Adenoid squamous cell carcinoma of the vulva. Cancer 33:224–227

Levin W, Goldberg G, Altaras M et al. (1986) The use of concomitant chemotherapy and radiotherapy prior to surgery and advanced stage of carcinoma of the vulva. Gynecol Oncol 25:20–25

Lindeque BG, Nel AE, Du Toit JP (1987) Immune deficiency and invasive carcinoma of the vulva in a young woman: a case report. Gynecol Oncol 26:112–118

Lister UM, Akinla O (1972) Carcinoma of the vulva in childhood. J Obstet Gynaecol Br Commonw 79:470–473

Lowe D, Fletcher CDM (1984) Eosinophils in squamous cell carcinoma of the oral cavity, external genitalia and anus: clinical correlations. Histopathology 8:627–632

Lundwell F (1961) Cancer of the vulva: a clinical review. Acta Radiol [Suppl] 208:105

Lunin AB (1949) Carcinoma of the vulva: a review of 50 cases. Am J Obstet Gynecol 57:742–747

Macafee CHG (1962) Some aspects of vulva cancer. J Obstet Gynecol Br Commonw 69:177–195

Marcus SL (1960) Multiple squamous cell carcinoma involving the cervix, vagina, and vulva: the theory of multicentric origin. Am J Obstet Gynecol 80:802–812

Melfetano JH, Piver MS, Tsukada Y et al. (1985) Univariate and multivariate analyses of 5 year survival, recurrence, and inguinal node metastases in stage I and II vulvar carcinoma. J Surg Oncol 30:124–131

Merrill JA, Ross NL (1961) Cancer of the vulva. Cancer 14:13–20

Mickal A, Andonie JA, Dougherty CM (1966) Squamous cellcarcinoma of the vulva. Obstet Gynecol 28:670–674

Monaghan JM, Hammond IG (1984) Pelvic node dissection in the treatment of vulval carcinoma – is it necessary? Br J Obstet Gynaecol 91:270–274

Monaghan JM, Lindeque G (1986) Vulvar carcinoma in pregnancy. Br J Obstet Gynaecol 93:785–786

Morley GW (1976) Infiltrative carcinoma of the vulva: results of surgical treatment. Am J Obstet Gynecol 124:874–888

Morris JM (1977) A formula of selective lymphadenectomy: its application to cancer of the vulva. Obstet Gynecol 50:152–158

Nadji M, Ganjei P, Renneys NS et al. (1984) Immunohistochemistry of vulvar meoplasms: a brief review: Int J Gynecol Pathol 3:41–50

Nichols CE, Bonney WA (1973) Carcinoma of the vulva producing hy¡percalcemia. Obstet Gynecol 42:58–61

Niebyl JR, Grandy R, Friedrich EG Jr (1975) Vulvar carcinoma with hypercalcemia. Obstet Gynecol 45:343–348

Nobler MP (1972) Efficacy of perineal teletherapy portal in the management of vulvar and vaginal cancer. Radiology 103:393–397

Palmer JP, Sodugori MG, Reinhard MC (1949) Carcinoma of the vulva: report of 313 cases. Surg Gynecol Obstet 88:435–440

Parry-Jones E (1960) Lymphatics of the vulva. J Obstet Gynaecol Br Commonw 67:919–928

Phillips B, Buchsbaum HJ, Lifshitz S (1981) Pelvic exenteration for vulvovaginal carcinoma. Am J Obstet Gynecol 141:1038–1044

Piver MS, Xynos FP (1977) Pelvix lymphadenectomy in women with carcinoma of the clitoris. Obstet Gynecol 49:592–595

Podratz KC, Symmonds RE, Taylor WF et al. (1983) Carcinoma of the vulva: analysis of treatment and survival. Obstet Gynecol 61:63–74

Punnonen R, Grönroos M, Lindgren I (1977) The value of p32 in the diagnosis of various vulvar lesions. Gynecol Oncol 5:187–188

Rahman MS, Rahman J, Al-Sibai MH (1982) Carcinoma of the vulva in pregnancy, case report. Br J Obstet Gynaecol 89:244–246

Renziehausen VK (1974) Zur Kryotherapie des Vulvakarzinoms. Zentralbl Gynäkol 96: 1121–1129

Rutledge FN (1965) Cancer of the vulva and vagina. Clin Obstet Gynecol 8:1051–1079

Rutledge F, Smith JP, Franklin EW (1970) Carcinoma of the vulva. Am J Obstet Gynecol 106:1117–1130

Saltzstein SL, Woodruff JD, Novak ER (1956) Postgranulomatous carcinoma of the vulva. Obstet Gynecol 7:80–90

Sawyer KC, Baker WG, McClure HE (1949) A case of carcinoma of the vulva involving only the prepuce and clitoris. West J Surg Obstet Gynecol 57:589–591

Sengupta BS (1981) Carcinoma of the vulva in Jamaican women. Acta Obstet Gynecol Scand 60:537–544

Shafeek MA, Osman MI, Hussein AM (1979) Carcinoma of the vulva arising in condylomata acuminata. Obstet Gynecol 54:120–123

Shimm DS, Fuller AF, Orlow EL et al. (1986) Prognostic variables in the treatment of squamous cell carcinoma of the vulva. Gynecol Oncol 24:343–358
Shingleton HM, Fowler WC Jr, Palumbo L et al. (1970) Carcinoma of the vulva: influence of radical operation on cure rate. Obstet Gynecol 35:1–6
Smith FR, Pollack RS (1947) Carcinoma of the vulva: results of treatment and effects of special factors or results. Surg Gynecol Obstet 84:78–84
Sutton GP, Stehman FB, Ehrlich CE et al. (1987) Human papillomavirus deoxyribonucleic acid in lesions of the female genital tract: evidence of type 6/11 in squamous cell carcinoma of the vulva. Obstet Gynecol 70:564–568
Taussig FJ (1938) A study of lymph glands in cancer of the cervix and cancer of the vulva. Am J Obstet Gynecol 36:819–832
Taussig FJ (1940) Cancer of the vulva: an analysis of 155 cases. Am J Obstet Gynceol 40:764–779
Thomas G (1965) The role of radioactive phosphorous (P32) in the localisation of vulval lesions. Aust N Z J Obstet Gynecol 5:241–248
Thornton WN Jr, Flanagan WC Jr (1973) Pelvic exenteration in the treatment of advanced malignancy of the vulva. Am J Obstet Gynecol 117:774–781
Wallach RC (1975) Cryosurgery of advanced carcinoma. Obstet Gynecol 47:454–458
Way S (1948) The anatomy of the lymphatic drainage of the vulva. Ann R Coll Surg Engl 3:187–209
Way S (1954) Results of a planned attack on carcinoma of the vulva. Br Med J 2:780–782
Way S (1960) Carcinoma of the vulva. Am J Obstet Gynecol 79:682–697
Wilkinson EJ, Crocker BP, Friedrich EG Jr (1988) Two distinct pathologic types of giant cell tumor of the vulva: a report of two cases. J Reprod Med 33:519–522
Woodcock AS (1976) The etiology and pathology of cancer of the vulva. Clin Obstet Gynecol 3:201–216
Wright VC (1976) Carcinoma of the vulva. J Am Geriatr Soc 24:232–235
Zaino R, Husseinzadeh N, Mortel R et al. (1982) Improved histological grading system for squamous carcinoma of the vulva. Lab Invest 46:93A
zur Hausen H, Gissmann L, Schlenhafer JR (1984) Viruses in the etiology of human genital cancer. Prog Med Virol 30:170–186

Verrucous Carcinoma

Ackerman LV (1948) Verrucous carcinoma of the oral cavity. Surgery 23:670–678
Crowther ME, Shepherd JH, Fisher C (1988) Verrucous carcinoma of the vulva containing human papilloma virus 11: case report. Br J Obstet Gynaecol 95:414–418
De Graaff J, van der Harten JJ (1975) Ineffectiveness of verrucous carcinoma of the vulva. Eur J Obstet Gynecol Reprod Biol 5/6:327–330
Demian SD, Bushkin FL, Echevarria RL (1973) Perineural invasion and anaplastic transformation of verrucous carcinoma. Cancer 32:395–401
Foye G, Marsh MR, Minkowitz S (1969) Verrucous carcinoma of the vulva. Obstet Gynecol 34:484–488
Gallousis S (1972) Verrucous carcinoma: a report of three vulvar cases and review of the literature. Obstet Gynecol 40:502–507
Gissmann L, de Villiers EM, zur Hausen H (1982) Analysis of human genital warts (condyloma acuminata) and other genital tumors for human papillomavirus type 6 DNA. Int J Cancer 29:143–146
Gissmann L, Wolnik L, Ikenberg H et al. (1983) Human paillomavirus 6 and 11 DNA sequences in genital and laryngeal papillomas and in some cervical cancers. Proc Natl Acad Sci USA 80:560–563
Isaacs JH (1976) Verrucous carcinoma of the female genital tract. Gynecol Oncol 4:259–269
Japaze H, Dinh TV, Woodruff JD (1982) Verrucous carcinoma of the vulva: study of 24 cases. Obstet Gynecol 60:462–466
Jennings RH, Barclay DL (1972) Verrucous carcinoma of the cervix. Cancer 30:430–434

Judge JR (1969) Giant condyloma acuminatum involving vulva and rectum. Arch Pathol Lab Med 88:46–48

Kraus FT, Perez-Mesa C (1966) Verrucous carcinoma: clinical and pathologic study of 105 cases involving oral cavity, larynx and genitalia. Cancer 19:26–38

Lucas WE, Benirschke K, Lebherz TB (1974) Verrucous carcinoma of the female genital tract. Obstet Gynecol 119:435–440

Partridge EE, Murad T, Shingleton HM et al. (1980) Verrucous lesions of the female genitalia: 1 giant condylomata. Am J Obstet Gynecol 137:412–418

Powell JL, Franklin EW III, Niekerson JF et al. (1978) Verrucous carcinoma of the female genital tract. Gynecol Oncol 6:565–573

Prioleau PG, Santa-Cruz J, Meyer JS et al. (1980) Verrucous carcinoma: a light microscopic, autoradiographic and immunofluorescent study. Cancer 45:2849–2854

Rando RF, Sedlacek TV, Jean Hunt RN et al. (1986) Verrucous carcinoma of the vulva associated with an unusual type 6 human papilloma virus. Obstet Gynecol 67 [Suppl]:70–75

Selim MA, Lankerani MR (1979) Verrucous carcinoma of the vulva. J Reprod Med 22:93–96

Stehman FB, Castaldo TW, Charles EH et al. (1980) Verrucous carcinoma of the vulva. Int J Gynecol Obstet 17:523–525

Ubben K, Krzyzek R, Ostrow R et al. (1979) Human pailloma virus DNA detected in two verrucous carcinoma. J Invest Dermatol 72:195–210

Vayrynen M, Romppanen T, Koskela RE et al. (1981) Verrucous squamous cell carcinoma of the female genital tract: report of three cases and survey of the literature. In J Gynecol Obstet 19:351–356

Zaaijman CF, Slabber CF (1978) Verrucous carcinoma of the vulva. Br J Obstet Gynaecol 85:74–76

7 Basal Cell Carcinoma

Basal cell carcinoma constitutes 2%–4% of the vulval malignancies. Breen et al. (1975) found, on reviewing the literature, an incidence of one basal cell carcinoma for every 37 squamous cell carcinomas of the vulva. These tumours are also designated as rodent ulcers because of its infiltration and erosiveness of the neighbouring soft tissues, bone and cartilage if left untreated.

The age incidence is similar to that in squamous cell carcinoma and ranges from 34 to 90 years old with a mean of 64.8 year (Palladino et al. 1969). Vulval basal cell carcinoma occurs most commonly in the labium majus, followed by a relatively smaller group in the mons pubis, labium minus and clitoris. The lesions may be bilateral and multicentric.

7.1 Aetiology

The aetiology of vulval basal cell carcinoma is unknown. Syphilis, arsenicals, previous irradiation (Marcus 1960; Bean and Becker 1968; Breen et al. 1975) and chronic irritation (Ward 1956) have been suggested as factors.

7.2 Clinical Features

The patient complains of episodes of itching, mass with or without irritation, sometimes with a sore, ulceration, bleeding or chronic discharge. Some 20% of patients with vulval basal cell carcinoma shows second primaries in the genital tract and other sites (Palladino et al. 1969).

7.3 Pathological Features

Several macroscopic types of basal cell carcinoma may be seen: (a) solid, starting as a small firm nodule which later ulcerates, or rarely the tumour may be large and pedunculated (Dudzinski et al. 1984); (b) cicatrical, a superficial spreading lesion with central ulceration and scarring; (c) morphaic, a slowly growing, greyish-white to ivory-coloured plaque; and (d) erythrematoid, a pink to brownish granular patch with a distinct but irregular border. The lesion may be single or multiple, involving most commonly the labia majora, labia minora, clitoris (Ridley 1972) and mons pubis (Schueller 1965).

7.3.1 Microscopical Appearance

The cells of basal cell carcinoma show a striking resemblance to those of the basal layer of the epidermis and pilosebaceous adnexae. The neoplastic cells are round, oval and oblong in shape and contain hyperchromatic nuclei surrounded by a thin rim of cytoplasm without any spinous processes. Mitotic figures may be frequent. Occasional giant multinucleate tumour cells are seen. A variable number of lymphocytic infiltrations and desmoplastic reactions are seen in the dermis around the mass of tumour cells. Several histological types of basal cell carcinoma have been described: (a) solid consisting of irregular strands and nests of haphazardly arranged but closely packed cells. The peripheral layers of these nests and strands display a characteristic palisading by a single layer of neoplastic cells (Fig. 7.1); (b) cystic occurring when there is necrosis of the central part of the solid nests of tumour cells. It is, therefore, a variant of the solid variety (Fig. 7.2); (c) adenoid, a mass with strands and ribbons of tumour cells, enclosing a space resembling glands (Fig. 7.3); (d) morphaic in which the neoplastic cells form irregular columns traversing the dermis in all directions.

Scattered deposits of melanin pigments may be seen in all types. The stroma between the columns is dense and hyalinised. Occasionally, intra-tumoural localised amyloidosis (Hashimoto and Brownstein 1973; Meng 1983) and systemic amyloidosis (Lichtenstein and Lee 1980) associated with metastasising basal cell carcinoma have been noticed and are probably due to the aberrant functional activities of the tumour cells.

7.3.2 Baso-squamous Carcinoma

Foci of mature squamous cell are seen occasionally in the basal cell carcinoma with the formation of keratin pearls in the centre of the basal cell nests. These benign foci are to be differentiated from the aggressive baso-squamous carcinoma in which the squamous cell component shows central necrosis and anaplasia (Schueller 1965; Ward 1956). It is estimated that 5% of basal cell carcinoma are truly baso-squamous carcinoma (Breen et al. 1975).

7.4 Treatment

Local excision with deep and wide margins is the treatment advocated (Schueller 1965; Breen et al. 1975; Cruz-Jimenez and Abell 1975; Ambrosini et al. 1980) for the pure basal cell carcinoma, and radical vulvectomy with bilateral inguinal

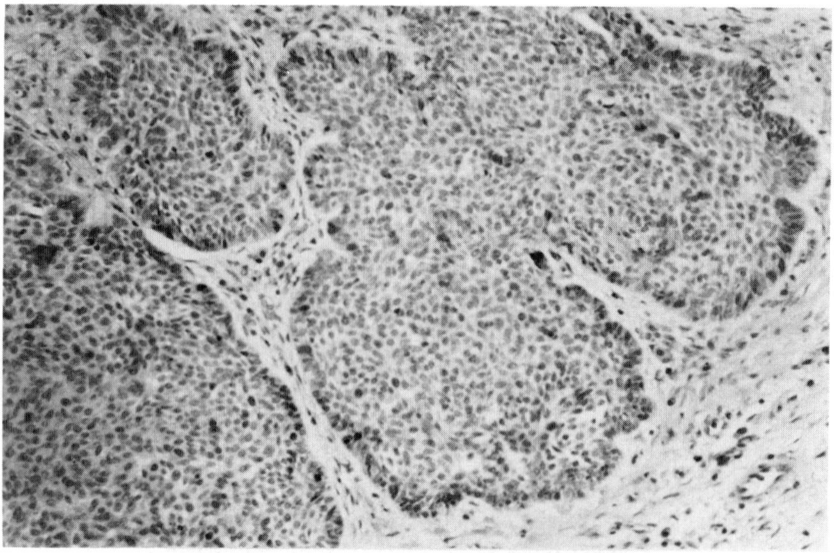

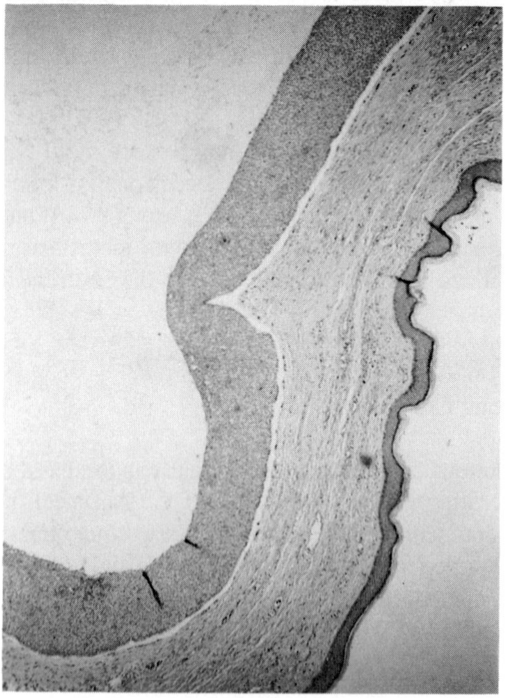

Fig. 7.1. Basal cell carcinoma: nests of basal cells displaying peripheral palisading

Fig. 7.2. Basal cell carcinoma cystic variant

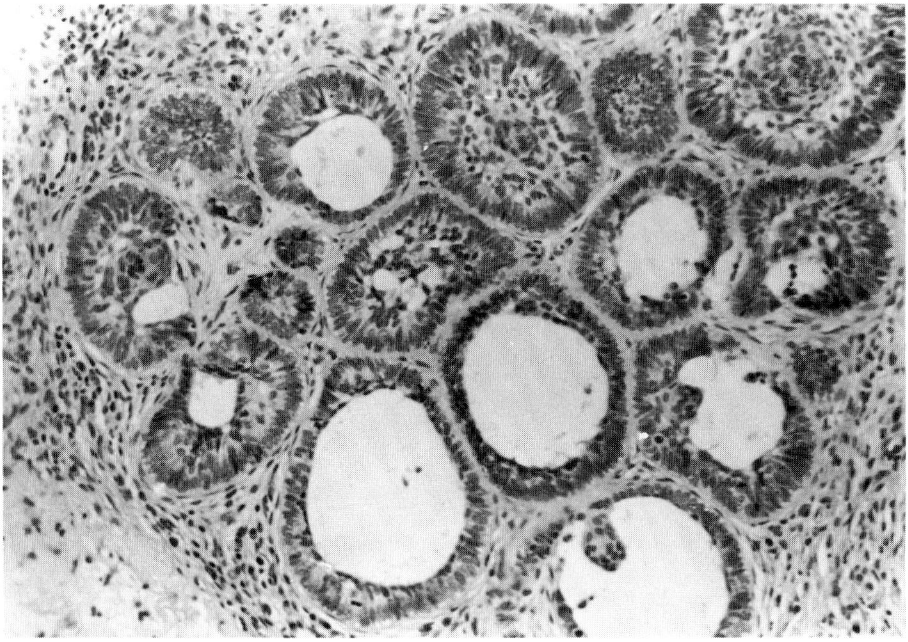

Fig. 7.3. Basal cells carcinoma: adenoid pattern with gland-like spaces

lymphadenectomy for baso-squamous carcinoma (Marcus 1960). Aggressive treatment has also been advocated for the large tumours that are locally destructive and have extended to the sub-cutaneous fat (Perrone et al. 1987). The patients are generally old, and the surgical morbidity should be carefully balanced against the ultimate benefit. Radiotherapy and electrocauterisation or cryosurgery are reserved as non-surgical modalities for patients with poor medical conditions and surgical risks (Breen et al. 1975; Zerner and Fenn 1979). Although chemotherapy has been used in the metastasising lesions in other sites, the ultimate prognosis has been bleak (Coker et al. 1983).

7.5 Biological Behaviour

The biological behaviour of the basal cell carcinoma appears to be variable. Although the prevalent opinion is that the basal cell carcinoma of the vulva is locally infiltrative and does not metastasise (Ackles and Pratt 1956; Schueller 1965; Palladino et al. 1969), there are several reported cases of metastases in the literature (Jimenez et al. 1975; Safai and Good 1977; Sworn et al. 1979; Hoffman et al. 1988). The incidence is indeed very low and ranges form 0.028% to 0.1% (Cotran 1961; Paver et al. 1973). Some authors hold that pure basal cell carcinomas of the vulva do not metastasise (Palladino et al. 1969). The reported metastases contained squamous elements and were therefore baso-squamous carcinoma (Marcus 1960).

Mixed carcinoma of the vulva with metastasis of the basal cell component to the inguinal nodes has also been noticed (Hoffman et al. 1988). Perrone et al. (1987) have suggested that a tumour in the advanced clinical stage, with invasion of the subcutaneous fat, urethra and vagina, tumour thickness more than 1 cm in diameter and morphoeic-like growth pattern is more likely to metastasise. According to Jacobs et al. (1982), an aggressive basal cell carcinoma tends to be ulcerated, is composed of small groups of cells displaying an irregular spiky appearance, does not show peripheral palisading, infiltrates in cords of 1–2 cells thick and has hyalinised stroma.

The recurrence rate is 5%–10% (Simkin and Fisher 1977) but may be as high as 21.5% (Palladino et al. 1969). This is thought to be due to the inadequate excision of the lesions (Nel 1957; Palladino et al. 1969; Marcus 1960).

References

Ackles RC, Pratt JP (1956) Basal cell carcinoma of the vulva. Am J Obstet Gynecol 72:1124–1126

Ambrosini A, Becagli L, Resta P et al. (1980) Basal cell carcinoma of the vulva. Eur J Gynaecol Oncol 1:16–128

Bean SF, Becker FT (1968) Basal cell carcinoma of the vulva. Arch Dermatol 98:284–286

Breen JL, Neubecker RD, Greenwald E et al. (1975) Basal cell carcinoma of the vulva. Obstet Gynecol 46:122–129

Coker D, Elias EG, Varavathana T et al. (1983) Chemotherapy for metastatic basal cell carcinoma. Arch Dermatol 119:44–50

Cotran RS (1961) Metastasising basal cell carcinomas. Cancer 14:1036–1040

Cruz-Jimenez PR, Abell MR (1975) Cutaneous basal cell carcinoma of the vulva. Cancer 36:1860–1868

Dudzinski MR, Askin FB, Fowler WC Jr (1984) Giant basal cell carcinoma of the vulva. Obstet Gynecol 63 [Suppl]:57–60

Hashimoto K, Brownstein H (1973) Localised Amyloidosis in basal cell epitheliomas. Acta Derm Venercol (Stockh) 53:331–339

Hoffman MS, Roberts WS, Ruffulo EH (1988) Basal cell carcinoma of the vulva with inguinal node metastases. Gynecol Oncol 29:113–119

Jacobs GH, Rippey JJ, Affini M (1982) Prediction of aggrtessive behavior in basal cell carcinoma. Cancer 49:533–537

Jimenez HT, Fenoglio CM, Richart RM (1975) Vulvar basal cell carcinoma with metastases. Am J Obstet Gynecol 121:285–286

Lichtenstein HL, Lee JCK (1980) Amyloidosis associated with metastasising basal cell carcinoma. Cancer 46:2693–2696

Marcus SL (1960) Basal cell and basal squamous carcinoma of the vulva. Am J Obstet Gynecol 79:461–469

Meng LM (1983) Localised amyloidosis in basal cell carcinoma: a pathologic study. Cancer 52:1833–1836

Nel RW (1957) Basal cell carcinoma of the vulva: review of the literature and report of a case. S Afr Med J 31:381–383

Palladino VS, Duffy JL, Bures GJ (1969) Basal cell carcinoma of the vulva. Cancer 24:460–470

Paver KK, Poyzer K, Burry N et al. (1973) The incidence of basal cell carcinoma and their metastases in Australia and New Zealand. Australas J Dermatol 14:53

Perrone T, Twiggs LB, Adcock LL et al. (1987) Vulvar basal cell carcinoma: an infrequently metastasising neoplasm. Int J Gynecol Pathol 6:152–165

Ridley CM (1972) Review of recent literature on diseases of the vulva. Br J Dermatol 87:163–170

Safai B, Good RA (1977) Basal cell carcinoma with metastasis. Arch Pathol Lab Med 101:317–331

Schueller EF (1965) Basal cell cancer of the vulva. Am J Obstet Gynecol 93:199–208

Simkin RJ, Fisher BK (1977) Basal cell epithelioma of the vulva. Obstet Gynecol 49:617–619

Sworn MJ, Hammond GT, Buchanan R (1979) Metastatic basal cell carcinoma of the vulva. Br J Obstet Gynaecol 86:332–334

Ward J (1956) Five cases of basal cell carcinoma of the vulva. J Obstet Gynaecol Br Emp 65:697–705

Zerner J, Fenn ME (1979) Basal cell carcinoma of the vulva. Int J Gynecol Obstet 17:203–205

8 Adenocarcinoma

Adenocarcinoma, either primary or metastatic, is an uncommon malignancy of the vulva. The most common primary is adenocarcinoma of Bartholin's gland origin. The other possible primaries are: (a) sweat and sebaceous glands, (b) paraurethral glands, (c) Minor vestibular glands, (d) ectopic tissues in the vulva (breasts, endometriosis, misplaced cloacal tissue) and (e) embryonic rests, Gartner's duct remnants.

When a primary adenocarcinoma is diagnosed in the vulva, the most likely site of origin is Bartholin's gland. Adenocarcinoma arising in other structures is extremely rare, and most of those reported so far have been diagnosed by presumptive evidence of anatomical locations. When the tumour is localised and small, the anatomical location is helpful, but in a larger lesion occupying a wide area of the vulva, localisation of the primary site of origin becomes impossible. The histological appearances are unreliable, as there are not distinctive histological featutres for most of these adenocarcinomas. For clinical purposes, such diagnoses are less important because all these lesions are to be treated radically like other common vulval malignancies.

8.1 Adenocarcinoma Arising in the Sweat Glands

8.1.1 Apocrine Gland

Primary adenocarcinoma arising in the apocrine glands of the vulva without an association with Paget's disease is extremely rare. Controversies still surround the histogenesis of Paget's disease. From time to time, apocrine gland carcinoma has been thought to be the primary site of origin of Paget's disease (Plachta and Speer 1954; Boehm and Morris 1971), while others have suggested that the apocrine gland carcinoma is due to invasion by malignant cells of epidermal origin (Taki and Janovski 1961). In the earlier literature, several low grade adenocarcinomas not associated with Paget's disease were reported (Folsome 1940; Lovelade and Waugh 1941; McDonald 1941). Novak and Stevenson (1945) rejected many of these as representing benign hidradenoma. None showed any infiltration, metastasis or recurrence after local excision. Judging from the clinical behaviour and histopathological appearances, Novak and Stevenson (1945), however, accepted one report of Eichenberg (1934) as genuine adenocarcinoma. The lesion occurred in the labium majus of a 30-year-old woman and metastasised to the regional inguinal lymph nodes. Novak added two patients of this own, a 60-year-old woman with involvement of almost the whole vulva and a 41-year-old woman with a large, indurated and ulcerated lesion on the posterior part of the left labium. Subsequently, Lacy (1946) reported a tumour in a 67-year-old woman who presented with vaginal bleeding and discharge, and an indurated superficial ulcer overlying the Bartholin's gland. The tumour was composed of solid sheets of small malignant cells with hyperchromatic nuclei, numerous mitotic figures, areas of squamous differentiation and distinct invasion. The tumour persisted after local fulguration with cautery but did not metastasise. In these reports, there was no attempt to differentiate between the eccrine and apocrine origin of these carcinomas. From the descriptions, it appears that some of them could belong to apocrine gland carcinoma.

Apocrine gland carcinoma is extremely rare but nonetheless can occur in areas bearing apocrine glands (Baes and Suurmond 1970; Warkel and Helwig 1978). Histologically, these tumours display a glandular arrangement with papillary formations, cystic dilatations, and decapitation secretion of the lining epithelial cells which contain abundant eosinophilic cytoplasm and diastase-resistant, PAS-positive granules. These tumours are locally invasive and spread to the regional lymph nodes (Futrell et al. 1971).

8.1.2 Eccrine Gland

Adenocarcinoma arising in the eccrine sweat gland is also very rare. Of the four distinct histological types of eccrine adenocarcinoma, viz. eccrine porocarcinoma, syringoid eccrine carcinoma, mucinous eccrine carcinoma and clear cell eccrine carcinoma (Mehregan et al. 1983), eccrine porocarcinoma is the most common variety and has been reported to occur also on the vulva (Gartmann 1985; Donna et al. 1978; Wick et al. 1985). Webb and Beswick (1983) reported a mucinous eccrine carcinoma of the vulva in association with vulval Paget's disease. Histologically, these tumours are characterised by the presence of well-defined islands of anaplastic cells within the acanthotic epidermis, presence of glycogen granules within the cytoplasm of tumour cells, lack of keratinisation and foci of duct-like lumina (Mehregan et al. 1983). The neoplastic cells may be arranged in cords, acini, and solid nests and infiltrate the dermis. The epidermis may be ulcerated.

Ultrastructurally, the peripheral layer of acini are anchored to the collagen by pseudopodia. The cells display poorly formed desmosomes, many ribosomes, glycogen-like granules, moderately developed mitochondria and characteristic bundles of microfilaments in the perinuclear zone (Rich et al. 1981; Fukuma et al. 1986). The nuclei with multiple nucleoli show indentation of the nuclear membranes (Rich et al. 1981; Fukuma et al. 1986).

They are usually asymptomatic and discovered accidentally (Webb and Beswick 1983). Recently, Fukuma et al. (1986) noticed an elevated level of alpha subunit of chorionic gonadotropin in a 69-year-old patient who presented with abdominal pain, pink vaginal discharge and swelling of the right labia. The patient had metastases to the right subclavian lymph nodes.

Eccrine sweat gland carcinomas tend to recur but metastases to the regional lymph nodes or distant sites are rare. Paget's disease of the vulva has been thought to originate from eccrine sweat gland carcinoma (Koss et al. 1968: Belcher 1972).

Although some individualisation of treatment is desirable, radical surgery may be considered, as these tumours can metastasise to the regional nodes.

8.2 Sebaceous Gland Carcinoma

Sebaceous gland carcinoma is common in the eyelids where it arises from meibomian and infrequently from the zeisian glands. It is rare on the vulval skin. The patient described by Rulon and Helwig (1974) was a 31-year-old women who presented with an indurated plaque on the left labium minora for 6 months, and the one of Jacobs et al. (1986) presented, with a painful vulval lesion and dysuria for 1 year. Clinically, sebaceous gland carcinoma may present as a lump, plaque or a nodule usually greater than 1 cm in diameter. The cut surfaces are pink to yellow in appearance. Sebaceous gland neoplasms may be associated with internal malignancies and have been reported to be a component of what is known as Muir-Torre syndrome, comprising sebaceous neoplasms, keratoacanthomas, carcinomas of the larynx, duodenum, ampulla of Vater, colon and female genital tract (Muir et al. 1967; Torre 1968). The genital carcinoma may be of the vulva, cervix or endometrium (Jacobs et al. 1986).

8.2.1 Microscopical Appearance

Sebaceous gland carcinomas are composed of irregular lobules of sebaceous cells which are foamy due to the high lipid content of the cytoplasm. They are generally large and contain a centrally located, pyknotic nucleus. In a poorly differentiated tumour the cells are small and poor in lipid and display considerable nuclear pleomorphism. Fine lipid granules can be demonstrated in the cytoplasm in the frozen section tissue by oli red O. Rulon and Helwig (1974) classified these carcinomas into sebaceous carcinoma and basal cell carcinoma with sebaceous differentiation. The latter type is characterised by a solid or lacy growth pattern of basal cell carcinoma with multiple contacts with the superficial basal cell carcinoma. The sebaceous cells with bubbly cytoplasm are scattered within the basal cell carcinoma either singly or more commonly in groups. The tumour may show many microcystic spaces containing keratin or eosinophilic material.

The vulval tumour reported by Jacobs et al. (1986) was associated with Bowen's disease of the vulva. The sebaceous carcinoma was composed of lobules of sebaceous cells with nuclear pleomorphism, many mitoses, atypical keratinocytes and subepidermal in location. The tumour was attached to the superficial epidermis which displayed full thickness keratinocytic atypia, mitoses, multinucleation and focal dyskeratosis of typical Bowen's disease.

Sebaceous carcinoma of the eyelid metastasises (Boniuk and Zimmerman 1968), but of the other areas, recurrences and metastases are infrequent.

8.2.2 Treatment

The vulval tumour should be completely excised with wide excision margins.

8.3 Paraurethral Glands

See Part III.

8.4 Minor Vestibular Glands

Although adenoma has been described, carcinoma arising in the minor vestibular glands has not been reported.

8.5 Adenocarcinoma Arising in Ectopic Tissue

8.5.1 Breast

Malignant changes in ectopic vulval breast tissue are extremely rare. Only a few cases of adenocarcinoma complicating the vulval breast have so far been reported (Greene 1936; Hendrix and Behrman 1956; Guerry and Pratt-Thomas 1976; Guercio et al. 1984; Cho et al. 1985; Simon et al. 1988). The other possible instance reported by Hoogerland and Buchler (1979) was an 84-year-old woman who presented with unusual symptoms of erythema of the left thigh and inguinal area and soreness of the left labium.

8.5.1.1 Clinical Features

The patients are elderly, between 50 and 70 years of age, and present with vulval growth, vaginal bleeding discharge and pain.

8.5.1.2 Pathological Features

The tumours are hard nodules 1.5–20 cm, usually located on the labia. In one patient there was a history of right mastectomy (Guerry and Pratt-Thomas 1976).

8.5.1.3 Microscopical Appearance

The tumour shows similar histological features to pectoral breast carcinoma and consists of neoplastic ducts, acini, groups and cords of cells with irregular infiltrating margins, variable desmoplasia of typical duct carcinoma of the pectoral breast. The intraduct and scirrhous components may also be noticed. Vulval breast carcinoma has the potential to metastasise to the regional lymph nodes and distal sites (Greene 1936; Hendrix and Behrman 1956; Simon et al. 1988). Differential diagnosis from adnexal adenocarcinoma associated with Paget's disease and metastatic carcinoma from other primary sites including pectoral breast and melanoma when the tumour is poorly differentiated should be considered. Metastases from other primaries to the vulva are rare, and when present, tend to be multiple and expansile in nature (Cho et al. 1985). Also, the presence of an in situ component adjacent to the infiltrating lesions of the vulva and associated metastases to the regional nodes, if present, eliminate the possibility of a secondary deposit. Immunoperoxidase studies of the vulval tumour and metastatic nodes using monoclonal antibodies against guinea pig fat globules as well as analysis of the oestrogen hormone receptors can help to establish a breast origin (Cho et al. 1985; Simon et al. 1988).

8.5.1.4 Treatment

Patients are treated by radical vulvectomy with or without node dissection, radical hemivulvectomy with ipsilateral inguinal node dissection and wide local excision when an early diagnosis is made. With disseminated disease the prognosis is generally poor.

8.5.2 Endometriosis

Mesko et al. (1988) reported a clear cell adenocarcinoma developing in the focus of endometriosis within the canal of Nuck at the superior aspect of the right labia majora of a 57-year-old woman who 9 years earlier had had herniorrhaphy. The patient had skin recurrence, pelvic nodal metastases at 3 months' and lung metastases at 2 years' follow-up.

8.6 Adenocarcinoma Arising in Misplaced Cloacal Tissue

Tiltman and Knutzen (1978) described a firm rubbery papillary growth 2 cm in diameter arising in the external urethral meatus in a 50-year-old woman who presented with dyspareunia. The lesion was treated by modified radical vulvectomy and bilateral inguinal node dissection. Histologically, the tumour was a mucus-secreting adenocarcinoma with metastases to the left inguinal node. The neoplastic glands were lined by columnar epithelium, goblet cells and Paneth's cells. The mucin was a mixture of neutral, sulphated and non-sulphated acid mucopolysaccharide. The colonic type epithelium representing cloacal tissue was thought to be misplaced in the vulva during embryonic division of the cloaca by the urogenital fold. Vulval ulcer developing in what appeared to be heterotopic intestinal mucosa has recently been reported by Yeoh et al. (1987). It may be mentioned that mucinous adenocarcinoma can occasionally originate in the urinary tract (Aufderheide and Streitz 1974).

References

Aufderheide AC, Streitz JM (1974) Mucinous adenocarcinoma of the renal pelvis. Cancer 167–173

Baes H, Suurmound D (1970) Apocrine sweat gland carcinoma. Br J Dermatol 83:843–846

Belcher RW (1972) Extramammary Paget's disease: enzyme histochemical and electron microscopic study. Arch Pathol 94:59–64

Boehm F, Morris J (1971) Paget's disease and apocrine gland carcinoma of the vulva. Obstet Gynecol 38:185–192

Boniuk K, Zimmerman LE (1968) Sebaceous carcinoma of the eyelid, eyebrow, and orbit. Trans Am Acad Ophthalmol Otolaryngol 72:619–642

Cho D, Buscema J, Rosenshein NB et al. (1985) Primary breast cancer of the vulva. Obstet Gynecol 66 [Suppl]:79–81

Donna A, Lampertico P, Torchio B (1978) Hidradenoma papilliferum of the vulva – case report and review of literature. Pathologica 70:359–375

Eichenberg HE (1934) Hidradenoma vulvae. Z Geburtshilfe Gynäkol 109:358–375

Folsome CE (1940) Tumors of the vulva. JAMA 114:1499–1503

Fukuma K, Inoue S, Tamaka N et al. (1986) Eccrine adenocarcinoma of the vulva producing alpha subunit of glycoprotein hormones. Obstet Gynecol 67:193–296

Futrell JW, Krueger GR, Chretien PB et al. (1971) Multiple primary smeat gland carcinoma. Cancer 28:686–691

Gartmann H (1985) Eccrine porocarcinoma. Z Hautkr 1:555–562

Greene HJ (1936) Adenocarcinoma of supernumerary breasts of the labia majora in a case of epidermoid carcinoma of the vulva. Am J Obstet Gynecol 31:660–663

Guercio E, Cesone P, Saracino A et al. (1984) Adenocarcinoma occurring in an aberrant mammary gland located in the vulva. Minerva Ginecol 36:315–319

Guerry RL, Pratt-Thomas HR (1976) Carcinoma of supernumerary breast of vulva with bilateral mammary cancer. Cancer 38:2570–2574

Hendrix RC, Behrman SJ (1956) Andenocarcinoma arising in a supernumerary mammary gland in the vulva. Obstet Gynecol 8:238–241

Hoogerland DL, Buchler DA (1979) Inflammatory carcinoma of the vulva. Gynecol Oncol 8:240–245

Jacobs DM, Sandles LG, Leboit PE (1986) Sebaceous carcinoma arising from Bowen's disease of the vulva. Arch Dermatol 122:1191–1192

Koss LG, Ladinsky S, Brockunier A Jr (1968) Paget's disease of the vulva: report of 10 cases. Obstet Gynecol 31:513–525

Lacy GR Jr (1946) Hydradenoma and hydradenoid carcinoma of the vulva. Am J Obstet Gynecol 51:268–271

Lovelady SB, Waugh JM (1941) Adenocarcinoma of the vulva. Am J Obstet Gynecol 42:304–309

McDonald JR (1941) Apocrine sweat gland carcinoma of the vulva. Am J Clin Pathol 11:890–897

Mehregan AH, Hashimoto K, Rahbari H (1983) Eccrine adenocarcinoma: a clinicopathologic study of 35 cases. Arch Dermatol 11).104–114

Mesko JD, Gates H, McDonald TW et al. (1988) Clear cell (mesonephroid) adenocarcinoma of the vulva arising in endometriosis: a case report. Gynecol Oncol 29:385–391

Muir EG, Bell AJY, Barlow KA (1967) Multiple primary carcinoma of the colon, duodenum and larynx associated with keratoacanthomata of the face. Br J Surg 54:191–195

Novak E, Stevenson RR (1945) Sweat gland tumors of the vulva, benign (hidradenoma) and malignant (adenocarcinoma). Am J Obstet Gynecol 50:641–659

Plachta A, Speer F (1954) Apocrine gland adenocarcinoma and extramammary Paget's disease of the vulva. Cancer 7:910–9191

Rich PM, Okagaki T, Clark B et al. (1981) Adenocarcinoma of the sweat gland of the vulva: light and electron microscopic study. Cancer 47:1352–1357

Rulon DB, Helwig EB (1974) Cutaneous sebaceous neoplasms. Cancer 33:82–102

Simon KE, Dutcher JP, Runwicz CD et al. (1988) Adenocarcinoma arising in vulvar breast tissue. Cancer 62:2234–2238

Taki I, Janovski NA (1961) Paget's disease of the vulva: presentation and histochemical study of four cases. Obstet Gynecol 18:385–401

Tiltman AJ, Knutzen VK (1978) Primary adenocarcinoma of the vulva originating in misplaced cloacal tissue. Obstet Gynecol 51 [Suppl]:30–33

Torre D (1968) Multiple sebaceous tumours. Arch Dermatol 98:549–551

Warkel RL, Helwig EB (1978) Apocrine gland carcinoma and adenoma of the axilla. Arch Dermnatol 114:198–203

Webb JB, Beswick IP (1983) Eccrine hidradenocarcinoma of the vulva with Paget's disease: case report with a review of the literature. Br J Obstet Gynaecol 90:90–95

Wick MR, Goelner JR, Wolfe JT et al. (1985) Vulvar sweat gland carcinomas. Arch Pathol Lab Med 109:43–47

Yeoh G, Bannatyne P, Kosard S et al. (1987) Intestinal heterotopia: an unusual case of vulval ulceration, a case report. Br J Obstet Gynaecol 94:600–602

9 Paget's Disease

Vulval Paget's disease is an uncommon tumour which constitutes less than 5% of vulval neoplasms (Breen et al. 1978). Its approximate frequency has been estimated to be of the order of 19 Paget's disease per 1000 carcinomas of the vulva (Taylor et al. 1975).

It is considered to be a distinctive type of intra-epithelial neoplasia (Creasman et al. 1975) with a protracted clinical course. In contrast to the extra-mammary Paget's disease, vulval Paget's disease has a different natural history, survival statistics, recurrence rates and incidence of related or underlying carcinoma (Fetherston and Friedrich 1972). It has been described as a benign intra-epithelial disease which can recur locally and become invasive (Friedrich et al. 1975).

9.1 Clinical Features

The age of the patients ranges between 45 and 85 years old with an average of 65 years. The youngest patient reported was 24 years old (Stapleton 1984). The usual presenting symptoms are pruritus, irritation, tenderness and burning sensation. The average duration of symptoms is 1 year (Breen et al. 1978). A small number of patients are asymptomatic. The most common sites of the lesion are the labia (one or both may be affected; Fig. 9.1). The lesion may also involve the clitoris, urethra and an extensive area over the mons pubis, inguinal region, inner aspect of thigh and perineum. Paget's disease of the vulva is frequently multicentric. It is a demarcated, red, thickened area with some induration and excoriation, or with a fine velvety appearance. It may also be eczematoid, red and weepy lesion interspaced with white patches.

9.2 Microscopical Appearance

The epidermis is thickened and acanthotic with hyperkeratosis and parakeratosis. The characteristic appearance of the lesion is due to the presence of large cells with granular, pale or vacuolated cytoplasm and vesicular nuclei scattered in the epidermis (Fig. 9.2) and sometimes in the pilosebaceous units in which the cells tend to be at the basal locations. Taki and Janovski (1961) noticed these cells in the

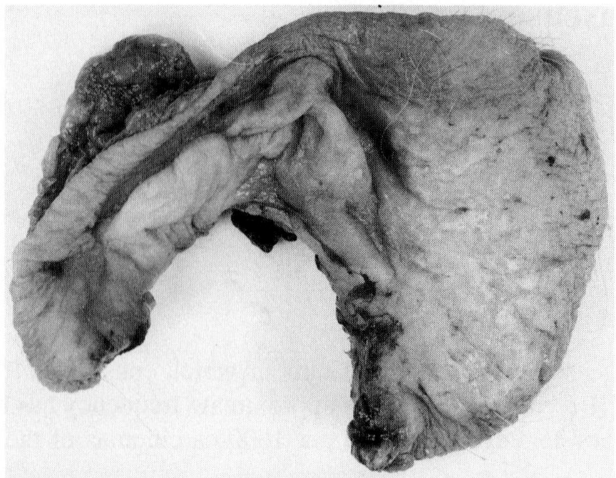

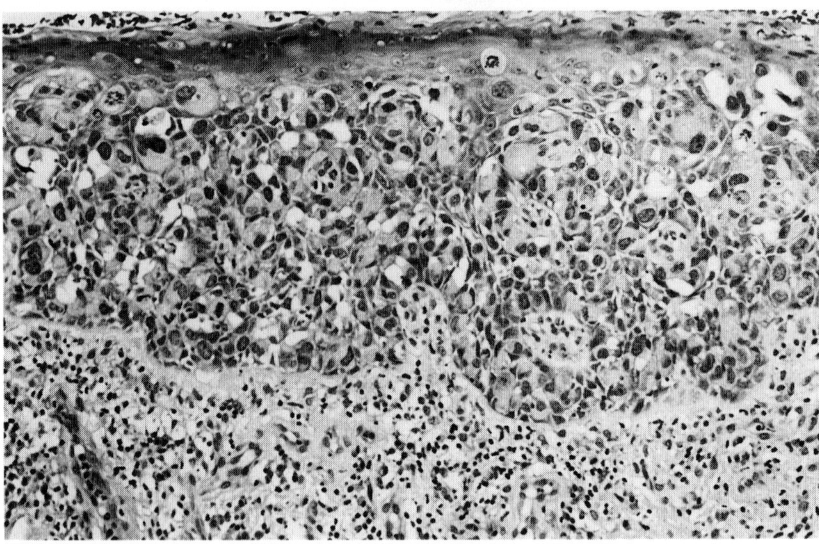

Fig. 9.1. Paget's disease: wide area of thickening on the labia

Fig. 9.2. Paget's disease: large, vacuolated cells scattered in the epidermis

acini and ducts of the apocrine glands in 46.4% and 39.1% of patients, respectively. The cells do not possess prickles (Huber et al. 1951) and are seen either singly or in groups, most often in the parabasal location and at dermo-epidermal junctions. Upward extension of these cells into the epidermis is also frequent, and the cells sometimes occupy the whole thickness including the rete pegs. A tendency to gland formation with true lumina within the epidermis by the tumour cells can occasionally be a conspicuous feature (Fig. 9.3). The large, vacuolated cells are also seen in pagetoid melanoma, but gland formation is not a common feature of the latter (Helwig and Graham 1963). The lumina may, however, be artefactual in

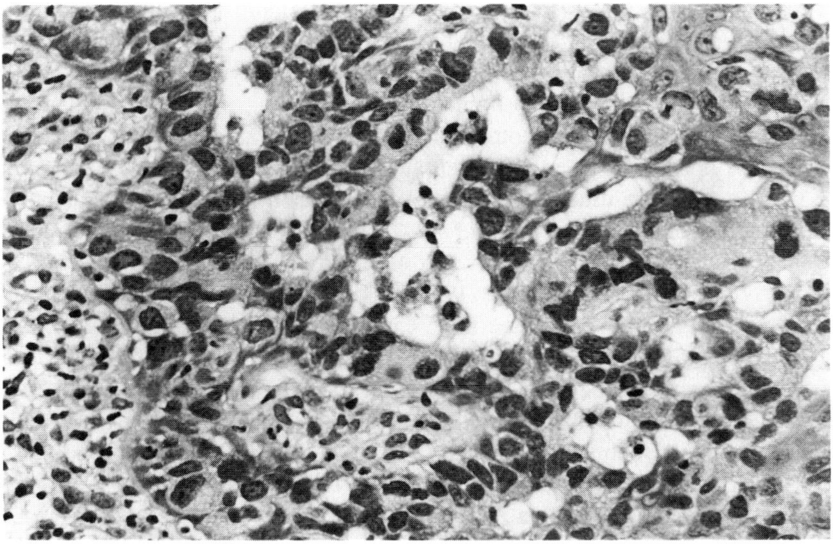

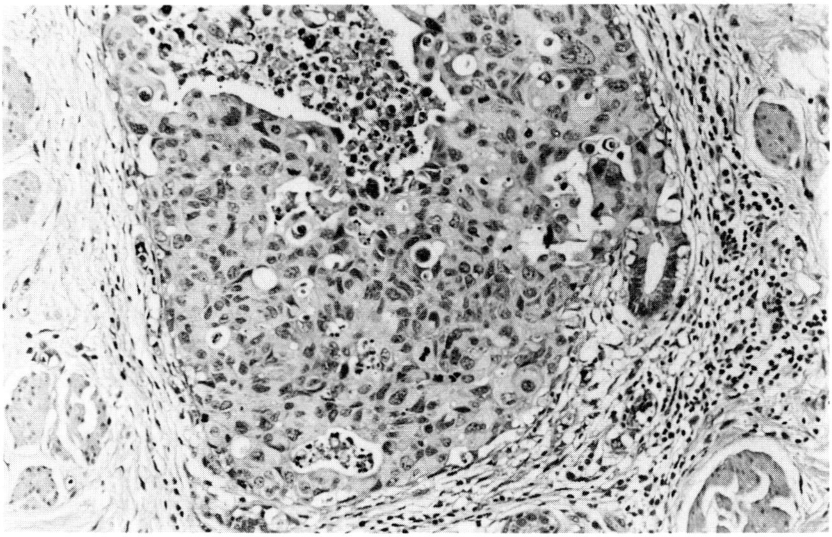

Fig. 9.3. Paget's disease: gland-type lumina within the epidermis

Fig. 9.4. Paget's disease: an adenocarcinomatous focus in the sweat gland

many cases and are not reliable indicators of Paget's disease. The cells of melanoma react positively to antibody to S-100 protein whereas Paget's cells are non-reactive (Glasgow et al. 1987). The neoplastic cells are PAS-positive, which is resistant to diastase digestions. Mitoses are sparse. Plasma cells, lymphocytes and mast cells in the dermis are always present in Paget's disease (Koss et al. 1968). Occasionally, Paget's cells contain melanin granules which may be positive for Fontana-Mason as well as DOPA-oxidase (Janovski 1962). The melanin is mainly perinuclear in distribution and can be distinguished from melanocytes by the positive reaction of Paget's cells for neutral, acid and sulphated mucopolysaccharides with PAS/D, alcian blue, mucicarmine and colloidal iron stains (Janovski 1962).

The underlying adenocarcinoma involving the sweat glands may show well-formed acini or may be poorly differentiated, consisting of a solid cluster of small cells with a scanty to moderate amount of cytoplasm and round vesicular or hyperchromatic nuclei (Fig. 9.4).

Controveries still surround the origin of Paget's cells and their relationship to the underlying adenocarcinoma. In 1958 Falkinburg et al. (1958) commented that "in about only one-half of the recorded cases has it been possible to demonstrate underlying sweat gland malignancy, although with study by serial sections, it might have been demonstrated in all". Several other reports (Weiner 1937; Dockerty and Pratt 1952; Paget et al. 1954; Plachta and Speer 1954; Helwig and Graham 1963; Koss et al. 1968; Boehm and Morris 1971; Lee et al. 1977; Webb and Beswick 1983) confirmed this association. It has been thought that Paget's cells arise in the underlying adenocarcinoma and subsequently invade the epidermis (Huber et al. 1951; Dockerty and Pratt 1952; Webb and Beswick 1983). The finding of Paget's disease in the epidermis over a metastatic deposit from breast carcinoma (Greenwood and Minkowitz 1971) and in association with sweat gland carcinoma in the knee region (de Blois et al. 1984) lends some support to the adenocarcinomatous origin of Paget's cells. In patients with Paget's disease in which an adenocarcinoma is present, assigning its origin to an eccrine (Lennox and Pearse 1954; Koss et al. 1968; Belcher 1972; Ferenczy and Richart 1972; Roth et al. 1977; Webb and Beswick 1983) or apocrine (Weiner 1937; Dockerty and Pratt 1952; Plachta and Speer 1954; Demopoulos 1971; Caputo et al. 1975; Mazoujian et al. 1984) sweat gland is difficult. Tamaki et al. (1985) have recently suggested on the basis of immunohistochemical studies that Paget's cells are of apocrine gland origin. Breen et al. (1978), in a review of 98 patients including 13 of their own, found only 25 with apocrine or eccrine gland involvement. There are still others who could not find this association (Fetherston and Friedrich 1972; Vogel and Ayers 1970; Fenn et al. 1971), and it was concluded that Paget's cells were epidermal (Eton and Parker 1958; Kaufman et al. 1960; Vogel and Ayer 1970), probably from the intermediate rather than the basal or prickle cells (Taki and Janovski 1961). Zaino (1984) reported Paget's disease in a squamous cyst lining a retroperitoneal teratoma in which apocrine or eccrine sweat glands were not present. Some authors hold the view that Paget's disease may originate from epithelial structures (Woodruff 1955) derived from the stratum germinativum and postulate that neoplastic changes may simultaneously occur in the basal cells as well as the appendages. If this is the case, one does not have to postulate a metastasis from malignancy either of the epidermis or of the underlying glands (Casper 1948; Helwig and Graham 1963; Fenn et al. 1971; Fetherston and Friedrich 1972; Breen et al. 1978).

9.3 Special Studies

Bussolati and Pich (1975) detected human casein in Paget's cells as well as in the intraductal carcinoma of the nipple and suggested the possible origin of Paget's cells in intraductal carcinoma of the nipple, sweat or sebaceous gland carcinoma in the anogenital area or from in situ modification of epidermal cells. Carcinoembryonic antigen has also been demonstrated in the in situ and invasive carcinomas of Paget's disease as well as in lymph node metastases (Nadji et al. 1982, 1984; Ordonez et al. 1987). In one immunohistochemical study of Paget's cells, reaction to the human fat globule membrane antigen was positive and to CEA was variable (Vanstapel et al. 1984); the lesion was found to be an extension from the sweat gland carcinoma. Using GCDFL-15, a marker for the apocrine gland, Mazoujian et al. (1984), on the other hand, demonstrated that the cells were of apocrine origin. It has been shown in another study (Nagle et al. 1985) that cytokeratin antigen, KA4, which is not normally present in the vulval epidermis, is found in Paget's cells and luminal cells of eccrine and apocrine ducts and glands, pointing to the phenotypical relationship among the vulval Paget's cells, breast, eccrine and apocrine epithelium. Moll and Moll (1985) noted that cytokeratins of Paget's cell were different from those of the keratinocytes and ductal cells of the skin and related to the cytokeratins of apocrine and eccrine sweat glands. It has also been shown that Paget's cells react positively for cytokeratin 54 kDa, the cells of Bowen's disease for cytokeratins 57 and 66 KD, whereas the melanoma cells do not react for any cytokeratin (Shah et al. 1987).

A metabolic study with tritiated thymidine (Woodruff and Pauerstein 1966) revealed a strikingly increased activity of the normal-appearing epithelial cells around the pagetoid groups, which themselves, on the other hand, were much less active. It was suggested that the normal-looking cells were actively involved in the neoplastic transformation. The observations and inferences from the ultrastructural studies are also not consistent. Several studies demonstrated tonofilaments and desmosomes to indicate squamous celll characteristics of Paget's cells (Fetherston and Friedrich 1972; Sagami 1963). The presence of glycogen, scarcity of organelles, formation of acini, presence of intercellular canaliculi and convoluted plasma membranes containing microvilli were suggested to indicate eccrine derivation (Koss and Brockunier 1969; Belcher 1972; Ferenczy and Richart 1972). The observations, on the other hanbd, that the cells contained electron-lucent cytoplasm with prominent Golgi apparatus, abundant rough-surfaced vesicular endoplasmic reticulum and numerous intra-cytoplasmic vacuoles could be interpreted as evidence of apocrine characteristics (Demopoulos 1971). Neilson and Woodruff (1972) also noticed secretory vesicles, mitochondria, ferritin-like granules and membrane junctional structures, which are indicative of apocrine cell differentiation. Occasional giant mitochondria, rare desmosomes between Paget's cells and keratinocytes, abundant cytoplasmic organelles, microvilli and thick bundles of filaments not connected to the plasma membrane were observed in one study and considered to be alterations of keratinocytes to Paget's cells (Medenica and Sahihi 1972). Roth et al.

(1977) thought that the cells probably originated from the secretory portion of either apocrine or eccrine type of sweat glands.

In the karyotype analysis of Paget's disease, 55% of the cells were found to contain a diploid number of chromosomes (Katayama et al. 1972), whereas another investigator noted an aneuploid constitution (Sachs 1970).

While the controversies continue, some authors tend to believe that the histogenesis and natural history of vulval Paget's disease are not uniform. It is more likely that it can arise in any of the ways postulated in various studies. Biologically, the disease appears to be two entities – one is intra-epithelial and remains as such for many years before invasion (Hart and Millman 1977) and may recur after excision, and the other is invasive with a high risk of metastases. The former is associated with long survival (Parmley et al. 1975) whereas the outlook of the latter is poor, with a fatal outcome (Boehm and Morris 1971). Separation between the intra-epithelial and invasive forms purely on the basis of histological appearances or differentiation cannot be made, although variations in the degree of differentiation can be seen in the latter form of the disease from anaplasia with small undifferentiated cells to moderate differentiation with the formation of acinar structures (Parmley et al. 1975). The invasive and metastatic lesions are often adenocarcinoma (Dockerty and Pratt 1952; Plachta and Speer 1954), but typical Paget's cells can also be seen in the metastatic deposits (Hart and Millman 1977). Jones et al. (1979) concluded that the extra-mammary Paget's disease is more than one entity.

The incidence of recurrence in vulval Paget's disease has been reported to be as high as 30%, and recurrences have been noted 3 months to 10 years after surgery or radiotherapy (Taki and Janovski 1961; Tsukada et al. 1975). The review of Breen et al. (1978) revealed an average recurrence rate of 12.4% in 98 patients. Clinically adequate resection may not often guarantee against further recurrence, which can develop even in the skin graft following radical resection (Beecham 1976). This should not be an argument against surgery, which is undoubtedly the most effective treatment available for the condition. Whether the recurrences are due to "field change" (Fetherston and Friedrich 1971) or to the intra-epidermal migration of Paget's cells (Adamsons and Reisfield 1963) in which many authors believe, is still a matter of speculation.

9.4 Prognosis

The prognosis is very good when the disease is limited to the epidermis. No death occurred in 62 patients with in situ lesions (Breen et al. 1978) whereas 10 of 26 patients with underlying apocrine gland carcinoma did not survive 5 years (Boehm and Morris 1971).

There is a high incidence of association with other carcinomas, an incidence varying from 17% to 40% of patients (Helwig and Graham 1963; Fenn et al. 1971; Taylor et al. 1975). The incidence of association is highest with breast carcinoma (Breen et al. 1978), while carcinoma of the cervix, vulva, vagina, endometrium, gall bladder, urinary bladder and basal cell carcinoma, melanoma, liver cell carcinoma and Bartholin's gland adenocarcinoma have also been found (Tchang et al. 1973; Friedrich et al. 1975; Breen et al. 1978; Degefu et al. 1986). The majority of the associated carcinomas are adenocarcinoma (Tuck and Williams 1985), but squamous cell carcinoma of the cervix (Milne et al. 1966) and transitional cell carcinoma of the urinary bladder and ureter (Fukutani et al. 1987) have also been recorded.

An altered immune status in the integument with increased susceptibility to neoplastic processes has been suggested by Friedrich et al. (1975), who noticed from in vitro blast transformation studies the depression of the T-cell response to phytohemagglutinin and concavalin A and the depression of B-cell activity with pokeweed mitogen in a patient with vulval Paget's disease associated with breast carcinoma. In vivo skin tests with mumps antigen, PPD, streptokinase and streptodornase were negative (Friedrich et al. 1975).

9.5 Treatment

The important factors considered responsible for recurrences are frequent multicentricities, diffuseness of the lesion as well as the presence of Paget's cells along the basal layer beyond the clinically apparent border and in the appendages (Parmley et al. 1975; Taylor et al. 1975). The extent of histologically demonstrable disease is in fact far wider than its clinical extent (Gunn and Gallagar 1980). Surgical excisions therefore need to include these areas with a wide healthy skin margin. Frozen sections can be used to define a tumour-free area during surgery (Stacy et al. 1986). The removed specimen is examined meticulously to exclude Paget's cells in the excision margin and underlying adenocarcinoma. When an underlying adenocarcinoma is discovered, radical vulvectomy with inguinal or inguinopelvic lymphadenectomy depending on the site of the lesion should be undertaken (Tsukada et al. 1975). The limited experiences with radiotherapy have shown variable results from poor (Koss et al. 1968; Fetherston and Friedrich 1972) to a good response (Creasman et al. 1975; Parmley et al. 1975). In some patients, local recurrences may be treated by re-excision with a wide normal skin margin, topical use of 5-fluorouracil (Fetherston and Friedrich 1972) and bleomycin (Watring et al. 1978).

References

Adamsons K Jr, Reisfield D (1963) Observations on intradermal migration of Paget's cells. Am J Obstet Gynecol 90:1274–1280

Beecham CT (1976) Paget's disease of the vulva: recurrences in skin grafts. Obstet Gynecol 47 [Suppl]:55–58

Belcher RW (1972) Extramammary Paget's disease: enzyme histochemical and electron microscopic study. Arch Pathol 94:59–64

Boehm F, Morris JM (1971) Paget's disease and apocrine gland carcinoma of the vulva. Obstet Gynecol 38:185–192
Breen JL, Smith CI, Gregori CA (1978) Extramammary Paget's disease. Clin Obstet Gynecol 21:1107–1115
Bussolati G, Pich A (1975) Mammary and extramammary Paget's disease – an immunohistochemical study. Am J Pathol 80:117–128
Caputo R, Pich A, Alfam V (1975) Immunofluorescence detection of casein in human mammary dysplastic and neoplastic tissues. Virchows Arch [A] 356:15–21
Casper WA (1948) Paget's disease of the vulva. Arch Dermatol Syphilol 57:668–678
Creasman WT, Gallager HS, Rutledge F (1975) Paget's disease of the vulva. Gynecol Oncol 3:133–148
De Blois GG, Patterson JW, Hunter SB (1984) Extramammary Paget's disease arising in knee region in association with sweat gland carcinoma. Arch Pathol Lab Med 108:713–716
Degefu S, O'Quinn AG, Dhurandar AN (1986) Paget's disease of the vulva and urogenital malignancies: a case report and review of the literature. Gynecol Oncol 25:347–354
Demopoulos RI (1971) Fine structure of the extramammary Paget's cells. Cancer 27:1202–1210
Dockerty MB, Pratt JH (1952) Extramammary Paget's disease: a report of four cases in which certain features of histogenesis were exhibited. Cancer 5:1161–1168
Eton B, Parker RA (1958) The nature of Paget's disease of the vulva: a study of two cases, one with and one without underlying carcinoma. J Obstet Gynaecol Br Empire 65:284–287
Falkinburg LW, Hoey WO, Providence RI (1958) Paget's disease of the vulva: a report of a case and review. Am J Obstet Gynecol 75:189–194
Fenn ME, Morley GW, Abell MR (1971) Paget's disease of the vulva. Obstet Gynecol 38:660–670
Ferenczy A, Richart RM (1972) Ultrastructure of perianal Paget's disease. Cancer 29:1141–1149
Fetherston WC, Friedrich EG Jr (1972) The origin and significance of vulvar Paget's disease. Obstet Gynecol 39:735–744
Friedrich EG Jr, Wilkinson EJ, Steingraeber PH et al. (1975) Paget's disease of the vulva and carcinoma of the breast. Obstet Gynecol 46:130–134
Fukutani K, Kawabe K, Niijima T et al. (1987) Transitional cell carcinoma of the urinary tract associated with vulvar Paget's disease: a report of two cases. Urol Int 42:71–73
Glasgow BJ, Al-Jitawi S, Cochran AJ (1987) Antibody too S-100 protein aids the separation of pagetoid melanoma from extramammary Paget's disease. J Cutan Pathol 14:223–226
Greenwood SM, Minkowitz S (1971) Paget's disease in metastatic breast carcinoma. Arch Dermatol 104:312–315
Gunn RA, Gallager HS (1980) Vulvar Paget's disease: a tophographic study. Cancer 46:590–594
Hart WR, Millman JB (1977) Progression of intraepithelial Paget's disease of the vulva to invasive carcinoma. Cancer 40:2333–2337
Helwig EG, Graham JH (1963) Anogenital extramammary Paget's disease: a clinicopathological study. Cancer 16:387–403
Huber CP, Gardiner SH, Michael A (1951) Paget's disease of the vulva. Am J Obstet Gynecol 62:778–792
Janovski NA (1962) DOPA-oxidase and P32 uptake in extramammary Paget's disease of the vulva. Gynecologia (Basel) 153:354–368
Jones RE Jr, Austin C, Ackerman AB (1979) Extramammary Paget's disease: a critical examination. Am J Dermatopathol 1:101–132
Katayama KP, Woodruff JD, Jones HW Jr et al. (1972) Chromosomes of condyloma acuminata, Paget's disease, in-situ carcinoma and malignant melanoma of the human vulva. Obstet Gynecol 39:346–356
Kaufman RH, Boice EH, Knight WR III (1960) Paget's disease of the vulva. Am J Obstet Gynecol 79:451–454

Koss LG, Brockunier A Jr (1969) Ultrastructural aspects of Paget's disease of the vulva. Arch Pathol 87:592–600

Koss LG, Ladinsky S, Brockunier A Jr (1968) Paget's disease of the vulva: report of 10 cases. Obstet Gynecol 31:513–525

Lee SC, Roth LM, Ehrlich C et al. (1977) Extramammary Paget's disease of the vulva. Cancer 39:2540–2549

Lennox B, Pearse AGE (1954) Histochemical characterisation of the specific cells in Paget's disease of the vulva. J Obstet Gynaecol Br Emp 61:758–761

Mazoujian G, Pinkus GS, Haagensen DE (1984) Extramammary Paget's disease – evidence for an apocrine origin: an immunoperoxidase study of gross cystic disease fluid protein-15, carcinoembryonic antigen and keratin protein. Am J Surg Pathol 8:43–50

Medenica M, Sahihi T (1972) Ultrastructural study of a case of extramammary Paget's disease of the vulva. Arch Dermatol 105:236–243

Milne JA, Mainer J, Phillips DL (1966) Carcinoma of the cervix uteri presenting as Paget's disease of the vulva with note on the pathogenesis of the latter. J Obstet Gynaecol Br Commonw 75:258–263

Moll I, Moll R (1985) Cells of extramammary Paget's disease express cytokeratins different from those of epidermal cells. Lab Invest 84:3–8

Nadji M, Morales AR, Girtanner RE et al. (1982) Paget's disease of skin: a unifying concept of histogenesis. Cancer 50:2203–2206

Nadji M, Ganjei P, Penneys NS et al. (1984) Immunochemistry of vulvar neoplasms: a brief review. Int J Gynecol Pathol 3:41–50

Nagle RB, Lucas DO, McDanial K et al. (1985) New evidence linking mammary and extramammary Paget's cells to a common phenotype. Am J Clin Pathol 83:431–438

Neilson D, Woodruff JD (1972) Electron microscopy in in-situ and invasive vulvar Paget's disease. Am J Obstet Gynecol 113:719–732

Ordonez NG, Awatt H, Mackay B (1987) Mammary and extramammary Paget's disease: an immunochemical and ultrastructural study. Cancer 59:1173–1183

Paget GE, Rowley HA, Woodcock AS (1954) Paget's disease of the vulva: report of a case. J Pathol Bacteriol 67:256–259

Parmley TH, Woodruff JD, Julian CG (1975) Invasive vulvar Paget's disease. Obstet Gynecol 46:341–346

Plachta A, Speer FD (1954) Apocrine gland adenocarcinoma and extramammary Paget's disease of the vulva. Cancer 7:910–919

Roth LM, Lee SC, Ehrlich CE (1977) Paget's disease of the vulva: a histogenetic study of five cases including ultrastructural observations and review of the literature. Am J Surg Pathol 3:193–206

Sachs H (1970) Cytophotometrische Messungen an Zellen des Morbus Paget der Mamille und der Vulva. Arch Gynäkol 209:256–261

Sagami S (1963) Electron microscopic studies in Paget's disease. Med J Osaka Univ 14:173–187

Shah KD, Tabibzadeh SS, Gerber MA (1987) Immunohistochemical distinction of Paget's disease from Bowen's disease and superficial spreading melanoma with the use of monoclonal cytokeratin antibodies. Am J Clin Pathol 88:689–695

Stacy D, Burrell MO, Franklin EW III (1986) Extramammary Paget's disease of the vulva and anus: use of transoperative frozen section margin. Am J Obstet Gynecol 155:519–523

Stapleton JJ (1984) Extramammary paget's disease of the vulva in a young black woman: a case report with histogenetic confirmation by immunostaining. J Reprod Med 29:444–446

Taki I, Janovski NA (1961) Paget's disease of the vulva: presentation and histochemical study of four cases. Obstet Gynecol 18:385–402

Tamaki K, Hino H, Ohara K et al. (1985) Lectin binding sites in Paget's disease. Br J Dermatol 113:17–24

Taylor PT, Stenwig JT, Klausen H (1975) Paget's disease of the vulva: a report of 18 cases. Gynecol Oncol 3:46–60

Tchang F, Okagaki T, Richart RM (1973) Adenocarcinoma of Bartholin's gland associated with Paget's disease of the vulvar area. Cancer 31:221–225
Tsukada Y, Lopez RG, Pickeren JW et al. (1975) Paget's disease of the vulva: a clinicopathological study of eight cases. Obstet Gynecol 45:73–78
Tuck SM, Williams A (1985) Paget's disease of the vulva complicated by bladder carcinoma: case report. Br J Obstet Gynaecol 92:416–418
Vanstapel M-J, Gatter KC, Wolf-Peeters CD et al. (1984) Immunohistochemical study of mammary and extramammary Paget's disease. Histopathology 8:1013–1023
Vogel EH, Ayers MA (1970) Primary epidermal Paget's disease of the vulva. Obstet Gynecol 36:284–286
Watring WG, Roberts JA, Lagasse LD et al. (1978) Treatment of recurrent Paget's disease of the vulva with topical bleomycin. Cancer 41:10–11
Webb JB, Beswick IP (1983) Eccrine hidradenocarcinoma of the vulva with Paget's disease: case report with a review of the literature. Br J Obstet Gynaecol 90:90–95
Weiner HA (1937) Paget's disease of the skin and its relation to carcinoma of apocrine glands. Am J Cancer 31:373–403
Woodruff JD (1955) Paget's disease of the vulva: review, report of two cases. Obstet Gynecol 5:175–186
Woodruff JD, Pauerstein CJ (1966) Differential metabolic activity in Paget's cells and associated epithelia of the vulva. Obstet Gynecol 28:663–669
Zaino RJ (1984) Paget's disease in a retroperitoneal teratoma. Hum Pathol 15:622–624

10 Naevi and Melanoma

10.1 Lentigo and Pigmented Naevi

Pigmented naevi, although not commonly noticed, are not infrequent on the vulva. It has been estimated that vulval naevi constitute about 0.1% of all cutaneous naevi (Pack and Oropeza 1967). Lentigo is a flat or macular brown lesion, frequently seen on the vulva of elderly women. It is asymptomatic and resembles freckles.

10.1.1 Microscopical Appearance

The basal layer of squamous epithelium is replaced in linear fashion by uniformly regular, normal-looking melanocytes which do not invade either the superficial epidermis or the dermis.

10.1.2 Treatment

Biopsy and excision of the lesion is probably advisable in view of the fact that malignant melanomas constitute the second most frequent malignancies of the vulva.

Melanosis of the Vulva. Vulval melanosis consists of a hyperpigmented, flat, brown patch with irregular margins. It may be mistaken clinically for a melanoma (Sison-Torre and Ackerman 1985). Microscopical appearances are unalarming, hyperpigmentation of the epidermis with an increase in the normal melanocytic cells without atypia.

10.2 Junctional Naevus

Junctional naevi are probably the most common naevi on the vulva (Allen and Spitz 1953). It is a flat, pale brown, smooth, usually hairless mole which on histological examination shows clusters of round and enlarged melanocytes at the dermo-epidermal junctions (Fig. 10.1). The cells may have abundant and occasionally vacuolated cytoplasm and contain fine granules of melanin. Atypia and mitoses in these cells are considered pre-invasive changes.

10.3 Compound Naevus

This brown, papular lesion consists microscopically of clusters of naevus cells at the dermo-epidermal junctions and free naevus cells in the underlying dermis (Fig. 10.2). It transforms infrequently to malignancy by virtue of the junctional component.

10.4 Intradermal Naevus

This is the common mole and may be flat, raised or polypoidal. Microscopically, it is composed of nests and cords of naevus cells (Fig. 10.3) without any contact with the superficial epidermis. The cells are uniform, round and oval with a thin rim of cytoplasm. The superficial cells may contain melanin which are sparse in the deeper level. The cells do not display any atypia. Occasionally a mild degree of histological atypia may occur in pregnancy (Foucar et al. 1985) and should not alarm the clinician or pathologist.

10.5 Spitz Naevus

Also known as juvenile melanoma, this histologically worrisome lesion occurs predominantly in children. It is a variant of the compound naevus and consists predominantly of spindle cells, which tend to be arranged in whorls. In some lesions, the cells are predominantly epithelioid with many bizarre giant cells. Mitotic figures may be frequent. The nesting arrangement of the naevus cells is considered to be a diagnostic clue (Allen 1963) with artefactual cleavages at the dermo-epidermal junctions. The superficial epidermis often displays pseudo-epitheliomatous hyperplasia, and the rate pegs are elongated. Stromal oedema, presence of dilated capillaries within and around the lesion and inflammatory cells are common features.

In some lesions cellular pleomorphism, many mitoses and large nests of cells may appear alarming and masquerade as nodular melanoma. An absence of abnormal mitoses, lack of significant epidermal spread and presence of mature naevus cells at the base of the lesion (Weedon and Little 1977) are helpful differentiating features. The pinkish, diastase-resistant, PAS-positive globules described by Kamino et al. (1979) in the epidermis of the Spitz naevus are also helpful diagnostic clues.

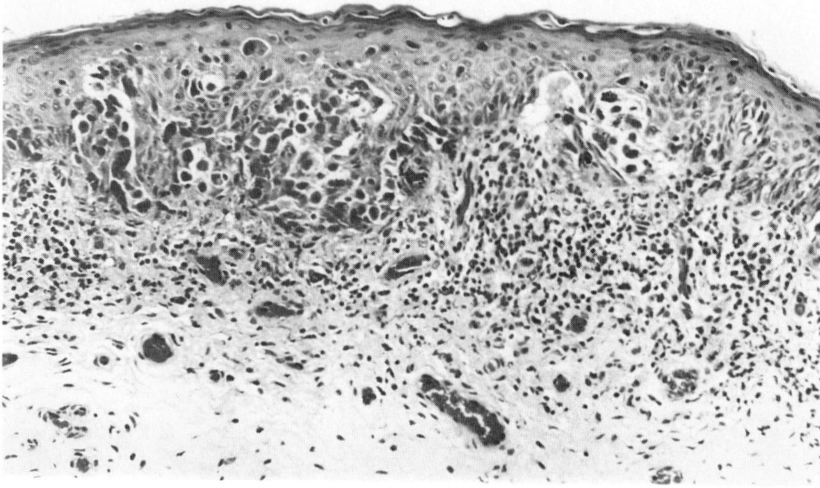

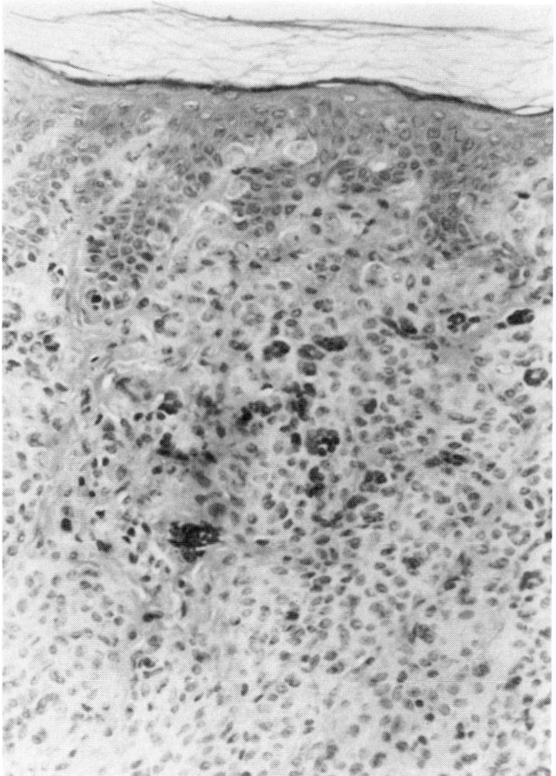

Fig. 10.1. Junctional naevus: nests of melanocytes at the dermo-epidermal junction

Fig. 10.2. Compound naevus: junctional naevus and clusters of naevus cells in the dermis

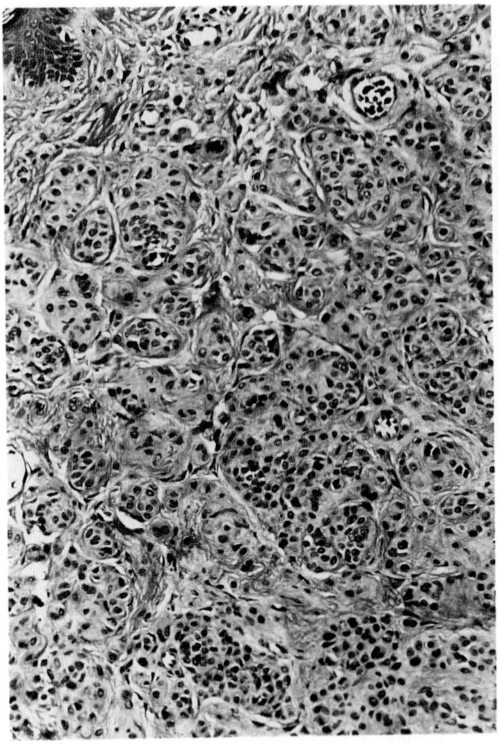

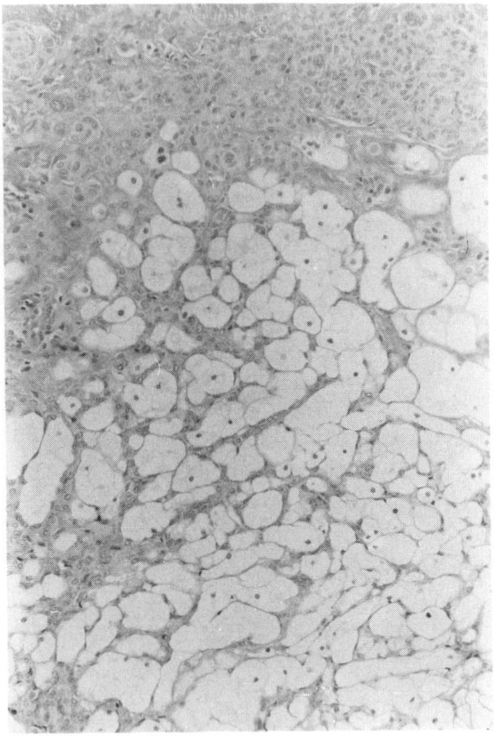

Fig. 10.3. Intradermal naevus: nests of naevus cells in the dermis

Fig. 10.4. Balloon cell naevus: large vacuolated cells containing pyknotic nuclei

10.5.1 Treatment

Excision is adequate treatment. A 9-year-old girl with a clitoral lesion was reported to be free of the disease 7 years after surgical excision (Hulagu and Erez 1973).

10.6 Balloon Cell Naevus

Balloon cell naevus is a rare variety of naevus characterised histologically by the predominance of large, vesicular clear cells. The naevus can occur in any part of the body but commonly appears in the head and neck region as a pale brown, raised nodule of average diameter 3–4 mm. It is seen very rarely on the vulval skin. Schrader and Helwig (1968) found only one case of vulval balloon cell naevus in the files of the Armed Forces Institute of Pathology.

10.6.1 Microscopical Appearance

The component cells of the balloon cell naevus are larger than the common naevus cells and contain abundant clear cytoplasm and central nuclei (Fig. 10.4). The cytoplasm is voluminous and frequently contains fine granules of melanin pigment which are usually distributed at the periphery. Multinucleate balloon cells can occasionally be seen in some lesions.

10.6.2 Treatment

All pigmented lesions of the vulva should be excised and subjected to histological examination.

10.7 White Sponge Naevus

White sponge naevus is an autosomally dominant hereditary disorder characterised by white sponge plaques affecting predominantly the oral mucosa. It can also affect the nasal, oesophageal, laryngeal and vaginal mucosa. Lesions occurring in the vulva have also been reported (Buchholz et al. 1985; Sayag et al. 1985). It is a sponge-like lesion with a well-delineated, whitish margin occurring on the mucosa of the labia minora (Buchholz et al. 1985).

Microscopically, the lesion shows irregular hyperplasia and papillomatosis of the epidermis with pronounced hydropic degeneration of the epidermal cells including the cells of the rete pegs. There is a layer of parakeratosis on the surface.

10.7.1 Treatment

The sponge naevus is benign, and Buchholz et al. (1985) recommend surgical removal of the extra-oral lesions. Improvement with penicillin treatment has also been reported (Alinovi et al. 1983).

10.8 Atypical Melanocytic Hyperplasia

Atypical melanocytic hyperplasia is a controversial term which has been used and interpreted differently by different workers. It is generally believed that during the process of development, many melanomas progress through several phases. In the initial phase there is melanocytic hyperplasia, which is characterised by an increase in the number of slightly enlarged melanocytes disposed individually along the basal layer of the epidermis. In the next phase, which is that of atypical melanocytic hyperplasia, the melanocytes not only increase in number but also become atypical and spread horizontally along the basal plate. Some melanocytes may even escend higher in the epidermis (Kerl et al. 1982). The subsequent phase is of melanoma-in-situ, which displays cytological atypia characteristic of melanoma but lacks invasion (Fig. 10.5). A vertical growth phase follows after an interval of time, and the lesion becomes invasive.

Bordell and Santa Cruz (1985) have described five phases of evolution. In phase 1, there is hyperplasia of the melanocytes but no atypia. Phase 2 is melanocytic dysplasia characterised by atypical melanocytic hyperplasia with cytological and pattern atypia as well as a stromal reaction consisting of lamellar fibrosis, vascular proliferation and lymphocytic infiltration. The next phase is melanoma-in-situ. In phase 4 the lesion becomes invasive, and in phase 5 lymph node and visceral metastases are seen. In the above two schema of evolution of melanoma, atypical melanocytic hyperplasia and dysplasia have been used synonymously.

There is also no unanimity about the lesion designated as the borderline melanomas. Atypical melanocytic hyperplasia has been included in this category by some workers while being excluded by others. It appears that the confusion will persist until a suitable definition is agreed upon by the workers in this field.

Cochran (1983) divided melanocytic proliferations into two groups – one in which the increase of melanocytes is a benign and self-limiting process, and another in which proliferation continues with increasing morphological atypia and neoplastic spread. The former group includes simple lentigo and junctional naevus, while the latter consists of dysplastic naevus, atypical melanocytic hyperplasia (superficial spreading melanoma-in-situ), lentigo maligna and acral-lentiginous melanoma-in-situ. Cochran (1983) has advocated the separation of benign lesions from those with malignant potential on the basis of cytology, disposition in the epidermis, alteration in the structure, extent and cytology of the papillary dermis beneath the melanocytic abnormalities.

It is apparent that atypical melanocytic hyperplasia is the phase of early neoplastic change. The change probably occurs more commonly de novo in the skin with ultimate evolution into a superficial spreading melanoma (Sagebiel 1979) than in association with a pre-existing benign naevus. Recognition and treatment of the lesion in this stage ensures a complete cure.

10.9 Melanoma

Melanoma is the second most common malignancy of the vulva (Phillips et al. 1982) and constitutes about 10% of all vulva cancers (Morrow and Rutledge 1972; Smith and Pollack 1947). Up to 1980, fewer than 400 cases of female genital melanomas had been reported in the world literature (Bastable et al. 1980). Although the female genitalia constitute only 1% of the total body surface, about 18% of melanomas occur in this organ, and approximately 3%–5% of malignant melanomas in women occur on the vulva (Christensen et al. 1987).

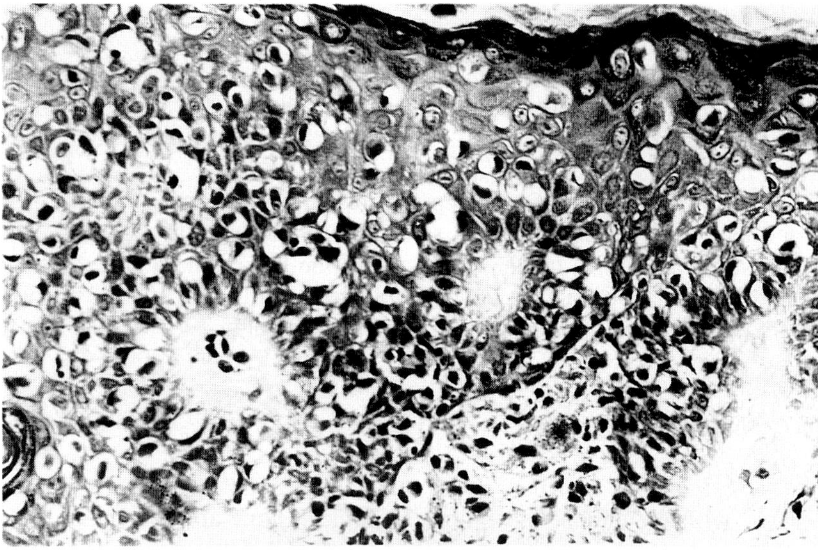

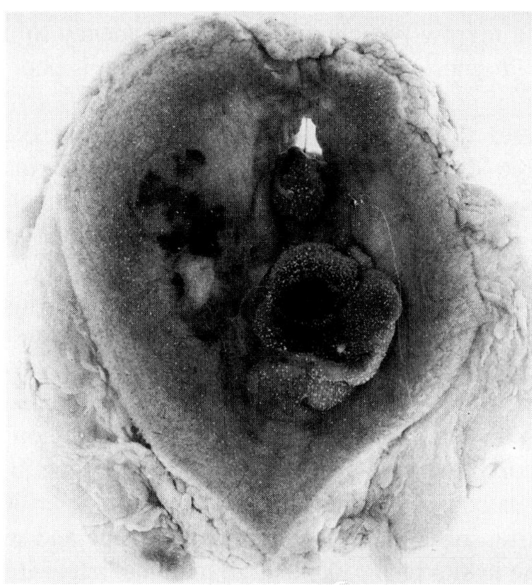

Fig. 10.5. Atypical melanocytic hyperplasia: atypical melanocytes in the epidermis

Fig. 10.6. Malignant melanoma: dark brown nodule in the labia minora

10.9.1 Clinical Features

The age of the patient ranges from 15 (Ariel 1981) to 94 years old (Karlen et al. 1975) with peak incidence occurring in the 6th decade. Some patients with female genital tract melanoma have a familial background of malignant melanoma (Gleicher et al. 1979).

The common symptoms are a lump, bleeding, pruritus and a rapidly growing mole and less common burning pain, swollen legs and lump in the groin.

Most commonly, vulval melanomas occur in the labia minora and clitoris, 81% being in the mucous portion of the vulva (Morrow and DiSaia 1976). Involvement of the adjacent areas may obscure the initial site of origin.

10.9.2 Pathological Features

The lesion is a grey, brown or black pigmented nodule 0.5–8 cm in diameter (Fig. 10.6) with or without ulceration. Multiple lesions are uncommon. An occasional tumour may become polypoidal, measuring 4–5 cm in diameter. It is generally supported on a narrow pedicle and shows a tendency to ulcerate and bleed (Byrne et al. 1963). Prognosis of these polypoid tumours is poor (McGovern et al. 1983).

Clark and associates (1969) and McGovern (1970) have classified cutaneous melanomas into three major morphological types: lentigo maligna, superficial spreading melanoma and nodular melanoma, which are distinct in their histological appearances and biological behaviour. Most melanomas are now known to evolve through a prolonged in situ phase in which they grow radially along the epidermis before they assume a vertical growth phase and invade the dermis. The lentigo maligna or Hutchison's freckle which occurs in sun-exposed areas and has a prolonged intra-epidermal growth phase is not seen in the vulva.

The superficial spreading melanoma, the most common type of vulval melanoma, begins as a small pigmented lesion which may mimic a common junctional naevus in the in situ and early invasive phases (Silvers and Halperin 1978), and as it increases in size, it becomes elevated with distinct irregularities in the margins and displays a spectrum of colours: tan, grey, black, blue and white. This type of melanoma also has an in situ phase like lentigo maligna before it becomes invasive.

10.9.2.1 Microscopical Appearance

The superficial spreading melanoma shows in its radial or in situ growth phase a large number of atypical melanocytes distributed in single cells in a pagetoid pattern and small nests within the epidermis and at the dermo-epidermal junctions. These cells are large, pale and epithelioid and possess abundant cytoplasm with fine granules of melanin and a large irregular nucleus with prominent nucleoli. The vertical growth phase of the invasive lesion is characterised by atypical large melanocytes first invading the papillary and later the reticular dermis. When two or more cell types different from the cells of the radial growth phase make up the vertical growth component, the lesion is likely to metastasise (Clark et al. 1975). Pagetoid invasion of the whole thickness of the epidermis may resemble closely Paget's disease of the vulva, from which melanoma has to be distinguished. Histochemically, the cells of Paget's disease are mucicarcmine and PAS-positive and immunohistochemically S-100-negative (Glasgow et al. 1987). In some lesions, the neoplastic melanocytes are spindle-shaped and grouped around the dermo-epidermal junctions. Mitoses may be a few or many. A dense band of inflammatory cells consisting of lymphocytes, plasma cells, mast cells, histocytes as well as melanophages is almost always seen in the dermis.

Nodular melanoma occurs as a smooth-surface, polypoid or raised nodule of 1–2 cm in average diameter, with uniform blue grey, blue black or purplish blue colour, either arising in association with a pre-existing mole or most commonly in normal skin (Mihm et al. 1975). The lesion grows rapidly and does not have an invasive phase, being invasive from early phase. Ulceration of nodular melanoma is not uncommon.

In a typical lesion, small nests of atypical melanocytes aggregate to form a large nodule filling the papillary dermis and later extending to the reticular dermis or even to the subcutaneous fat. The cells vary in size and form and may be spindle-shaped or cuboidal. Infiltrations by the inflammatory cells at the dermo-epidermal junctions may or may not be present. To differentiate the nodular melanoma from the vertical growth phase of the superficial spreading type, limit of the intra-epidermal component to three rete ridges is taken as a diagnostic criterion for the former.

Nodular melanoma arises as localised proliferations of intra-epidermal melanocytes which grow rapidly vertically to the dermis (Fig. 10.7), and as such atypical melanocytes are not seen in the epidermis adjacent to the focus of invasion. The base of the large polypoid tumour is usually seen at the interface between the papillary and reticular dermis (Clark et al. 1969).

The cells of the invasive melanomas of the vulva may vary histologically, as in cutaneous melanomas, from oval, spindle-shaped (Fig. 10.8) to extremely pleomorphic forms and are arranged in nests and diffuse sheets. Mitotic figures are usually frequent.

Chung et al. (1975) have described squamous mucosal melanoma which involves the mucous surface of labia minora and resembles histologically malignant lentigo melanoma. It spreads laterally along the basal layer of the epidermis and sometimes along the outer sheath of nearby hair follicies. The component cells are vacuolated and less frequently pigmented (Chung et al. 1975). The recently reported acral-lentiginous melanoma (De Palo et al. 1986) and malignant melanoma of the mucous membrane (Kato et al. 1987) occurring in the vulva are likely to be similar lesions. Although these lesions bear some resemblance to malignant lentigo melanoma (LMM), they are thought to differ both histologically and biologically. While LMM is an actinically induced and biologically slow growing lesion, the mucous membrane melanoma, acral and plantar lentiginous melanoma are non-actinic and more aggressive (Arrington et al. 1977). Histologically, the mucous membrane melanoma is psoriasiform in its radial growth phase, and has

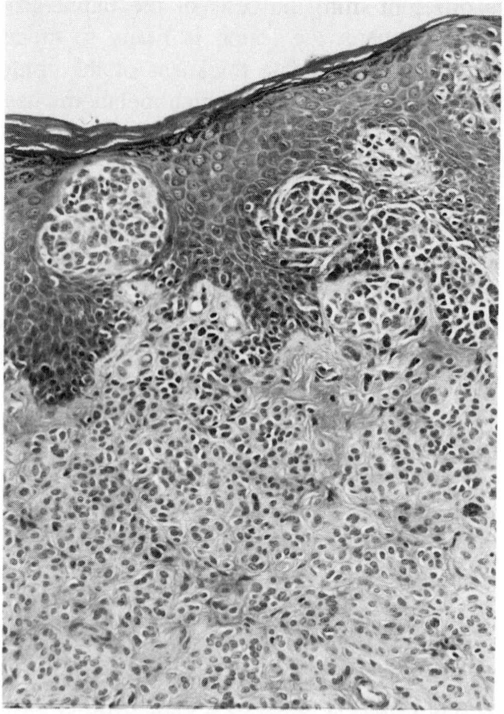

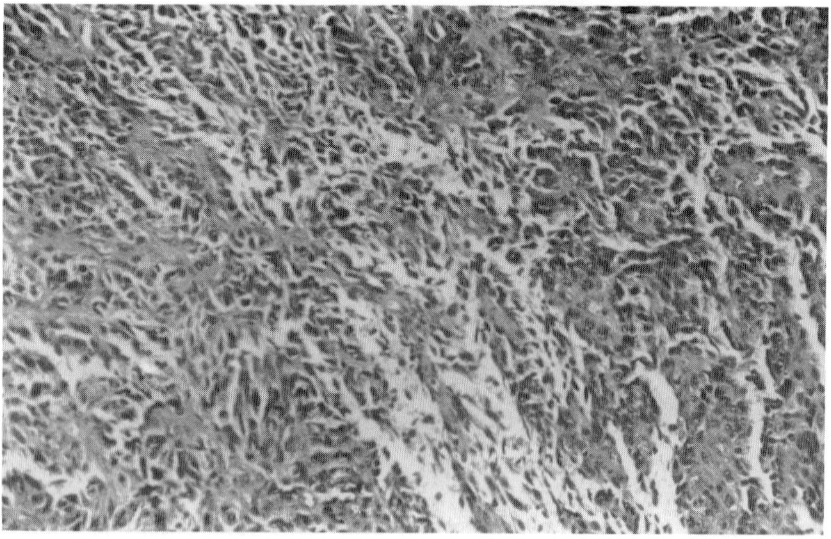

Fig. 10.7. Malignant melanoma: intra-epidermal nests and diffuse sheets of malignant melanocytes in the dermis

Fig. 10.8. Malignant melanoma: diffuse sheets of spindle cells to be differentiated from spindle cell carcinoma

a spindle cell component, prominent desmoplasia and common level 4 invasion in the vertical growth phase (Coleman et al. 1980).

Neurotropic Melanoma. A neuroma-like tumour composed of neoplastic spindle cells with hyperchromatic nuclei, prominent nucleoli and pale cytoplasm arranged in small and broad fascicles in the dermis is called neurotropic melanoma. This variant of melanoma has also been reported in the vulva (Warner et al. 1982). It shows direct contact with lentiginous melanocytic proliferations and junctional components of the superficial epidermis and invades the cutaneous nerves (neurotropic). Because of the formation of fascicles similar to desmoplastic melanoma, its neural character, neurotropism and association with the melanocytic dysplasia of superficial epidermis, neurotropic melanoma has been thought to be a variant of desmoplastic melanoma (Reed and Leonard 1979). Neurotropic melanoma tends to infiltrate diffusely with inconspicuous margins. Risk of incomplete excision and recurrences are high (Warner et al. 1982).

10.9.3 Staging

Although the FIGO classification and staging system of vulval cancer has been indicated to be adequate also for vulval melanomas (Morrow and Rutledge 1972), its correlation with the recent classification formulated by the International Body on Melanoma (McGovern et al. 1973) and other workers in this field (Clark et al. 1969; Breslow 1970) as well as with the biological behaviour of cutaneous melanoma of the vulva (Silvers and Halperin 1978) has been found to be unsatisfactory. While the FIGO staging takes into account the size and extent of the lesion and clinical assessment of the nodes, the recent classification emphasises the depth of invasion as the most important criterion for the assessment of prognosis. In a few recent reports on vulval melanomas (Jaramillo et al. 1985; Podratz et al. 1983), the assessment of prognosis by the FIGO staging system has been found to be of little value.

Clark et al. (1969) and McGovern (1970) found that the microstaging based on the measurement of depth of invasion below the basement membrane shows a strong correlation with survival rate and that there was an inverse relationship between the tumour thickness and the survival rate. These workers defined five levels according to the presence of tumour cells. In level I, the tumour cells are confined to the epidermis; in level II, tumour cells invade up to the papillary dermis; in level III, tumour cells extend up to the junction between the papillary and reticular dermis; in level IV, tumour cells extend to the reticular dermis; and in level V the tumour cells invade the sub-cutaneous tissue. According to Breslow (1970), combined tumour thickness and stage of invasion was a better indicator of prognosis than either parameter alone. Baltzer et al. (1986) found that the tumour thickness multiplied by the number of mitoses per square millimeter was also a good prognostic indicator. Clark et al. (1975) felt that level III lesions of one cell type and lesions less than 0.76 mm in thickness were unlikely to metastasise.

The mortality rate in level II lesions were 8.3%, rising through 35.2% in level III, 46.1% in level IV to 52% in level V lesions (Clark et al. 1969). This staging system, which has been found to be very significant in predicting the prognosis (Phillips et al. 1982; Podratz et al. 1983; Jaramillo et al. 1985) is considered of limited value in assessing vulval melanoma owing to the lack of well-defined papillary dermis in much of the vulval skin and its absence in the labia (Chung et al. 1975). Chung et al. (1975) used a separate staging system in which the tumour was intra-epithelial in level I, penetrated up to 1 mm into the dermis in level II, between 1 and 2 mm in level III, beyond 2 mm into the fibromuscular tissue in level IV, and into the fat in level V. These workers observed a greater mean depth (7.3 mm) of invasion by nodular melanoma than the squamous mucosal melanoma (4.1 mm) and superficial spreading melanoma (3.3 mm). While no patients with level III lesions died, mortality was 60% with levels II and IV and 80% with level V lesions. The mortality rate was 80% in nodular, 55% in squamous mucosal and 43% in superficial spreading melanomas (Chung et al. 1975).

There is a strong correlation between the level of invasion and occurrence of lymp node metastases in the cutaneous melanomas; the incidence is 4% in level II, 7% in level III, 25% in level IV and 70% in level V lesions (Wanebo et al. 1975). A report of a similar correlative study on vulval melanomas is at present not available, but nodal metastases clearly indicate a poorer outcome. In one series (Das Gupta and D'Urso 1964), 35% of the patients with vulval melanomas were noted to have positive lymph nodes when first seen.

10.9.4 Survival

The 5-year survival rate for vulva melanomas varies in different series from 25% (Karlen et al. 1975) to 50% (Morrow and Rutledge 1972), with mean survival of 35% (Chung et al. 1975). In the series of Edington and Monaghan (1980) the 5-year survival rate was only 8%. Malignant melanoma, nevertheless, is known to be unpredictable (Beller et al. 1986), and 5-year survival does not indicate a cure. Superficial spreading melanoma tends to bear a better prognosis than nodular melanoma (Itala et al. 1986), although Bailet et al. (1987) noted distal recurrence of superficial spreading melanoma which was in stage II and was removed locally with a wide margin.

10.9.5 Treatment

Before any treatment is planned, histological assessment of the type of lesion and the depth of invasion is essential. In the light of recently available information, one can only stress that recognition of the lesion in the in situ phase and its removal gives the best result. The cure rate is 100% with the level I lesion. Wide local excision with a margin 2 cm from the circumference of tumour has been advocated as definitive surgery for the lesion with a depth of less than 0.76 mm. Although on rare occasions, a lesion with less than 0.76 mm invasion was reported to recur distally after wide local excision (Bailet et al. 1987), radical vulvectomy was not found to improve survival rate over local therapy (Rose et al. 1988). With a more invasive tumour, a 5-cm tumour-free margin has been recommended (Silvers and Halperin 1978). Davidson et al. (1987) have advocated radical surgery for bulky primary disease and extensive local recurrence which cannot be controlled with more conservative excision.

The value of prophylactic node dissection has been debated for a long time. Generally, gynaecologists favour radical vulvectomy and bilateral groin node dissection as the best mode of treatment (Chung et al. 1975; Bouma et al. 1982; Karlen et al. 1975; Yackel et al. 1970; Morrow and Rutledge 1972), although the efficacy of the removal of the regional nodes in the treatment of melanomas at other locations has been questioned (Sim et al. 1978). Because melanomas are commonly located in the anterior vulva, and clitoral involvement is common, routine pelvic node dissection has been recommended (Morrow and DiSaia 1976; Symmonds et al. 1960). Although this has been claimed to improve the ulcimate outlook, some workers have doubted its efficacy (Silvers and Halperin 1978; Jaramillo et al. 1985). In advanced lesions involving the vagina, urethra and bladder, exenterative surgery has been recommended in the absence of distant metastases (Morrow and DiSaia 1976; Byrne et al. 1963). Melanomas are generally known to be radio-resistant, but in recent years, some success has been achieved with this mode of treatment (Habermatz and Fischer 1976; Kim et al. 1982; Johanson et al. 1983), either as primary or as an adjuvant in cutaneous melanomas. Because of the severe reactions of vulval skin to radiation, this method of treatment has, however, not gained much acceptance. Nevertheless, there are some indications that with various modifications, radiation can have some role in the treatment of vulval malignancies.

In disseminated disease, chemotherapy (McKelvey et al. 1977; Hill et al. 1984; Gerner et al. 1973) and interferon (Creagan et al. 1984; Retsas et al. 1983) have been used with a variable response. With effective chemotherapeutic agents, responses up to 20% have been possible (Rumke 1981). Immunotherapy for recurrent melanoma with BCG (Gutterman et al. 1973), BCG immunotherapy with regional lymphadenectomy for lesions with metastatic regional nodes (Morton et al. 1974) and immunotherapy with *Corynebacterium parvum* (Lipton et al. 1983) have also been reported to achieve some good response.

References

Naevi

Alinovi A, Benoldi D, Pezzarossa E (1983) White sponge nevus: sucessful treatment with penicillin. Acta Derm Venered (Stockh) 63:83–85

Allen AC (1983) Juvenile melanomas. Ann NY Acad Sci 100:29–46

Allen AC, Spitz S (1953) Malignant melanoma: a clinicopathologic analysis of the criteria for diagnosis and prognosis. Cancer 6:1–45

Buchholz F, Schubert C, Lehmann-Willenbrock E (1985) White sponge naevus of the vulva. Int J Gynecol Obstet 23:505–507

Christensen WN, Friedman KJ, Woodruff JD et al. (1987) Histologic charactersitics of the vulvar nevocellular nevi. J Cutan Pathol 14:87–91
Foucar E, Bentley TJ, Laube DW et al. (1985) A histopathologic evaluation of nevocellular nevi in pregnancy. Arch Dermatol 121:350–354
Hulagu C, Erez S (1973) Juvenile melanoma of clitoris. Br J Obstet Gynecol 80:89–91
Kamino H, Misheloff E, Ackerman AB et al. (1979) Eosinophilic globules in Spitz's nevi: new findings and a diagnostic sign. Am J Dermatopathol 1:319–324
Pack GT, Oropeza P (1967) A comparative study of melanoma and epidermoid cancer of the vulva: a review of 44 melanomas and 58 epidermoid carcinomas (1930–1965). Rev Surg 24:305–324
Sayag J, Jancovici E, Lacroix J (1985) White sponge naevus genital exclusif. Ann Dermatol Venereol 112:759–760
Schrader WA, Helwig EB (1967) Balloon cell nevi. Cancer 20:1502–1514
Sison-Torre EQ, Ackerman AB (1985) Melanosis of the vulva: a clinical simulator of malignant melanoma. Am J Dermatopathol 7 [Suppl]:51–60
Weedon D, Little JH (1977) Spindel and epithelioid cell nevi in children and adults: a review of 211 cases of Spitz naevus. Cancer 40:217–225

Atypical Melanocytic Hyperplasia

Bordell RT, Santa Cruz DJ (1985) Borderline and atypical melanocytic lesions. Semin Diagn Pathol 2:63–86
Cochran AJ (1983) Histology of borderline and atypical cutaneous malignant melanoma. In: Rona M, Mackie S (eds) Malignant melanoma. Karger, Basel, pp 36–64
Kerl H, Hodl S, Kresbach H et al. (1982) Diagnosis and prognosis of the early stages of cutaneous malignant melanoma. Clin Oncol 1:433–453
Sagebiel RW (1979) Histopathology of borderline and early malignant melanomas. Am J Surg Pathol 3:543–552

Melanoma

Ariel IM (1981) Malignant melanoma of the female genital system: a report of 48 patients and review of the literature. J Surg Oncol 16:371–383
Arrington JH III, Reed RJ, Ichinose H et al. (1977) Plantar lentigenous melanoma: a distinctive variant of human cutaneous malignant melanoma. Am J Surg Pathol 1:131–143
Bailet JW, Figge DC, Tamini HK (1987) Malignant melanoma of the vulva: a case report of distal recurrence in a patient with a superficially invasive primary lesion. Ostet Gynecol 70:515–517
Baltzer J, Kurzl RY, Lohe KJ et al. (1986) Melanoma of the vulva. J Reprod Med 31:825–827
Bastable JH, Gompel C, Verhest A (1980) Malignant melanoma of the vulva. Diagn Gynecol Obstet 2:55–62
Beller U, Demopoulos RI, Beckman EM (1986) Vulvovaginal melanoma. J Reprod Med 31:315–319
Bouma J, Weening JJ, Elders A (1982) Malignant melanoma of the vulva: report of 18 caes. Eur J Obstet Gynecol Reprod Biol 13:237–250
Breslow A (1970) Thickness, cross sectional areas and depths of invasion in the prognosis of cutaneous melanoma. Ann Surg 172:902–908
Byrne TK Jr, Banner EA, Pratt JH et al. (1963) Polypoid malignant melanoma of the vulva: report of 2 cases and review of the literature. Am J Obstet Gynecol 86:724–749
Chung AF, Woodruff JM, Lewis JL Jr (1975) Malignant melanoma of the vulva: a report of 44 cases. Obstet Gynecol 45:638–646
Clark WH Jr, From L, Bernerdino EA et al. (1969) The histogenesis and biological behaviour of primary human malignant melanomas of the skin. Cancer Res 29:705–727
Clark WH, Ainsworth AM, Bernerdino EA et al. (1975) The developmental biology of primary human malignant melanomas. Semin Oncol 2:83–103

Coleman WP III, Loria PR, Reed RJ et al. (1980) Acral lentigenous melanoma. Arch Dermatol 114:773–776

Creagan ET, Ahmann DL, Green SJ et al. (1984) Phase II study of recombinant leucocyte A interferon (TIFN-aA) in disseminated malignant melanoma. Cancer 54:2844–2849

Das Gupta T, D'Urso J (1964) Melanoma of female genitalia. Surg Gynecol Obstet 119:1074–1078

Davidson T, Kissin M, Westbury G (1987) Vulvo-vaginal melanoma – should surgery be abandoned? Br J Obstet Gynaecol 94:473–476

De Palo G, Clemente C, Nava M et al. (1986) Melanoma of the vulva: a clinicopathologic study of 19 new cases. J Reprod Med 31:977–978

Edington PT, Monaghan JM (1980) Malignant melanoma of the vulva and vagina. Br J Obstet Gynaecol 87:422–424

Gerner RE, Moore GE, Didolkar MS (1973) Chemotherapy of disseminated malignant melanoma with dimethyl triazenoimidazole carboxamide and dactinomycin. Cancer 32:756–760

Glasgow BJ, Al-Jitawi S, Cochran AJ (1987) Antibody to S-100 protein aids the separation of Pagetoid melanoma from extramammary paget's disease. J Cutan Pathol 14:223–226

Gleicher R, Cohen CJ, Deppe G et al. (1979) Familial malignant melanoma of the female genitalia: a case report and review. Obstet Gynecol Surv 14:1–15

Gutterman JU, Mavligit G, McBridge C et al. (1973) Active immunotherapy with BCG for recurrent malignant melanoma. Lancet I:1208–1212

Habermatz HJ, Fisher JJ (1976) Radiation therapy of malignant melanoma: experience with high individual treatment doses. Cancer 38:2258–2262

Hill GJ, Krementz ET, Hill HJ (1984) Dimethyl triazeno imidazole carboxamide and combination therapy for melanoma. Cancer 53:1299–2305

Hulagu C, Erez S (1973) Juvenile melanoma of clitoris. J Obstet Gynaecol Br Commonw 80:89–91

Itala J, Di Piola GR, Rueda NG et al. (1986) Melanoma of the vulva. The experience of Buenos Aires University. J Reprod Med 31:836–838

Jaramillo BA, Ganjei P, Averette HE et al. (1985) Malignant melanoma of the vulva. Obstet Gynecol 66:398–401

Johanson CR, Harwood AR, Cummins BJ et al. (1983) O-7-21 radiotherapy in nodular melanoma. Cancer 51:226–232

Karlen JR, Piver MS, Barlow JJ (1975) Melanoma of the vulva. Obstet Gynecol 45:181–185

Kato T, Takematsu H, Tomita Y et al. (1987) Malignant melanoma of mucous membranes: a clinicopathologic study of 13 cases in Japanese patients. Arch Dermatol 123:216–220

Kim JH, Hahn EW, Ahmed SA (1982) Combination hyperthermia and radiation therapy for malignant melanoma. Cancer 50:478–482

Lipton A, Harvey HA, Lawrence B et al. (1983) Corynebaterium parvum versus BCG adjuvant immunotherapy in human malignant melanoma. Cancer 51:57–60

McGovern VJ (1970) The classification of melanoma and its relationship with prognosis. Pathology 2:85–98

McGovern VJ, Mihm MC, Bailly C et al. (1973) The classification of malignant melanoma and its histologic reporting. Cancer 32:1446–1457

McGovern VJ, Shaw HM, Milton GW (1983) Prognostic significance of a polypoid configuration in malignant melanoma. Histopathology 7:663–672

McKelvey EM, Luce JK, Talley RW et al. (1977) Combination chemotherapy with BIS chloethyl nitrosourea (BCNU), vincristine and dimethyl triazeno imidazole carboxamide (DTIC) in disseminated malignant melanoma. Cancer 39:1–4

Mihm MC Jr, Clark WH Jr, Reed RJ (1975) The clinical diagnosis of malignant melanoma. Sem Oncol 2:105–118

Morrow CP, DiSaia PJ (1976) Malignant melanoma of the female genitalia: a clinical analysis. Obstet Gynecol Surv 31:233–271

Morrow CP, Rutledge FN (1972) Melanoma of the vulva. Obstet Gynecol 39:745–752

Morton DL, Eilber FR, Holmes EC et al. (1974) BCG immunotherapy in malignant melanoma: summary of a seven year experience. Ann Surg 180:635–643

Phillips GL, Twiggs LBH, Okagaki T (1982) Vulvar melanoma: a microstaging study. Gynecol Oncol 14:80–88

Podratz KC, Gaffey TA, Symmonds RE et al. (1983) Melanoma of the vulva: an update. Gynecol Oncol 16:153–168

Reed RJ, Leonard DD (1979) Neurotropic melanoma: a variant of desmoplastic melanoma. Am J Surg Pathol 3:301–311

Retsas S, Preistman TJ, Newton KA (1983) Evaluation of human lymphoblastoid interferon in advanced malignant melanoma. Cancer 51:273–276

Rose PG, Piver S, Tsukada Y et al. (1988) Conservative therapy for melanoma of the vulva. Am J Obstet Gynecol 159:52–55

Rumke PH (1981) Malignant melanoma. In: Pinedo HM (ed) The E.O.R.T.C. cancer chemotherapy annual, 3rd edn. Excerpta Medica, Amsterdam, pp 397–408

Silvers DN, Halperin AJ (1978) Cutaneous and vulvar melanoma: an update. Clin Obstet Gynecol 21:1117–1133

Sim FH, Taylor WF, Ivins JC et al. (1978) A prospective randomized study of the efficacy of routine elective lymphadenectomy in management of malignant melanoma: preliminary results. Cancer 41:948–956

Smith FR, Pollack RS (1947) Carcinoma of the vulva. Surg Gynecol Obstet 84:78–84

Symmonds RE, Pratt JH, Dockerty MB (1960) Melanoma of the vulva. Obstet Gynecol 15:543–553

Wanebo HJ, Woodruff J, Fortner JG (1975) Malignant melanoma of the extremities: a clinicopathologic study using levels of invasion (microstage). Cancer 35:666–676

Warner TF, Hafez GR, Buchler DR (1982) Neurotropic melanoma of the vulva. Cancer 49:999–1004

Yackel DB, Symmonds RE, Kempers RD (1970) Melanoma of the vulva. Obstet Gynecol 35:625–631

11 Mesenchymal Tumours

11.1 Benign

11.1.1 Fibroma

Fibroma is a firm, subcutaneous nodule composed of fibrous tissue (Lovelady et al. 1942). The size varies from a few millimetres to several centimetres. When it is large, it becomes pedunculated. It has a smooth surface which may be ulcerated. Cochrane (1954) reported a fibroma 20 cm in diameter arising in the right labium majus of a 36-year-old woman. These large tumours can cause discomfort, pain and a dragging sensation. Smaller lesions are asymptomatic.

11.1.1.1 Microscopical Appearance

The tumour is covered by squamous epithelium and consists of interwoven bundles of fibrous tissue which may show hyaline and myxomatous changes.

11.1.1.2 Treatment

Treatment is excision.

11.1.2 Lipoma

Lipomas are subcutaneous, slow-growing tumours of fat cells. These are either pedunculated or sessile with the size varying from 5 to 8 cm. It occurs infrequently in the vulva. Two reported vulval lipomas were congenital (Tsoutsoplides 1980; Fukamizu et al. 1982). The other two occurred in a 29-year-old and a 35-year-old woman (DeLima Filho et al. 1969; Sen Gupta 1976). The common location is the labia majora, but they can also occur in the genito-crural folds (Folsome 1940).

Microscopically, lipomas are composed of mature fat cells (Fig. 11.1) with scattered bands of vascular fibrous connective tissue. The case reported by Sen Gupta (1980) was an angiolipoma. This tumour is composed of, besides fat cells, many small-sized vascular channels. It tends to be multiple.

11.1.2.1 Treatment

The vulval lipomas are excised mainly for cosmetic reasons and when the tumours produce discomfort.

11.1.3 Neurofibroma

Neurofibroma may present as solitary or multiple lesions as a component of von Recklinghausen's disease, which is transmitted as a Mendelian dominant with variable gene expression and characterised by café-au-lait spots, multiple dermal neurofibromas, skull and facial defects, optic glioma and in small number of cases mental handicap. While café-au-lait can be seen in almost all patients with neurfibromatosis (Haroka et al. 1988), the stigma of pigmented hamartoma of the uvea (Lisch nodules) is seen in only a few of them (Ricchardi 1981). The lesion may be multisystemic, and genital affliction may be the initial manifestation in some patients (Friedrich and Wilkinson 1985). The vulva is stated to be involved in 14% of cases (Schreiber 1963), and solitary neurofibroma of the vulva may be the only stigma (Venter et al. 1981) of the condition. Solitary neurofibroma may also occur unrelated to von Recklinghausen's disease. There are more than a dozen reported cases of vulval neurofibromatosis in which clitoral involvement (Haddard and Jones 1960; Kenny et al. 1966; Labardini et al. 1968; Messina and Strauss 1976; Schepel and Tolhurst 1981; Rink and Mitchell 1983; Hanaoka et al. 1988) was noticed. These cases are often misdiagnosed as pseudohermaphroditism.

Grossly, a neurofibroma is an unencapsulated tumour of firm and rubbery consistency with grey cut surfaces. The vulval neurofibromata are seen as small, firm, rubbery and unencapsulated polypoid nodules of 2.0 cm average diameter at any location on the vulval skin. Because of their slow growth and smaller size, the lesions are asymptomatic. On rare occasions they may become as large as 25 cm (Venter et al. 1981), and involve a wide area of the vulva, in which case complete surgical removal may be difficult (Friedrich and Wilkinson 1985).

11.1.3.1 Microscopical Appearance

The tumour is made of irregularly disposed, loosely textured and haphazardly arranged nerve tissues mingled with a variable amount of collagen (Fig. 11.2). There are focal or diffuse overgrowths of the cells of nerve sheaths, particularly of Schwann cells and fibroblasts. These involve both the endoneurium and perineurium, leading to distortion of the nerve bundles. Compact bundles of spindle cells arranged in parallel and in a wavy manner with variable hyalinised stroma may occasionally dominate the picture (Fig. 11.3). In some areas, myxoid changes are prominent. The nuclear regimentations are not a usual feature of the neurofibroma. Also, the thick-walled blood vessels which are seen in a schwannoma are rarely seen in a neurofibroma.

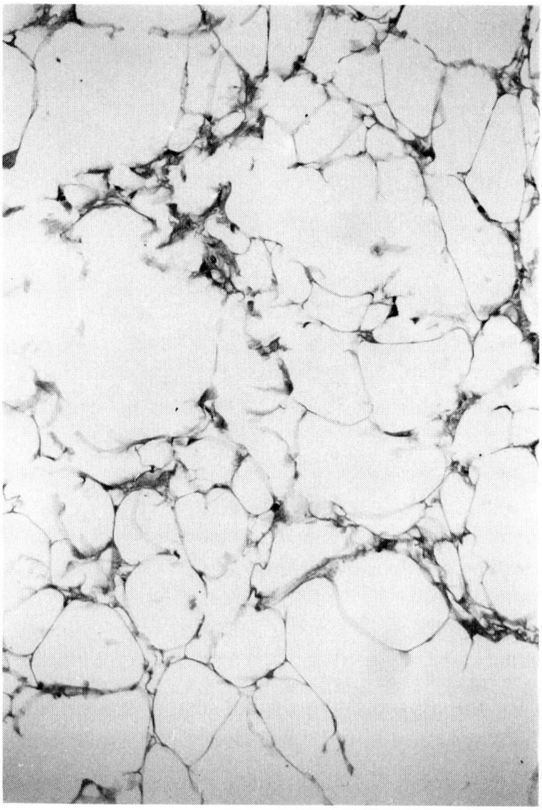

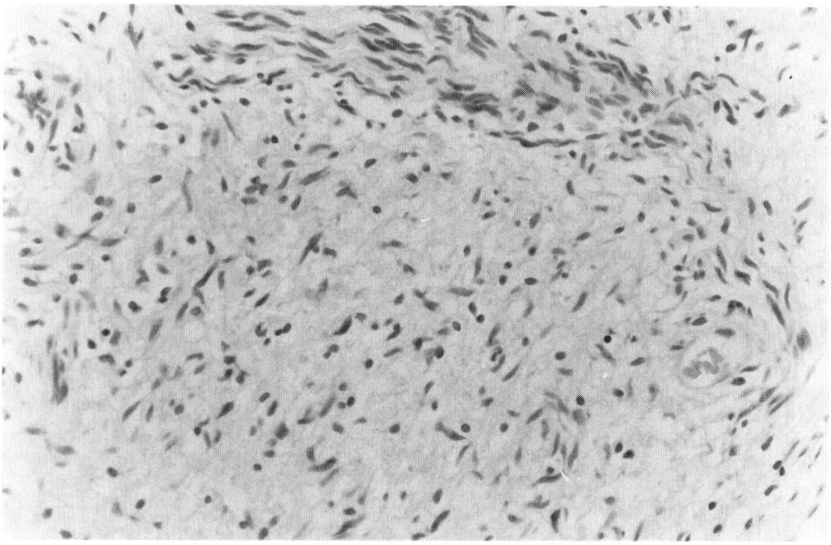

Fig. 11.1. Lipoma: composed of mature fat cells

Fig. 11.2. Neurofibroma

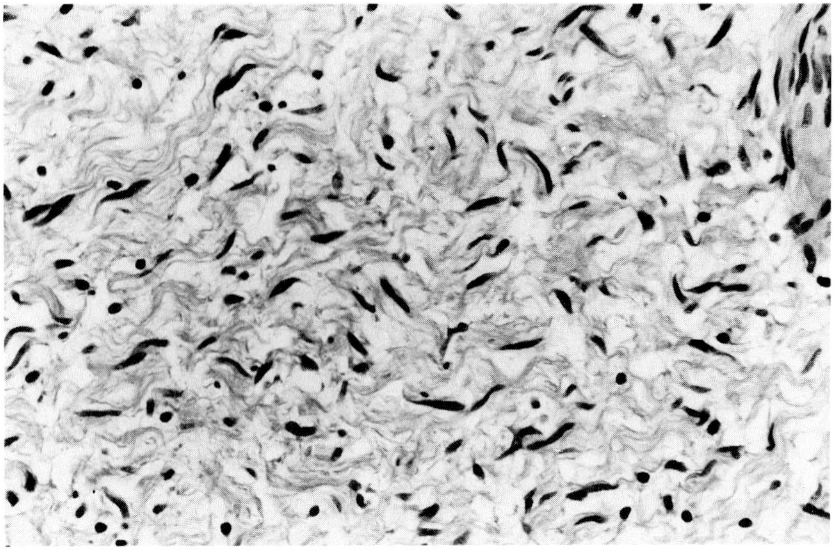

Fig. 11.3. Neurofibroma: loosely textured area

11.1.3.2 Treatment

Simple excision for the asymptomatic small lesion is adequate. With symptomatic multiple lesions, vulvectomy may be necessary (Kaufman and Gardner 1965).

11.1.4 Granular Cell Tumour (Myoblastoma)

Granular cell tumour is not an infrequent tumour of the vulva. Up to now approximately 60 patients have been reported. While the tumours are commonly found in the subcutaneous tissue of the trunk, arms, legs and face, 7% occur in the vulva (Birch and Sondag 1961; Svesko 1963). In some geographical areas, the tumour is said to be more common (Raju and Naraynsingh 1987) and tends to be multiple (Hutchins 1977) among the black population.

11.1.4.1 Clinical Features

The age of the patients with vulval lesions ranges from 6 years (Brooks 1985) to 70 years old (Coates and Hales 1973), the highest incidence occurring in the 2nd and 3rd decades. The tumour is a slow-growing, non-tender, sub-cutaneous, freely mobile and ocassionally pedunculated mass located in the labia, with a slight preponderance for the right side (Valentine and Thomas 1953; Ponnampalam 1968). The clitoris may occasionally be the primary site (Doyle and Hutchison 1968; Degefu et al. 1984; Slavin et al. 1986). The tumour may be multicentric in 2%–16% of cases (McSwain et al. 1980), and a vulval tumour may occur simultaneously

(Chiodi et al. 1957) or precede the occurrence at other locations (Gifford and Birch 1973). Of patients with multiple lesions 21% has vulval involvement (Lieb et al. 1979). The tumour is asymptomatic, but some patients may complain of itchiness and soreness in the area. Ulceration and bleeding occur rarely. Clinically, this tumour is often diagnosed as a lipoma, sebaceous cyst, fibroma or hidradenoma (Rubin 1959).

11.1.4.2 Pathological Features

The tumour is a round to oval, smooth to gently bosselated mass 0.5–5 cm in size and firm to hard in consistency. It is usually unencapsulated but may be partly capsulated by the surrounding compressed tissue. Ulceration is not a usual feature of a benign tumour (Radman and Bhagavan 1969). The cut surface, which varies from grey and grey-tan to yellowish in colour, is usually smooth and bulging. A portion of the skin is often attached to the specimen at surgical removal.

11.1.4.2.1 Microscopical Appearance

The tumour is composed of closely packed, large, polyhedral cells containing numerous, acidophilic, ill-defined granules in the cytoplasm and relatively small, centrally or eccentrically located, darkly stained, regular, round nuclei (Fig. 11.4). The tumour cells may also be spindle-shaped, containing a large number of granules (Fig. 11.5). A thin and delicate vascular stroma often surrounds the neoplastic cells, segregating them into nests of various sizes. Areas of single cells separated by thin strands of collagen fibres can be present. One unexplained feature is the pseudoepitheliomatous hyperplasia of the overlying squamous epithelium, which may be mistaken for squamous cell carcinoma (Horen and Stout 1943). Histochemically, the neoplastic cells are diastase-resistant and PAS-positive and contain esterase, acid phosphatase and lipase enzymes (Fisher and Wechsler 1962). Reticulin preparations demonstrate fine reticulin fibres around individual and nests of cells.

Immunohistochemical studies by Miettinen et al. (1984) have shown that the tumour contains vimentin, S-100 protein and neuron-specific enolase but lacks keratin, desmin, neurofilaments, glial fibrillary acid protein and lysosome. The tumour cells stained positively also for CEA (Shousha and Lyssiotis 1972).

The histogenesis of this tumour is still controversial. The original theory of myogenic origin by Abrikossoff (1926) has been replaced by different concepts based on histochemical, ultrastructural and immunochemical studies over the last 60 years. Ideas concerning origin from histiocytes (Azzopardi 1956), fibroblasts (Pearse 1950), mesenchymal cells (Moscovic and Azar 1967), a form of neurofibroma (Fust and Custer 1949), neural tissue (Ashburn and Rodger 1952) and Schwann cells (Fisher and Wechsler 1962) have been suggested from time to time. The neural theory of origin, although not conclusive, has been advocated during the past 3 decades with some degree of acceptance by pathologists. In a recent immunohistochemical investigation (Miettinen et al. 1984), this theory of origin

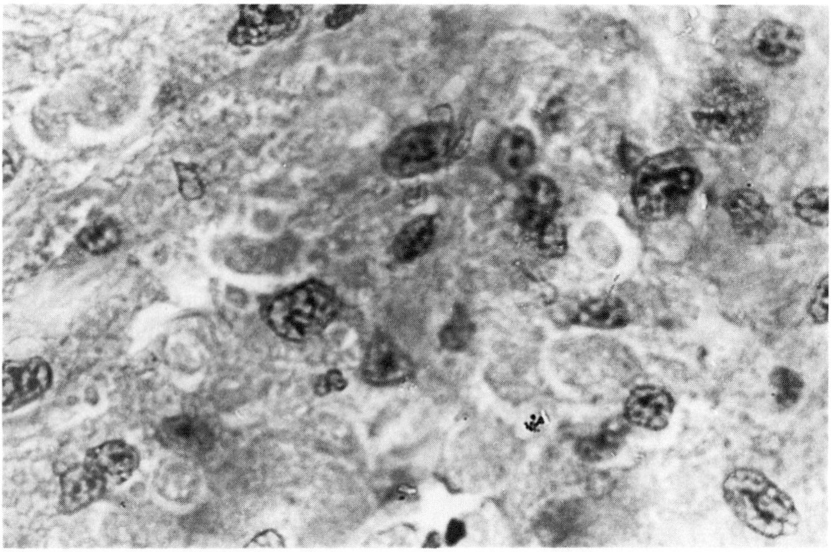

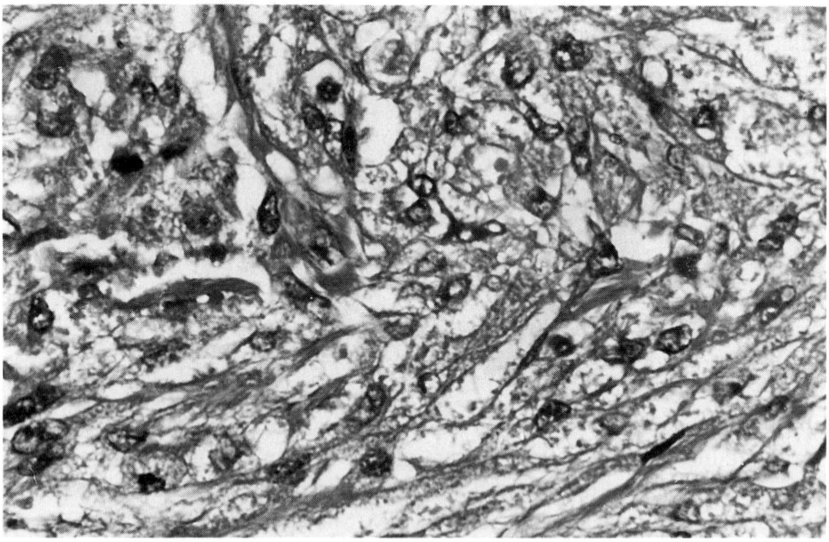

Fig. 11.4. Granular cell tumour: polyhedral cells containing granular cytoplasm

Fig. 11.5. Granular cell tumour: spindle-shaped cells with cytoplasmic granules

was questioned on the ground that the intermediate filament of the granular cell is vimentine and not the neurofilament type, and although a tumour cell like that of a schwannoma contains S-100 protein the granular cell is covered by laminin which does not cover the Schwann cells. The granular cells have been suggested to be uncommitted, nerve-related mesenchymal cells.

Ultrastructural studies (McSwain et al. 1980; Fisher and Wechsler 1962; Sobel et al. 1971; Miettinen et al. 1984; Garancis et al. 1970) reveal close approximation of cell borders with an occasional cell displaying intermediate type cell junctions. The cell cytoplasm contains abundant, membrane-bound, large and small granules, lysosomes, fewer mitochondria and rough endoplasmic reticulum and many fibres compatible with the intermediate filaments. The Golgi apparatus are inconspicuous, but some cells show prominent myelin figures. Cells with cytoplasmic granules may exhibit many lipid droplets. The nuclear membrane is often irregular and displays an invaginated contour. Basal lamina around the individual cell may occasionally be seen. Infrequently, non-myelinated nerve processes bordering a tumour cell are present.

11.1.4.3 Natural History and Treatment

The tumour grows slowly (Sadler and Dockerty 1951); sudden appearance and progressive growth of the tumour should be viewed with concern (Radman and Bhagavan 1969). Although from gross appearances the tumour appears well-circumscribed, it often shows a tendency to infiltrate the surrounding tissue. The tumour is known to recur, and a wide excision has, therefore, been recommended (Hanson and Beecham 1956; Winkelstein and Friedman 1958; Fliegner 1967; Dgani et al. 1978; Altaras et al. 1985). Surgical excision margins should be carefully examined for infiltrations. In the majority of cases, the tumour is benign and pursues a benign course, but the tumour can occasionally be malignant and metastasise. Such malignant tumours have been reported from the vulva (Sullivan et al. 1954; Robertson et al. 1981). From the histomorphology alone, it is difficult to distinguish between benign and malignant tumours (Robertson et al. 1981). Some authors advocate radical vulvectomy with bilateral inguinal and pelvic node dissection for the malignant tumours showing cellular pleomorphism (Lieb et al. 1979). Radiotherapy has not been found to be of any value (Lieb et al. 1979).

11.1.5 Neurilemmoma

Neurilemmoma is a slowly growing tumour occurring within or attached to the sheaths of peripheral nerves and is derived from the Schwann cells. In the original report, Stout (1935) stated that the genitourinary tract was, indeed, a rare site for this tumour. It is also an uncommon tumour of the vulva, and there are only about 50 tumours reported from this location. The tumour occurs usually in the labia majora (Bryan 1955) and clitoris (Migliorine and Amato 1978; Huang et al. 1983; Cheng 1966). The clitoral tumour may cause discomfort, pain and tenderness and may be mistaken as a sign of masculinisation. An increase in its size during pregnancy has occasionally been noticed. The patients are of a wide age range; the tumour has been reported in women between 17 and 71 years of age (Pece 1964). A high level of nuclear oestrogen receptors in pelvic neurofibroma and both cytoplasmic and nuclear progesterone receptors in a neurilemmoma tend to support the thesis of the hormone dependency of some of the neural tumours in women (Chetkowski et al. 1985).

11.1.5.1 Microscopical Appearance

The tumour is wrapped in a capsule of fibrous tissue of variable thickness. Two types of arrangment of the component cells have been described. In Antoni type A, the spindle cells are highly packed (Fig. 11.6) and arranged in parallel rows, interlacing bundles and whorls. A characteristic feature is the nuclear palisading – an arrangement of nuclei in parallel rows. In the Antoni type B arrangement, the tissue is oedematous, loosely textured and arranged without any pattern. Collection of oedema fluid leads to the formation of scattered microcysts. The blood vessels of the tumour often display hyaline thickening of the wall which, together with the features mentioned, serves as a diagnostic point. Mast cells are quite frequent in some tumours.

Heterologous epithelial differentiation with formation of glands may occasionally be encountered in this tumour (Fletcher et al. 1986).

The tumour is thought to arise from the Schwann cells. Ultrastructural features show predominant Schwann cell composition of the tumour (Erlandson and Woodruff 1982).

11.1.5.2 Treatment

Surgical excision is usually adequate.

11.1.6 Leiomyoma

Albeit rare, leiomyoma does occur in the vulva (Palermino 1964; Folsome 1940). The common sites of origin are the labia majora and less frequently the clitoris (Stenhever 1973). The tumour arises from the smooth muscles of the round ligament. Other possible sites of origin include the wall of blood vessels, myoepithelial cells of Bartholin's glands and erector pilorum of the skin. The tumour is usually asymptomatic but can produce a dragging sensation in the perineum if it is large in size, and bleeding and discharge if ulcerated.

Vulval leiomyoma can occasionally co-exist with leiomyoma at an other aite such as the oesophagus (Wahlen and Asted 1965) or uterus (Reed et al. 1973). Rare familial occurrence of vulval leiomyoma varies from a few millimetres to a predunculated large tumour which is firm in consistency and tends to ulcerate.

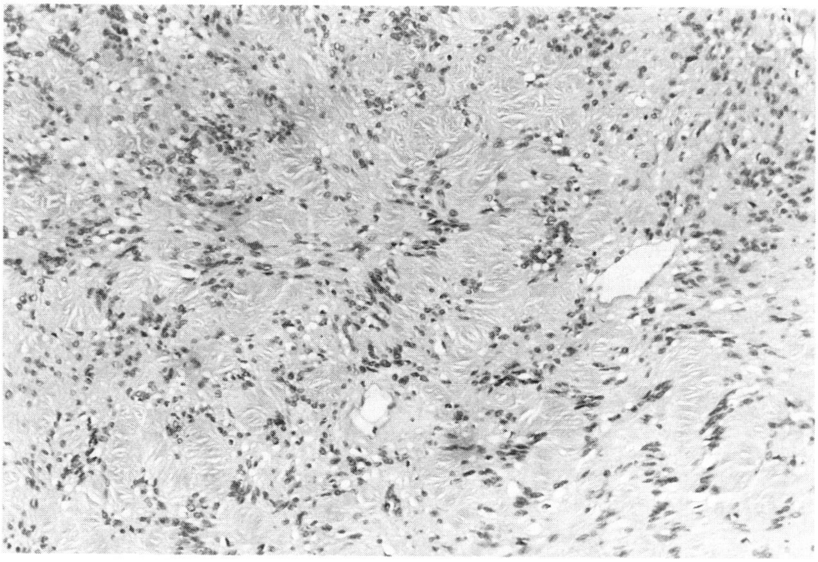

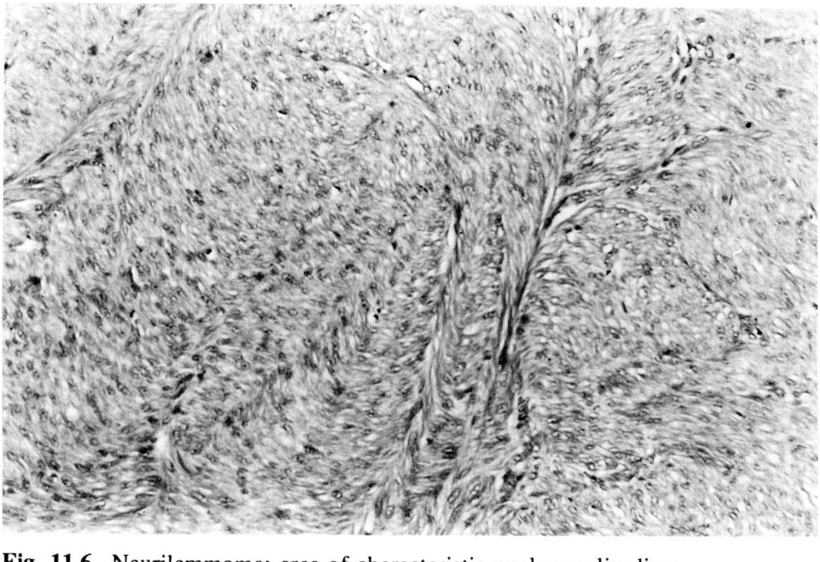

Fig. 11.6. Neurilemmoma: area of characteristic nuclear palisading

Fig. 11.7. Leimyoma: interlacing bundles of smooth muscles with a vague whorl

11.1.6.1 Microscopical Appearance

Leiomyomas are composed of elongated smooth muscle fibres containing a scanty to moderate amount of eosinophilic cytoplasm and elongated nuclei with round ends. The cells are arranged in whorled and interlacing bundles (Fig. 11.7) with a variable amount of intervening fibroblastic tissue. Mitoses are absent. In some tumours, the component cells are oval and epithelioid in shape, containing clear cytoplasm and round nuclei. This variant of the tumour labelled as epithelioid leiomyoma is common in the uterus but rare in the vulva; only one tumour has so far been reported (Aneiros et al. 1982) at this location.

The vascular leiomyomata show thick-walled vessels scattered within the tumour. Hyaline change is common. Abscess and haemorrhage can be seen in the ulcerated area.

11.1.6.2 Treatment

The treatment is excision.

11.1.7 Rhabdomyoma

The rhabdomyomas are benign tumours of the striated muscle cells known to occur at various sites (also see Vaginal rhabdomyoma). The lesions are conventionally divided into two groups – cardiac and extra-cardiac. The extra-cardiac rhabdomyomas are subgrouped into adult and fetal types, the latter occurring frequently in infants and children. The head and neck regions are common sites for the adult type and the post-auricular regions, for the fetal type (Dehner et al. 1972). The genital rhabdomyomas are more often of the fetal (Ceremsak 1969) than adult type. In the series of Di Sant'Agnese and Knowels (1980), the vulvovaginal region was the preferential site for the fetal type when occurring in adult women. In general, rhabdomyomas are uncommon tumours of the genitalia of adult women. Vulval tumours, which are less frequent than those of the vagina and cervix, occur as firm, grey-tan, circumscribed nodules of an average 2 cm in size at and around the introitus. The patients are usually in their 20s and 30s.

Microscopically, the adult type is composed of large round or polygonal cells with abundant eosinophilic cytoplasm and round to oval nuclei containing prominent nucleoli. Scattered strap and ribbon cells may be present, and some of them may show cross-striations. This variant is rich in connective tissue stroma. The fetal type can be cellular and myxoid (Di Sant'Agnese and Knowels 1980). The myxoid variant occurs commonly in the vulvovaginal region of adult women. The cellular variant is made up of bundles of immature spindle cells with very little stroma. The cells are arranged haphazardly or in regular bundles. A tendency to differentiation towards striated muscle is evidenced by the presence of occasional strap and ribbon cells. The myxoid variant is less cellular and contains abundant loose myxoid stroma. Mitoses are absent in both types.

At the ultrastructural level, rhabdomyoblasts display abundant cytoplasmic fibrils, focal electron dense material resembling Z lines, numerous mitochondria, abundant endoplasmic reticulum and scattered glycogen granules (Helliwell et al. 1988). Gold and Bossen (1976) observed cytoplasmic bodies, peripheral couplings and specialised cell to cell attachments in the adult rhabdomyomas. Immunohistochemically, the cells are positive for desmin and myoglobin.

11.1.7.1 Treatment

Rhabdomyomas recur very rarely (Anderson and Elling 1986). The treatment is surgical excision.

11.1.8 Fibrous Histiocytoma

Fibrous histiocytoma, also known as dermatofibroma and sclerosing haemangioma, occurs commonly in the skin of the limbs but can also occur at other sites, including the vulva. They are more common in women than men (Meister et al. 1978).

11.1.8.1 Gross Appearance

The tumour presents as a reddish-brown, circumscribed nodule 2–3 cm in average diameter.

11.1.8.2 Microscopical Appearance

The nodule is composed of biphasic histiocytes and fibroblasts with variable amounts of collagen and blood vessels. The fibroblastic cells and collagen may be arranged in storiform pattern (Fig. 11.8), loose-textured fascicles and occasionally in whorls. The tumour may also be composed of cells which are histiocytic in appearance and scattered in a collagenous or fibrous background. Touton type multinucleate giant cells in some tumours are a conspicuous feature. Haemosiderin and lipid are present in approximately 25% of all tumours. The tumour is not well-demarcated, and its peripheral margins blend gradually with the surrounding collagenous tissue. The superficial squamous epithelium is frequently hyperplastic, and the tumour is usually separated from it by a band of collagen.

Fibrous histiocytomas are considered to develop from the histiocytes which are facultative fibroblasts (Ozzello et al. 1963). The other cell types suggested include endothelial cells (Carstens and Schrodt 1974), undifferentiated cells (Saito and Caines 1977) and myofibroblasts (Churg and Kahn 1977).

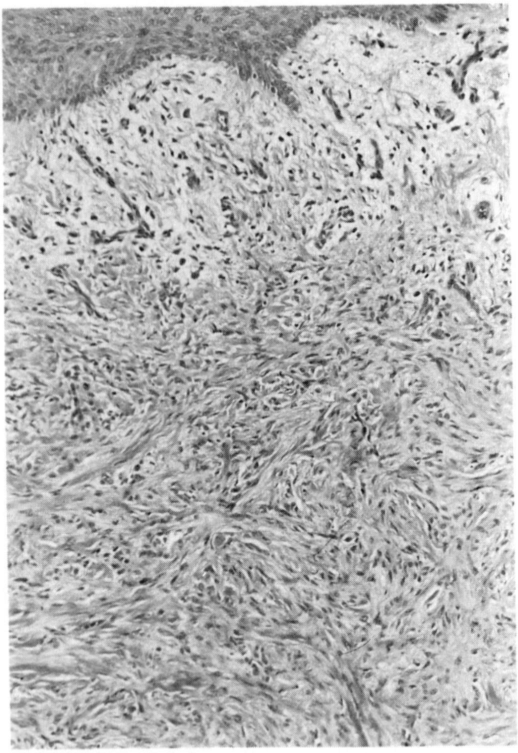

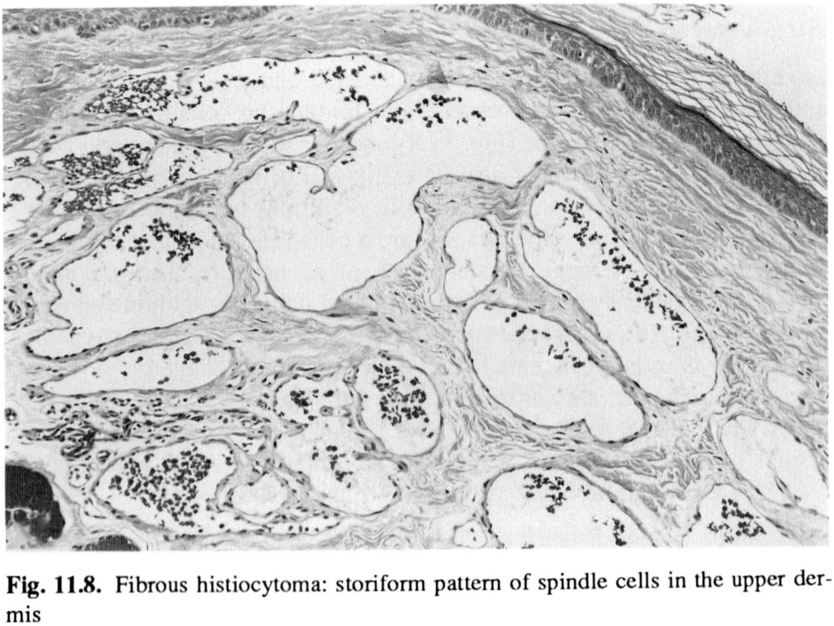

Fig. 11.8. Fibrous histiocytoma: storiform pattern of spindle cells in the upper dermis

Fig. 11.9. Haemangioma: dilated and intercommunicating veins

11.1.8.3 Treatment

Excision of the lesion is adequate.

11.1.9 Haemangioma

Haemangiomas are infrequent on the vulva. Folsome (1940) estimated that one case of haemangioma could be found per 1900 pelvic examinations. Whether haemangiomas are neoplasms or hamartomas is debatable. They are generally asymptomatic. The patient may occasionally complain of bleeding due to ulceration.

Haemangiomas are red-brown, maculopapular to lobulated, soft masses of a few millimeters to a few centimeters in size. Kaufman and Gardner (1965) classified haemanigomata into (1) port wine naevus, (2) strawberry mark (naevus vasculosus) and (3) covernous haemangioma (or angioma). The latter two types occur in the vulva. The strawberry haemanigomata are present at birth and may completely disappear over the years. Cavernous haemangioma, when large, may involve the vagina and distort the perianal region (Kaufman and Gardner 1965). The labia majora are a common site, but the clitoris may also be affected (Lovelady et al. 1941), when the lesion may be mistaken for adrenogenital syndrome (Kaufman-Friedman 1978).

11.1.9.1 Microscopical Appearance

The haemangiomata are composed of groups and clusters of capillaries and dilated intercommunicating veins located in the upper dermis (Fig. 11.9). The vascular spaces vary in size and are lined by prominent, round to oval and flattened endothelial cells. The supporting connective tissue between individual and groups of blood vessels are variable. Haemosiderin-laden macrophages can be seen in the lesions with repeated haemorrhage.

11.1.9.2 Treatment

Haemangiomata may remain static or disappear. Unless they are ulcerated, large or gradually increase in size, treatment is usually not necessary. Cryosurgery treatment using a carbon dioxide stick spaced 4–6 week apart can be used in the treatment of strawberry naevus (Kaufman and Gardner 1965).

11.1.10 Lymphangioma

Whether lymphangiomas, like haemangiomas, are true neoplasms is still debatable. Both types of lesion are known to occur in association with other malformations (Suringa and Ackerman 1970). They are solitary or multiple, ill-defined, firm or compressible nodules of average 1.5 mm in size.

Allen (Allen 1954) classified them into three groups – lymphangioma simplex, lymphangioma circumscriptum and lymphangioma cavernosum. This classification is not, however, universally accepted. Flanagan and Helwig (1977) divided them into two groups – lymphangioma circumscriptum and lymphanigoma cavernosum. The latter includes cystic hygroma. Lymphangioma circumscripta are enlarged groups of lymph vessels which are separated by scant intervening stroma and located immediately beneath the acanthotic epidermis (Fig. 11.10). Peachey et al. (1970) recognised three forms of lymphangioma circumscripta – classic, localised and spongy. The classic type occurs anywhere in the body and may be extensive. The localised form involves an area less than 1 cm, whereas the spongy form consists of more irregular lymphatic spaces in the upper dermis, with no protruberant subepidermal vesicles. The lymphangioma cavernosum is made of similar enlarged lymph vessels located deep in the subcutaneous tissue. The wall of the lymph vessels may be thick. The intervening stroma consists of compact or loose connective tissue (Flanagan and Helwig 1977), which may be compressed at the peripheral margins of the lesion.

Lymphangiomas are held to be developmental defects in which communication between the dermal lymphatic channels and the central lymphatic system failed to establish (Whimster 1976).

One should differentiate lymphangiomas, which are almost always congenital or develop soon after birth, from lymphangiectases which are acquired dilatations of lamphatic channels (Fisher and Orkin 1970). Lymphangiectases of the vulva have occasionally been noticed after pelvic exenteration (Robinowitz et al. 1977).

11.1.10.1 Clinical Features

Lymphangiomas are usually asymptomatic. They may occasionally involve the vagina and perineum, causing distortion and discomfort. Rarely, lymphangiomas have been reported to develop on the vulva as a complication of surgical treatment of cervical carcinoma (La Polla et al. 1985). Many of the post-surgical instances result from lymphatic obstruction and are more likely to be lymphangiectases rather than developmental disorders.

11.1.10.2 Microscopical Appearance

The nodules are composed of irregularly dilated lymphatic spaces lined by endothelial cells. The stroma between these spaces consists of very thin to moderately thick strands of colalgenous tissue.

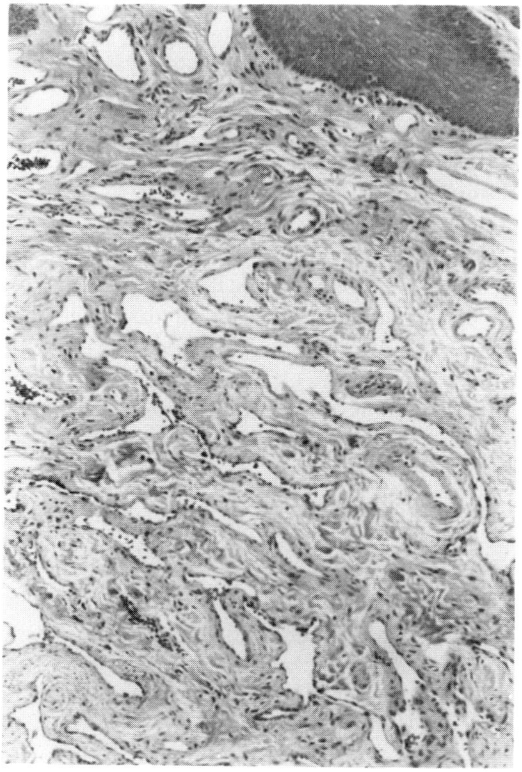

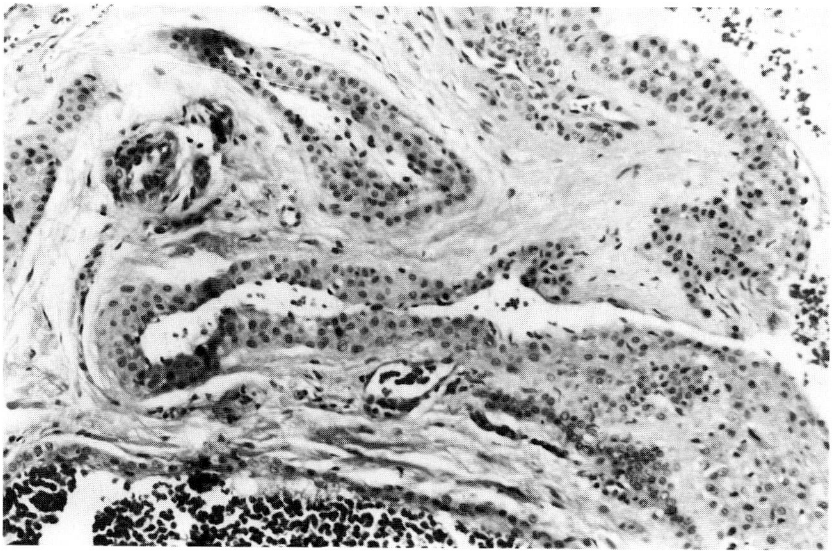

Fig. 11.10. Lymphangioma: irregular lymphatic spaces in the upper dermis

Fig. 11.11. Glomus tumour: epithelioid type cells in the wall of blood vessels

11.1.10.3 Treatment

Genital lymphangiomas rarely need any treatment unless they cause cosmetic problems.

11.1.11 Glomus Tumours

The glomus tumours which arise from the cells of arterio-venous anastomoses are most commonly seen in subungual locations. They have occasionally been found in the internal organs such as stomach, mediastinum, kidneys, vagina and uterus. Amongst them, the stomach is the site of predilection. Glomus tumours are infrequent on the vulva. Kohorn et al. (1986) found three cases previously reported in the German literature and added a case of their own. From this and other reports (Jagadha et al. 1985; Katz et al. 1986), it appears that glomus tumours are not as rare on the vulva as previously thought. The patients are adults and present for dyspareunia and intense vulval pain.

11.1.11.1 Gross Appearance

These tumours are usually small, round or ovoid nodules of an average 1.5 cm in size. They are usually single but may be multiple (Wood and Dimmick 1977). The cut surfaces are grey tan and myxoid.

11.1.11.2 Microscopical Appearance

Glomus tumours are composed of irregular vascular lumina which are lined by several layers of ovoid and round epithelioid type cells with a moderate amount of pale eosinophilic cytoplasm and central vesicular nuclei (Fig. 11.11). These cells are also present in the wall and perivascular location. Three morphological types have been described (Tsuneyoshi and Enjoji 1982): a vascular type which consists of many blood vessels and fewer glomus cells, a myxoid type in which the stroma is myxoid and a solid type in which the glomus cells are arranged in solid sheets and stroma is scant.

Ultrastructurally the glomus cells show myofilaments indicating a smooth muscle origin of the tumour.

The glomus tumours are said to arise from the cells of the glomus body, a thermoregulatory apparatus made of an afferent arteriole, a shunt Suquet-Hoyer canal and an efferent vein located in the dermis. They have, however, been noticed in locations where glomus bodies are not normally present. Many consider these lesions as developmental disorders and suggest that they occur as a result of an increase in the number of vessels accompanied by mural cells changing into proliferating glomus cells (Tsuneyoshi and Enjoji 1982).

11.1.11.3 Treatment

The lesion should be excised completely. Recurrences have been reported in lesions with margins extending into the surrounding tissue (Wood and Dimmick 1977).

11.1.12 Myxoma

Myxomas are tumours of primitive mesenchymal cells (Stout 1948). They are slow growing, unencapsulated, bulky, lobulated neoplasms which on their cut surface display a slimy and gelatinous appearance. These tumours occur commonly in the extremities but can also occur on the vulva (Borrow and Friedman 1956). In Stout's series of 148 cases of myxomas, 2 were from the labia majora (Stout 1948).

11.1.12.1 Microscopical Appearance

Myxomas consist predominantly of stellate and fusiform cells with mutliple, anastomosing, fibrillary processes in a setting of mucinous matrix. The tumour cells are bland and do not show any mitotic activities. Bands of thin collagen fibres may traverse the tumour in an irregular fashion. The tumour contains very few blood vessels, which are usually thin walled and inconspicuous. Myxomas are to be differentiated from the aggressive angiomyxomas (Steeper and Rosai 1983) which contain prominent, thick-walled blood vessels and foci of microhaemorrhages. Focal cutaneous mucinosis occurs in the vulval skin and is superficial in location.

Histogenesis of the myxoma cells is debatable. Enzinger (1965) expressed doubt about the origin of these tumours from primitive mesenchymal cells. He thought that the myxoma cells were altered mature fibroblasts that produced excess mucopolysaccharides.

11.1.12.2 Treatment

The tumour should be excised completely with tumour-free margins.

11.1.13 Ganglioneuroma

Ganglioneuromas, which consist of ganglion cells and nerve fibres, are rare, benign tumours of the sympathetic nervous system and occur mostly in the lumbar region, pelvis and adrenal medulla. Lovelady et al. (1941) mentioned an asymptomatic vulval nodule 1.5 cm in diameter in which Nissl's bodies could be demonstrated in the cells. He thought them to be ganglion cells. Ganglioneuromas of the skin are extremely rare and may represent an unusual manifestation of von Recklinghausen's neurofibromatosis or a hamartomatous neuroma (Lee et al. 1988).

References

Fibroma

Cochrane JB (1954) A case of fibroma of the vulva. J Obstet Gynaecol Br Emp 61:700–701

Lovelady SB, McDonald JR, Waugh JM (1942) Benign tumors of the vulva. Am J Obstet Gynecol 42:309–313

Lipoma

De Lima Filho OA, Cogliata AO, Reitzfeld G (1969) Lipoma of the vulva. Rev Paul Med 75:165–176

Folsome CE (1940) Benign and malignant tumors of the vulva. JAMA 114:1499–1503

Fukamizu H, Matsumato K, Inoue K et al. (1982) Large vulvar lipoma. Arch Dermatol 118:447

Sen Gupta S (1976) Angiolipoma of the labia majora. J Indian Med Assoc 66:40–41

Tsoutsoplides GC (1980) Surgical management of extensive congenital hemangiofibrolipoma. Am J Obstet Gynecol 130:260–261

Neurofibroma

Friedrich EG Jr, Wilkinson EJ (1985) Vulvar surgery for neurofibromatosis. Obstet Gynecol 65:135–138

Haddard HM, Jones HW Jr (1960) Clitoral enlargement simulating pseudohermaphroditism. Am J Dis Child 99:282–287

Haraoka M, Naito S, Kumazawa J (1988) Clitoral involvement by neurofibromatosis: a case report and review of literature. J Urol 139:95–96

Kaufman RH, Gardner HL (1965) Benign mesodermal tumors. Clin Obstet Gynecol 8:953–961

Kenny FM, Fetterman GH, Preeyasombat C (1966) Neurofibromata simulating a penis and labioscrotal gonads in a girl with von Recklinghausen's disease. Pediatrics 37:456–459

Lebardini MM, Kallet HA, Carney JC (1968) Urogenital neurofibromatosis simulating an intersex problem. J Urol 98:627–632

Messina AM, Strauss RG (1976) Pelvic neurofibromatosis. Obstet Gynecol 47 [Suppl]:63–66

Ricchardi VM (1981) Von Recklinghausen's neurofibromatosis. N Engl J Med 305:1617–1627

Rink RC, Mitchell ME (1983) Genitourinary neurofibromatosis in childhood. J Urol 130:1176–1179

Schepel JJ, Tolhurst DE (1981) Neurofibromata of clitoris and labium majus simulating a penis and testicle. Br J Plast Surg 34:221–223

Schreiber MM (1963) Vulvar von Recklinghausen's disease. Arch Dermatol 88:320–321

Venter PF, Rohm GF, Slabber CF (1981) Giant neurofibromatosis of the labia. Obstet Gynecol 57:128–130

Granular Cell Tumour

Abrikossoff A (1926) Über Myome ausgehend von der quergestreiften willkürlichen Muskulatur. Virchows Arch [A] 260:215–233

Altaras M, Jaffe R, Bernheim J et al. (1985) Granular cell myoblastoma of the vulva. Gynecol Oncol 22:352–355

Ashburn LL, Rodger RC (1952) Myoblastomas, neural origin. Am J Clin Pathol 22:440–448

Azzopardi JG (1956) Histogenesis of granular cell myoblastoma. J Pathol Bacteriol 71:85–94

Birch HW, Sondag DR (1961) Granular cell myoblastoma of the vulva: report of 4 cases. Acta Obstet Gynecol Scand 57:385–387

Brooks GG (1985) Granular cell myoblastoma of the vulva in a 6-year-old girl. Am J Obstet Gynecol 153:897–898

Chiodi NE, Siegel IA, Guerin PF et al. (1957) Granular cell myoblastoma of the vulva and lower respiratory tract. Obstet Gynecol 9:472–480
Coates JB III, Hales JS (1973) Granular cell myobalstoma of the vulva. Obstet Gynecol 41:796–799
Degefu S, Dhurandhar HN, O'Quinn AG et al. (1984) Granular cell myoblastoma of the clitoris during pregnancy. Gynecol Oncol 19:246–251
Dgani R, Czernobilsky B, Berstein R et al. (1978) Granular cell myoplastoma of the vulva. Report of 4 cases. Acta Obstet Gynecol Scand 57:385–387
Doyle WF, Hutchinson JR (1968) Granula cell myoblastoma of the clitoris. Am J Obstet Gynecol 100:589–590
Fisher ER, Wechsler H (1962) Granular cell myoblastoma: a misnomer. Cancer 15:936–954
Fliegner JRH (1967) Granular cell myoblastoma of the vulva. Aust NZ J Obstet Gynaecol 7:200–203
Fust JA, Custer RP (1949) On the histogenesis of the so called granularcell myoblastoma. Am J Clin Pathol 19:522–535
Garancis JC, Komorowski RA, Kuzma JF (1970) Granular cell myoblastoma. Cancer 25:542–550
Gifford RRM, Birch WH (1973) Granular cell myoblastoma of multicentric origin involving the vulva: a case report. Am J Obstet Gynecol 117:184–187
Hanson SH, Beecham CT (1956) Myoblastoma of the vulva. Am J Obstet Gynecol 71:190–198
Horen BC Jr, Stout AP (1943) Granular cell myoblastoma. Surg Obstet Gynecol 76:315–318
Hutchins CJ (1977) Granular cell myoblastoma of the vulva. Aust NZ J Obstet Gynaecol 17:117–119
Lieb SM, Gallousis S, Freedman H (1979) Granular cell myoblastoma of the vulva. Gynecol Oncol 8:12–20
McSwain GR, Colpitts R, Kreutner A et al. (1980) Granular cell myoblastoma. Surg Gynecol Obstet 150:703–710
Miettinen M, Lehtonen E, Lehtota H et al. (1984) Histogenesis of granular cell tumour – an immunohistochemical and ultrastructural study. J Pathol 142:221–229
Moscovic EA, Azar HA (1967) Multiple granular cell tumors (myoblastomas). Cancer 20:2032–2047
Pearse AG (1950) The histogenesis of granular cell myoblastoma (granular cell perineural fibroblastoma). J Pathol Bacteriol 62:351–362
Ponnampalam JT (1968) Granular cell myoblastoma of the vulva. J Obstet Gynaecol Br Commonw 75:976–977
Radman HM, Bhagavan BS (1969) Granular cell myoblastoma of the vulva. Obstet Gynecol 33:501–505
Raju GC, Naraynsingh V (1987) Granular cell tumour of the vulva. Aust NZ J Obstet Gynaecol 27:349–352
Robertson AJ, McIntosh W, Lamont P et al. (1981) Malignant granular cell tumour (myoblastoma) of the vulva: report of a case and review of the literature. Histopathology 5:69–79
Rubin AR (1959) Granular cell myoblastoma of the vulva. Am J Obstet Gynecol 77:292–297
Sadler WP, Dockerty MB (1953) Malignant myoblastoma vulvae. Am J Obstet Gynecol 61:1047–1055
Shousha S, Lyssiotis T (1979) Granular cell myoblastoma: positive staianing for carcinoembryonic antigen. J Clin Pathol 32:219–224
Slavin RE, Christie JD, Swedo J et al. (1986) Locally aggressive granular cell tumor causing priapism of the curs of the clitoris. Am J Surg Pathol 10:497–507
Sobel HJ, Marquet E, Avrin E et al. (1971) Granular cell myoblastoma. Am J Pathol 65:59–78
Sullivan TF, Melfetano J, Marsh MR (1954) Granular cell myoblastoma of the vulva. Am J Obstet Gynecol 67:687–690

Svesko VS (1963) Granular cell myoblastoma of the vulva. Am J Obstet Gynecol 87:143–144

Valentine FM, Thomas JR (1953) Granular cell myoblastoma of the labium majus. Am J Obstet Gynecol 65:213–216

Winkelstein LB, Friedman S (1958) Granular cell myoblastoma of the vulva. Am J Obstet Gynecol 75:325–326

Neurilemmoma

Bryan WE (1955) Neurilemmoma of the vulva. J Obstet Gynaecol Br Emp 62:949–950

Cheng WC (1966) Nerve tumour of the clitoris. J Obstet Gynaecol Br Commonw 73:1016–1017

Chetkowski R, Sakamoto H, McLusky N et al. (1985) Solitary pelvic neural tumors with high steroid content. Gynecol Oncol 20:43–52

Erlandson RA, Woodruff JM (1982) Peripheral nerve sheath tumors: electron mciroscopic study. Cancer 49:273–287

Fletcher CDM, Madziwa D, Hyderman E et al. (1986) Benign dermal Scwannoma with glandular elements – true heterology or a local 'organiser' effect? Clin Exp Dermatol 11:475–485

Huang HJ, Yamabe T, Tagawa H (1983) A solitary neurilemmoma of the clitoris. Gynecol Oncol 15:103–110

Migliorine A, Amato G (1978) Neurionoma of the clitoris. Minerva Ginecol 30:543–545

Pece G (1964) Nerve tumours of the vulva. J Obstet Gynaecol Br Commonw 71:643–645

Stout AP (1935) The peripheral manifestations of the specific nerve sheath tumor (neurilemmoma). Am J Cancer 24:751–796

Leiomyoma

Aneiros J, Beltran E, Del Moral RG et al. (1982) Epithelioid leimyoma of the vulva. Diagn Gynecol Obstet 4:351–355

Folsome CE (1940) Benign and malignant tumors of the vulva. JAMA 114:1499–1503

Palermino DA (1964) Leiomyoma of vulva. Obstet Gynecol 24:301–302

Reed WR, Walker R, Horowitz R (1973) Cutaneous leiomyomata with uterine leiomyomata. Acta Derm Venereol (Stockh) 53:409–416

Stenhever MA (1973) Leiomyoma of the clitoris. J Reprod Med 10:75–76

Wahlen T, Asted B (1965) Familial occurrence of coexisting leiomyoma of the vulva and oesophagus. Acta Obstet Gynecol Scand 44:197–203

Rhabdomyoma

Andersen CB, Elling F (1986) Adult rhabdomyoma of the oropharynx recurring three times within thirty five years. Acta Pathol Microbiol Immunol Scand [A] 94:281–284

Ceremsak AJ (1969) Benign rhabdomyoma of the vagina. Am J Clin Pathol 52:604–606

Dehner LP, Enzinger FM, Font RL (1972) Fetal rhabdomyoma: an analysis of nine cases. Cancer 30:160–166

Di Sant'Agnese PA, Knowels DM III (1980) Extracardiac rhabdomyoma: a clinicopathologic study and review of the literature. Cancer 46:780–789

Gold JH, Bossen EH (1976) Benign vaginal rhabdomyoma: alight and electron microscopic study. Cancer 37:2283–2294

Helliwell TR, Sissons MCJ, Stoney PJ (1988) Immunochemistry and electron microscopy of head and neck rhabdomyoma. J Clin Pathol 41:1058–1063

Fibrous Histiocytoma

Carstens PHB, Schrodt GR (1974) Ultrastructure of sclerosing hemangioma. Am J Pathol 77:377–382

Churg AM, Kahn LB (1977) Myofibroblasts and related cells in malignant fibrous and fibrohistiocytic tumors. Hum Pathol 8:205–218

Meister P, Konrad E, Krauss F (1978) Fibrous histiocytoma a histological and statistical analysis of 155 cases. Pathol Res Pract 162:361–379

Ozzello L, Stout AP, Murray MR (1963) Cellular characteristics of malignant histocytomas and fibrous xanthomas. Cancer 16:331–344

Saito R, Caines MJ (1977) Atypical fibrous histocytoma of the humerus: a light and electron microscopic study. Am J Clin Pathol 68:409–415

Haemangioma

Folsome CE (1940) Benign and malignant tumors of the vulva. JAMA 114:1499–1503

Kaufman RH, Gardner HL (1965) Benign mesodermal tumors. Clin Obstet Gynecol 8:953–961

Kaufman-Friedman K (1978) Haemangioma of clitoris confused with adrenogenital syndrome. Plast Reconstr Surg 62:452–454

Lovelady SB, McDonald JR, Waugh JM (1941) Benign tumors of vulva. Am J Obstet Gynecol 42:309–313

Lymphangioma

Allen AC (1954) The skin. Mosby, St Louis, p 967

Fisher I, Orkin M (1970) Aquired lymphangioma (lymphangiectasis): report of a case. Arch Pathol 101:k230–233

Flanagan BP, Helwig EB (1977) Cutaneous lymphangioma. Arch Dermatol 113:24–30

La Polla J, Foucar E, Leshin B et al. (1985) Vulvar lymphangioma circumscriptum: a rare complication of therapy of squamous cell carcinoma of the cervix. Gynecol Oncol 22:363–366

Peachey RDG, Lim CC, Whimster IW (1970) Lymphangioma of skin: a review of 65 cases. Br J Dermatol 83:519–527

Robinowitz R, Churchill BM, Alexis MY et al. (1977) Acquired vulvar lymphangiectasis in a child. Urology 10:459–460

Suringa DWR, Ackerman AB (1970) Cutaneous lymphangiomas with dyschondroplasia (Maffucci's syndrome). Arch Dermatol 101:472–747

Whimster IW (1976) Pathology of lymphangioma circumscriptum. Br J Dermatol 94:473–486

Glomus Tumour

Jagadha V, Srinivasan K, Panchacharan F (1985) Glomus tumor of clitoris. NY State J Med 85:611

Katz VL, Askin FB, Barbara B (1986) Glomus tumor of the vulva: a case report. Obstet Gynecol 63 [Suppl]:43–45

Kohorn EI, Merino MJ, Goldenhersh M (1986) Vulvar pain and dyspareunia due to glomus tumor. Obstet Gynecol 63 [Suppl]41–42

Tsuneyoshi M, Enjoji M (1982) Glomus tumor: a clinicopathologic and electron microscopic study. Cancer 50:1601–1607

Wood W, Dimmick JE (1977) Multiple infiltrating glomus tumors in children. Cancer 40:1680–1685

Myxoma

Borrow ML, Friedman S (1956) Myxoma of the vulva: report of a case. Obstet Gynecol 7:708–709

Enzinger FM (1965) Intramuscular myxoma: a review and follow up study of 34 cases. Am J Clin Pathol 43:104–113

Speeper TA, Rosai J (1983) Aggressive angiomyxoma of the female pelvis and perineum: report of nine cases of distinctive type gynecologic soft tissue neoplasm. Am J Surg Pathol 7:463–474

Stout AP (1948) Myxoma, the tumor of primitive mesenchyme. Ann Surg 127:706–709

Ganglioneuroma

Lee JY, Martinez AJ, Abell E (1988) Ganglioneuromatous tumor of the skin: a combined heterotopia of ganglion cells and hemartomatous neuroma. J Cutan Pathol 15:58–61

Lovelady SB, McDonald JR, Waugh JM (1941) Benign tumors of vulva. Am J Obstet Gynecol 42:309–313

11.2 Malignant

11.2.1 Sarcoma

11.2.11 General Consideration

In the earlier literature, classification of the soft tissue sarcomas of the vulva used to be based solely on cellular features (Bernstein 1939) rather than on a histogenetic concept. In later report, the classification was even broader (Nolan 1957), but the trend had somewhat changed and inclined more towards histogenesis. There is still, however, no uniformity in the use of terminology while reporting about vulval sarcomas. The main reason may be that they are very rare; another reason may be the unfamiliarity of the clinician and gynaecological pathologists with soft tissue sarcomas in general.

Sarcomas constitute 1.5%–3% of all malignant tumours of the vulva (Cramer et al. 1974; Davos et al. 1976; DiSaia et al. 1971; Gallup et al. 1976; Lundwall 1961). Of the various types of sarcoma, leiomyosarcomas appear to be the most common type (DiSaia et al. 1971). In the earlier literature these tumours used to be labelled as fibromyosarcomas and were considered to be the most common of all sarcomas (Priore et al. 1966). In later reports on vulval sarcomas, fibrohistiocytic sarcomas comprised the predominant group (Davos and Abell 1976).

11.2.1.2 Leiomyosarcoma

Many of the leiomyosarcomas of the vulva belong to the superficial group which arises in the subcutaneous tissue (Stout and Hill 1958). Some of the tumours are said to arise from the wall of blood vessels (Fields and Helwig 1981) and round ligaments. Leiomyosarcomas constitute about 1% of all vulval malignancies (Gompel and Silverberg 1977). They arise in the labia, posterior fourchette and area of Bartholin's glands (Davos and Abell 1976), in that order of frequency.

The patients are usually between 40 and 80 years old, with the median age about 45 years.

11.2.1.2.1 Clinical Features

The common symptoms are local discomfort, dyspareunia, slowly growing indolent tumour (DiSaia et al. 1971) or a rapidly growing painful mass and pruritus. Duration of symptoms varies generally from a few months to 1 year.

11.2.1.2.2 Gross Appearance

The leiomyosarcomas are firm, well-circumscribed, nodular or lobulated tumours with a greatest diameter ranging from 2 to 10 cm. The poorly delineated tumours are likely to be infiltrative (Tavassoli and Norris 1979). The cut surfaces of well-differentiated tumours are greyish-white in colour and display the irregular, whorled appearance of benign leimyomas. The poorly differentiated tumours may be soft and fleshy due to haemorrhage and necrosis. Some tumours may have shiny and myxoid areas.

11.2.1.2.3 Microscopical Appearance

The tumour consists of interlacing bundles of elongated cells with eosinophilic cytoplasm, hyperchromatic, blunt-ended nuclei forming whorls and interdigitating fascicles (Figs. 11.12, 11.13). Longitudinal striations can be demonstrated in the cytoplasm of well-differentiated tumours. In a moderately differentiated tumour, the atypical and hyperchromatic nuclei tend to be lobulated. Cellular pleomorphism is marked in the poorly differentiated tumours, with increased mitoses and diminished cytoplasmic striations. Mitotic figures are always present in the leiomyosarcomas and vary from one to several per 10 high power fields. Some tumours are very vascular and display focal and diffuse areas of haemorrhage. Areas of necrosis and haemorrhage are more pronounced in a poorly differentiated tumour. Myxoid changes can be seen in some tumours.

Immunohistochemically, the tumour cells are positive for vimentin, desmin and muscle-specific actin (Denk et al. 1983; Swanson et al. 1988), and about 50% of the tumours express epithelial membrane antigen and cytokeratin (Miettinen 1988).

Ultrastructurally, the cells show cytoplasmic filaments with focal condensation, marginal plaques and focal production of basal lamina (Knapp et al. 1984; Hashimoto et al. 1986).

11.2.1.2.4 Treatment

Radical vulvectomy with bilateral inguinal lymphadenectomy should be the initial treatment. Although leiomyosarcomas of the vulva are slow growing, these tumours have a tendency to recur and metastasise. According to Tavassoli and Norris (1979), neoplasms that are larger than 5 cm with infiltrating margins and 5 or more mitotic figures per 10 high power fields are likely to recur unless controlled by total excision. However, the biological behaviour of these tumours may be quite unpredictable (Varela-Duran et al. 1979), and a tumour appearing benign may recur and metastasise, assuming aggressive behaviour. The risk of haematogenous dissemination is, indeed, higher subsequent to recurrences (Audet-Laponte et al.

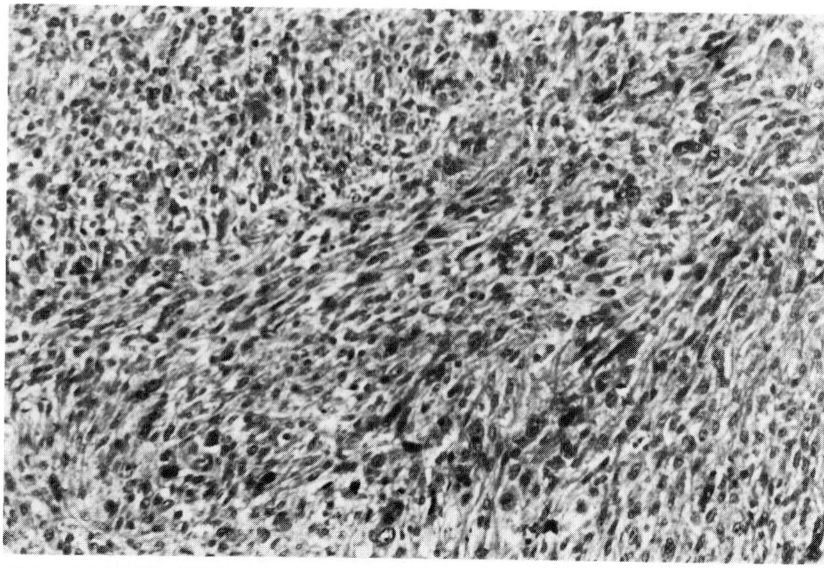

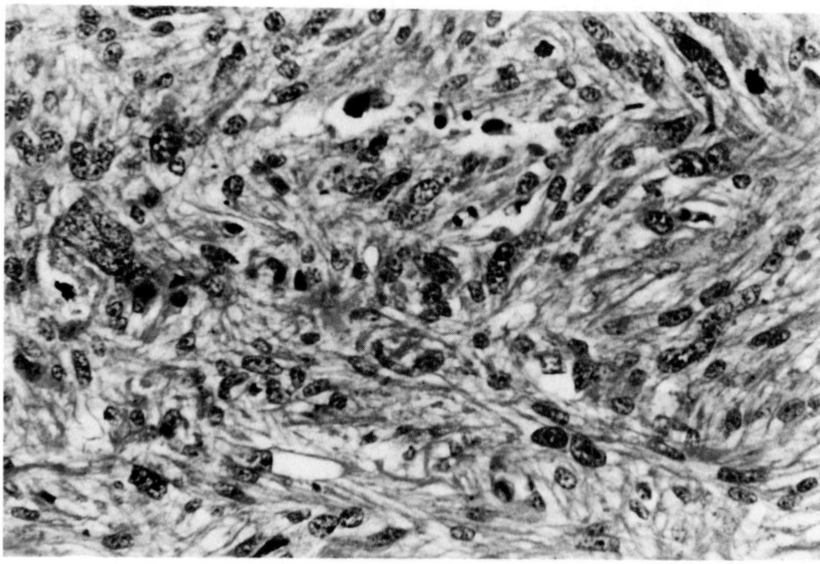

Fig. 11.12. Leiomyosarcoma: bundles of pleomorphic, elongated smooth muscle cells with hyperchromatic nuclei

Fig. 11.13. Leiomyosarcoma: high power view

1980). It is generally held that the subcutaneous leiomyosarcomas tend to recur and metastasise (Dahl and Angervall 1974; Swanson et al. 1988). According to Davos and Abell (1976), leiomyosarcomas of the vulva have the least favourable prognosis. Extensive or radical surgery soon after diagnosis and more superficially located tumours tend to offer a favourable outlook.

11.2.1.3 Malignant Fibrous Histiocytoma

Malignant fibrous histiocytomas, which have been labelled variously as myxofibrosarcomas, malignant fibrous xanthomas (O'Brien and Stout 1964) and fibroxanthosarcomas (Merkow et al. 1971; Kempson and Kyriakos 1972), are the second most common sarcomas of the vulva (Davos and Abell 1976). They occur commonly in the lower extremities, followed by the upper extremities and retroperitoneum (Weiss and Enzinger 1978). While the majority of these tumours are situated within the skeletal muscles, others occur superficially in the subcutis. The female genital tract is an uncommon site (Hensley and Friedrich 1973; Davos and Abell 1976; Taylor et al. 1985; Santala et al. 1987). Histogenetically, malignant fibrous histiocytomas are believed to arise from undifferentiated mesenchymal cells. The aetiology of this tumour is unknown. A few of these tumours have been noted to develop at a site of radiation (Halpern et al. 1984), metal implant (Lee et al. 1984) or previous surgical sites (Inoshita and Youngberg 1984) or produced by experimental injection of methyl-benzathracene (Sakamoto 1986).

11.2.1.3.1 Clinical Features

The patients are generally elderly, in their 60s and 70s. These tumours are uncommon in individuals below 40 years old. The age of the patients with vulval lesions ranges between 30 and 80 years. The presenting symptoms are pailful vulval nodule, ulcerated mass, gradually enlarging tumour, soreness, itchiness and haemorrhage. The common location is the labia majora, but others such as labia minora, clitoris, posterior fourchette and deep vulval tissue adjacent to the Bartholin's gland can also be involved (Santala et al. 1987).

11.2.1.3.2 Gross Appearance

Malignant fibrous histiocytoma is an unencapsulated, firm, nodular mass with a distinctly yellowish-grey appearance on the cut surface. Marked myxoid changes, necrosis and haemorrhages may be noticed in some tumours. The vulval tumour is generally a circumscribed nodule or an ulcer of 1–6 cm in diameter.

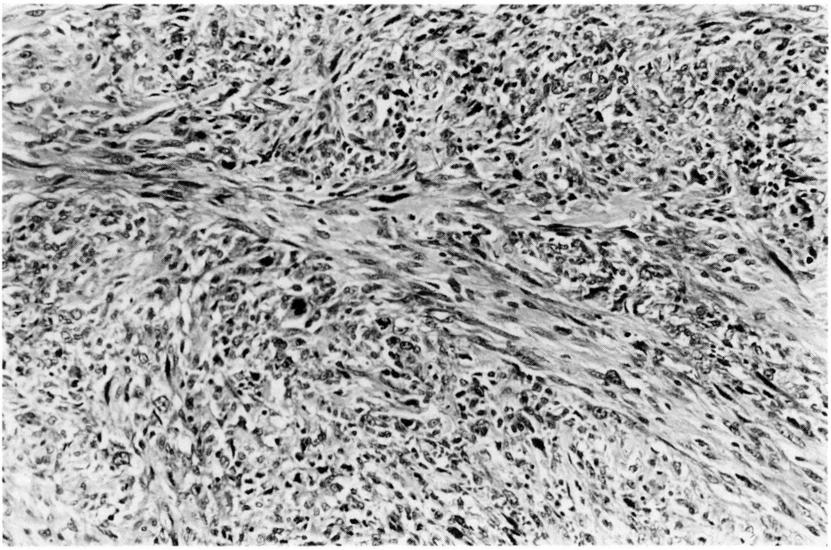

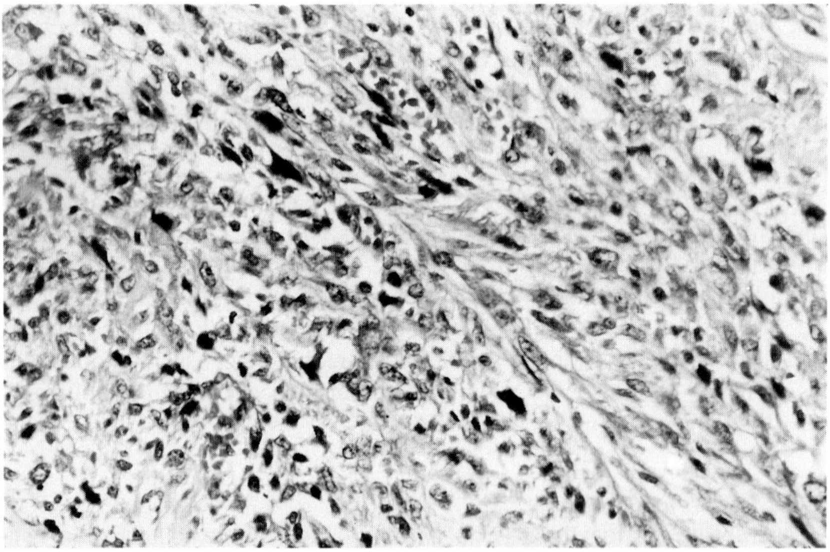

Fig. 11.14. Malignant fibrous histiocytoma: bundles of pleomorphic spindel cells

Fig. 11.15. Malignant fibrous histiocytoma: high power view

11.2.1.3.3 Microscopical Appearance

There are three cell types, spindle cells, round or oval cells and benign and malignant giant cells (Bertoni et al. 1985), that make up the tumours. Several morphological variants of malignant fibrous histiocytomas have been recognised, namely, storiform-pleomorphic, myxoid, giant cell, inflammatory and angiomatoid (Enzinger and Weiss 1983). The most common is the storiform-pleomorphic variant, which displays a characteristic storiform pattern of spindle cells admixed with pleomorphic histiocytes and multinucleate giant cells (Figs. 11.14, 11.15). Mitoses are fequent. The myxoid variant is composed predominantly of myxoid stroma rich in acid mucopolysaccharides and areas of spindle cells and giant cells arranged loosely in a storiform pattern. The giant cell type consists of a mixture of both benign and malignant giant cells. Many of the giant cells are similar to the osteoclasts and associated with mononuclear stromal cells. There are also areas of a storiform-pleomorphic arrangement of the spindle cells. The inflammatory variant displays pronounced inflammatory cell infiltrates consisting of neutrophils, plasma cells and lymphocytes. Occasionally, collections of foam cells in the tumour make it focally xanthomatous (Kearney et al. 1980). The angiomatoid variant shows cyst-like spaces filled with blood, solid areas of fibrohistiocytic tumour cells, haemosiderin pigments and inflammatory cells. The vulval tumours reported appear to be of pleomorphic-storiform and myxoid variants. None of the reports, however, clearly delineate the histological types.

Ultrastructural studies by Fu et al. (1975) demonstrated five cell types – fibroblast-like, histiocyte-like, immature cells resembling stem cells, xanthomatous and multinucleate giant cells. They concluded that the tumours were of stem cell rather than histiocytic origin. Hoffman and Dickersin (1983) did not observe any malignant histiocytes in their series. They thought that these tumours were derived from fibroblasts and myofibroblasts.

Immunohistochemical studies (Kindblom et al. 1982) suggest dual fibroblastic and histiocyte origin. The cells react positively for ferritin, Al-antitrypsin and lysozymes, which are markers for histiocytes, as well as for vimentin, a marker for mesenchymal cells. Other studies also have confirmed a positive reaction for vimentin (Lawson et al. 1987).

11.2.1.3.4 Prognosis

Prognosis has been correlated with the histological type, tumour size, location and depth. Angiomatoid fibrous histiocytomas generally bear a better prognosis than other types (Santa-Cruz et al. 1981), whereas the inflammatory type is aggressive (Kyriakos and Kempson 1976). Large, deep seated, thigh tumours are often histologically highly malignant (Bertoni et al. 1985; Rydholm and Syk 1986). According to Kearney et al. (1980), the location rather than the histological subtypes was more important. The patients with superficial tumours have a better prognosis than with deep tumours; patients with distally located tumours fare better than with proximal ones (Kearney et al. 1980).

11.2.1.3.5 Treatment

Malignant fibrous histiocytomas metastasise by haematogenous and lymphatic routes and have a high local recurrence rate (Weiss and Enzinger 1978) which varies from 20% to 50% (Markhede et al. 1982). Haematogenous spread occurs mainly to the lungs. About 17% of the lesions spread to the regional lymph nodes (Kearney et al. 1980). Similar risks exist also with the vulval tumours (Hensley and Friedrich 1973). Although radical vulvectomy has been recommended for treating vulval sarcomas (DiSaia et al. 1971), wide local excision has been found effective for vulval malignant fibrous histiocytomas (Taylor et al. 1985; Malfetano et al. 1986). Santala et al. (1987) recommended groin dissection in addition to surgery. Radiotherapy has not offered encouraging results in advanced local disease (Hensley and Friedrich 1973).

11.2.1.4 Fibrosarcoma

In the earlier literature, fibrosarcoma used to be mentioned as the most common soft tissue sarcoma of the body because of the fact that almost all spindle cell tumours were diagnosed as fibrosarcoma. This is also the reason why in the earlier literature fibrosarcomas were the most common malignant soft tissue tumours of the vulva (Priore et al. 1966). It is now apparent that many of these so-called fibrosarcomas were malignant fibrous histiocytomas or heterogeneous in origin. Nowadays the diagnostic criteria for differentiating types of spindle cell tumours have been largely defined, and fibrosarcoma as a separate malignant soft tissue entity is being recognised with somewhat more confidence. The cells of fibrosarcomas are uniform, spindle or fusiform in shape and lie shoulder to shoulder in a fasciculated or herring bone pattern. They possess scanty cytoplasm, slender nuclei and indistinct cell boundaries. Depending upon the degree of differentiation, variable reticulin fibres can be seen between the individual cells. Mitotic figures vary from area to area in the same tumour. Uniform cellular organisation is an important feature of a well-differentiated fibrosarcoma. Although giant cells may be seen, they are never conspicuous.

The aetiology of these tumours is uncertain. Fibrosarcomas have been noted to develop in the chronic sinus tract (Morris and Lucas 1964), after radiation therapy (Schwartz and Rothstein 1968; Oberman and Oneal 1970) and at the site of a plastic vascular graft (Burns et al. 1972).

11.2.1.4.1 Clinical Features

Fibrosarcomas occur in patients with a wide age range; the peak incidence is between 40 and 60 years old (Bizer 1971). The tumours occur predominantly in the trunk and extremities; the lower are more favoured than the upper. The tumours are deep sub-cutaneous in the majority of patients. The symptoms are mostly due to the lump and its pressure effects. Rare retroperitoneal fibrosarcomas are known to produce hypoglycemia.

The vulval tumour presents as a rapidly growing, painful lump or pruritic mass on one of the labia majora, clitoris (Keller 1951; DiSaia et al. 1971) or mons veneris (Woodruff and Brack 1958).

11.2.1.4.2 Gross Appearance

The tumours are round to oval masses 5–10 cm in diameter with a lobulated surface. They are firm, grey and circumscribed but unencapsulated. The cut surface is grey-white to fleshy in appearance with foci of haemorrhage and necrosis.

The vulval tumours are usually circumscribed and may grow up to the size of a grapefruit (Keller 1951).

11.2.1.4.3 Microscopical Appearance

As mentioned earlier, the tumour is composed of spindle cells arranged in a herring bone pattern with a variable amount of intercellular reticulin and collagen. The neoplastic spindle cells are uniform in size and shape. Mitotic figures are always seen. The tumour is unencapsulated and forms a pseudocapsule due to compression of the surrounding tissues. Sheets of tumour cells may be seen outside the pseudocapsule indicating infiltrative borders.

On electron microscopic studies, Gonzalez-Crussi (1970) observed two embryonic cell types – one with clear cytoplasm containing tenous filamentous structures, round mitochondria with short cristae, less rough endoplasmic reticulum, a polysomic configuration of the ribosomes and no junctional complex, and the other with aggregated filaments, free ribosomes and rough and smooth endoplasmic reticulum. These were interpreted as features of embryonic fibroblasts.

11.2.1.4.4 Prognosis

Prognosis of these tumours has been correlated with the histological grade, which is based on cellularity, mitosis, degree of anaplasia and production of ground substance (Heller and Sieber 1950; Pritchard et al. 1974). While Pritchard et al. (1974) graded fibrosarcomas into 4 grades, Mackenzie (1964) grouped them into 3 following the criteria based on nuclear appearance, mitotic figures, amount of intercellular substance and cellularitiy, although he recognised that there were borderline cases which could be graded only with difficulty. The 5-year survival rate was 83% in grade 1 and only 30% in grade 3 tumours (Mackenzie 1964). Pritchard et al. (1974) observed a great improvement of prognosis with aggressive treatment. The tumours tend to recur, and the recurrences are common with incompletely excised tumours. When the tumour metastasises, it is usually via haematogenous routes. Lymph node metastasis is rare although in some series it varied from 0.5% (Pritchard et al. 1974) to 8% (Stout 1948). Local recurrences predispose to distant metastases (van der Werf-Messing and van Unnik 1965).

11.2.1.4.5 Treatment

It is generally agreed that radical surgery is the treatment for fibrosarcoma. The recurrence rate is high with local excision (Bizer 1971). The patient with a vulval tumour treated initially by local excision suffered repeated recurrences and finally widely spread metastases (Davos and Abell 1976), while the patient treated initially by radical vulvectomy with pelvic and inguinal lymphadenectomy was tumour-free for at least 4 years (DiSaia et al. 1971). Chemotherapy, where radical surgery cannot be undertaken, must be tried (Soule and Pritchard 1977).

11.2.1.5 Liposarcoma

Liposarcomas were thought to be the most common soft tissue sarcomas (Enzinger and Winslow 1962) of adults, but their incidence is now considered to be much lower (Evans 1979). They are, however, one of the most common malignant tumours of soft tissue (Spittle et al. 1971) with an incidence ranging from 5% (Evans 1979) to 30% (Krall et al. 1981). Their occurrence on the female external genitalia has been noticed only rarely (Gompel and Silverberg 1977). In two large series on the vulval soft tissue sarcomas (DiSaia et al. 1971; Davos and Abell 1976), lipoosarcomas were not even mentioned.

11.2.1.5.1 Clinical Features

Liposarcomas occur commonly in the extremities and retroperitoneum. The lower extremity, especially the thigh, is more favoured than the upper (Reszel et al. 1966). While the benign lipomas arise commonly in subcutaneous tissue, liposarcomas show a predilection for deeper soft tissues (Pack and Pierson 1954). The patients are usually male and in their 50s (Kindblom et al. 1975). Liposarcomas are not common among children (Castleberry et al. 1984). The age of the patients with vulval liposarcomas varies between 15 (Brooks and LiVolsi 1987) and 60 (Genton and Maroni 1987) years old. The usual complaint of these patients is a slowly or rapidly growing lump in the perineum (Gondos and Casey 1982) or labium majus (Taussig 1937).

11.2.1.5.2 Gross Appearance

The vulval tumours vary between 4 and 18 cm in diameter. Detailed gross descriptions of these tumours are, however, not available. In general, liposarcomas tend to be oval with their major axis parallel to the longitudinal axis of the muscle (Kindblom et al. 1975). They appear well circumscribed but are unencapsulated and often infiltrative. Cut surfaces display variable appearances somewhat reflecting histological subtypes from lobular yellow-grey lipomatous (well-differentiated), jelly-like translucent (myxoid) to grey-white and grey-brown (round cell and pleomorphic) (Kindblom et al. 1975). Haemorrhage and necrosis are prominent in some tumours.

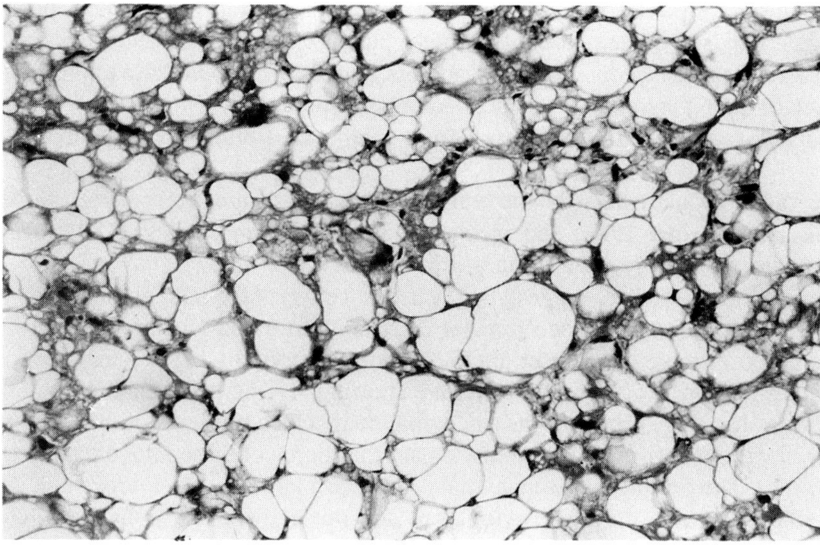

Fig. 11.16. Liposarcoma: scattered lipoblasts within the tumour

11.2.1.5.3 Microscopical Appearance

Enzinger and Weiss (1982) classified liposarcomas into (i) myxoid, (ii) well-differentiated, (iii) round cell and (iv) pleomorphic variants. The myxoid variant is the most common histological type, composed of lipoblasts in varying stages of differentiation, a rich plexiform capillary network and abundant myxoid matrix. The cells may be round or stellate, containing fat and vacuoles. They may be univacuolated (signet ring), multivacuolated with peripherally pushed nuclei (Lockerne) or sometimes simply multivacuolated (mulberry) (Hashimoto and Enjoji 1982). Cellularity of this variant varies. Mitosis is rare.

Well-differentiated liposarcomas fall into lipoma-like, inflammatory, sclerosing and dedifferentiated sub-types. In the lipoma-like subtype, the fat cells are similar to mature fat cells of lipoma with the exception of scattered pleomorphic cells and uni- and multivacuolated lipoblasts (Fig. 11.16). In the inflammatory form, in addition to the lipoma-like fat cells, occasional atypical cells with hyperchromatic nuclei or lipoblasts, many lymphocytes and plasma cells are seen. The sclerosing type is recognised by lipoma-like areas alternating with broad fibrous and myxoid areas in the same tumour. Atypical, pleomorphic cells and lipoblasts are common. The dedifferentiated liposarcoma shows areas of poorly differentiated cells often resembling malignant fibrous histiocytoma and occasionally fibrosarcoma (Evans 1979).

Round cell liposarcomas are composed of round cells with vesicular nuclei which may simulate lymphoma. These variants are less vascular and contain less intercellular myxoid material. The recognition of the lipoblasts is the clue for diagnosis. Evans (1979) preferred to group this type with the myxoid variant.

Pleomorphic liposarcomas, as the name suggests, present pleomorphic pictures and are composed of numerous, extremely pleomorphic, bizarre and giant, multivacuolated lipoblasts. Many of them possess abundant acidophilic cytoplasm reminiscent of rhabdomyoblasts. Typical lipoblasts may be absent in some of these liposarcomas, making differentiation from malignant fibrous histiocytomas difficult.

The histological details of the vulval liposarcomas are not precise. Myxoid (Brooks and LiVolsi 1987) and pleomorphic (Gondos and Casey 1982) variants have, however, been recognised in a few reports.

Ultrastructural studies suggest that various cell types could give rise to this neoplasm: undifferentiated perivascular cells (Battifora and Nunez-Alonso 1980), brown adipose tissue (Legace et al. 1979), non-fat-storing mesenchymal cells and fat-storing adipocytes or both (Bolen and Thorning 1984). It is generally believed that the fat-forming, primitive mesenchymal cells which are recognised ultrastructurally in various stages of differentiation are the source of these tumours (Russouw et al. 1986). The primitive mesenchymal cells have a large nucleo-cytoplasmic ratio, organelle-sparse and lipid-free cytoplasm, and nuclei with finely dispersed chromatin and occasional nucleoli. The early lipoblasts contain irregular lipid droplets, well-developed nucleoli and Golgi zones and are rich with many mitochondria, intermediate filaments and rough endoplasmic reticulum. Glycogen and many micropinocytic vesicles are also noticed. Junctional complexes are not found. In the mid-stage lipoblasts contain many non-membrane-bound lipid droplets, small mitochondria, lysosomes, polyribosomes, intermediate filaments and external lamina. The nuclei are irregular and eccentrically located. The late lipoblasts show monovacuolar cytoplasm with small, incompletely fused, lipid droplets compressed against the plasma membrane, few mitochondria and an oval nucleus (Rossouw et al. 1986).

11.2.1.5.4 Biological Behaviour and Prognosis

These tumours tend to recur most often due to incomplete excision. Some 70% of the lesions treated by local excision show evidence of recurrence (Reszel et al. 1966). Histological differentiation of the tumour is an important prognostic factor. The less differentiated tumours tend to metastasise, and in one series (Enterline et al. 1960) the least differentiated tumours metastasised in 86% patients. Generally, the patients with myxoid and well-differentiated liposarcomas have a better prognosis with a 5-year survival rate approaching almost 100% (Enzinger and Winslow 1962; Kindblom et al. 1975). Prognosis with the round cell and pleomorphic types is considered to be poor. The size of the tumour and treatment modality also contribute to the overall prognosis (Reitan et al. 1985). One patient with low grade vulval myxoid liposarcoma died of local recurrence (Brooks and LiVolsi 1987), and another patient with probable dedifferentiated liposarcoma died of metastases (Taussig 1937).

The overall survival of liposarcoma has been estimated to be about 65% (Spittle et al. 1971).

11.2.1.5.5 Treatment
Radical excision should be the first choice in treating liposarcomas (Enzinger and Weiss 1982). Adjunct radiotherapy and chemotherapy have been used with variable results (Spittle et al. 1971). The number of the vulval liposarcomas reported is very small for any meaningful comments. Radical surgery for vulval sarcoma (Davos and Abell 1976) and adjunct radiotherapy (Brooks and LiVolsi 1987) have been recommended.

11.2.1.6 Epithelioid Sarcoma

Epithelioid sarcoma, which was first described by Enzinger (1970), is an uncommon, distinctive tumour of soft tissue occurring in the extremities, chiefly in the hands of young adults, involving the skin, superficial fascia, tendons and nerves. The tumour grows slowly with a tendency to extend proximally along the fascial plane, has a high recurrence rate and eventually metastasises.

11.2.1.6.1 Clinical Features
The tumour occurs in patients with a wide age range. Epithelioid sarcoma is an uncommon tumour of the vulva (Piver et al. 1972; Gallup et al. 1976; Hall et al. 1980). Patients with vulval tumours are typically in their 2nd and 3rd decades and present with a gradually enlarging, asymptomatic mass or ulcer on the vulva. The tumour may be painful as it grows bigger. The common location is the labium majus.

11.2.1.6.2 Gross Appearance
The tumour is characteristically nodular but may be ovoid and bosselated. The size of the individual nodule varies from 0.5 to 2.5 cm; the multinodular tumour may be as large as 10 cm (Prat et al. 1978). Cut surfaces are glistening grey and white to grey-tan in appearance, with central areas of necrosis and haemorrhage.

11.2.1.6.3 Microscopical Appearance
The tumour nodules are composed predominantly of large, round and polygonal cells with distinctly eosinophilic cytoplasm and vesicular nuclei and prominent nucleoli. The cells resemble epithelioid cells of a granuloma and are arranged in pseudocarcinoma, melanoma, angiosarcoma and undifferentiated sarcoma-like patterns (Santiago et al. 1972). Bands of hyalinised collagen traverse between and separate the tumour nodules, groups and cords of tumour cells. Occasional cells are binucleate. Mitotic figures are always seen, but nuclear pleomorphism is minimal. Plump spindle cells with hyperchromatic nuclei are also noticed in varying proportions. The infiltrating cells at the margin of the tumour tend to be spindle-shaped, forming cords. Central necrosis is common. Irregular spaces and clefts which are seen in some areas of tumours result from necrosis and fixation artefacts. Lymphocytic infiltrations are common at the marginal zone.

The histogenesis of this tumour is debatable. Primitive mesenchymal cells (Enzinger 1970), fibrohistiocytic cells (Fisher and Horvat 1972) and myofibroblasts (Blewitt et al. 1983) have been suggested to be the cells of origin. Ultrastructural studies, on the other hand, have suggested synovial cells as the parent cells (Frable et al. 1973; Gabbiani et al. 1972; Miettinen et al. 1982). Immunohistochemically, the neoplastic cells show positive reactions for cytokeratin, epithelial membrane antigens (Manivel et al. 1987) and vimentin (Miettinen et al. 1982; Meis et al. 1988).

11.2.1.6.4 Natural History and Treatment

The majority of the tumours display a slow and relentless progression (Soule and Enriquez 1972) and have a high recurrence rate. Distant metastases follow after repeated recurrences. The vulval tumour spreads to the inguinal lymph nodes (Gallup et al. 1976). The prognosis is generally poor with local recurrence, vascular invasion and nodal metastases (Prat et al. 1978). At least three-quarters of the patients are likely to develop lung metastases when vascular or nodal invasion occurs.

Early diagnosis and wide, en block excision or radical vulvectomy with lymphadenectomy have been recommended (Hall et al. 1980). The role of radiotherapy and chemotherapy is uncertain (Hall et al. 1980; Bloustein et al. 1976). Shimm and Suit (1983), however, achieved a low recurrence rate with combined radiation and surgery.

11.2.1.7 Malignant Schwannoma

Malignant schwannomas commonly occur in the extremities, neck, trunk and paravertebral areas (Ghosh et al. 1973; Guccion and Enzinger 1979; Storm et al. 1980). They are uncommon soft tissue tumours but have been reported in the vulva under the names malignant schwannoma, neurofibrosarcoma and neurogenous sarcoma. The general tendency is to call these tumours "malignant schwannomas" as they are believed to arise from the Schwann cells. Others prefer the name "peripheral nerve sheath tumour" (Erlandson and Woodruff 1982), as the histogenesis of the tumour is not that certain. Malignant schwannomas occur ab initio as solitary lesions in a major nerve trunk or complicate von Recklinghausen's disease. This complication has been estimated to occur in from 5% (Ducatman et al. 1986) to 15% of patients (Vieta and Pack 1951). In a series of 115 cases, Ghosh et al. (1973) found that 74% of malignant schwannomas were solitary in the nerve trunk and 36%, in association with von Recklinghausen's disease. Multiple lesions are uncommon. All the reported lesions on the vulva are solitary.

Malignant schwannomas have been reported to arise at a previously irradiated site (Ducatman and Scheithauer 1983) and in ganglioneuromas (Chandrasoma et al. 1986; Fletcher et al. 1988).

11.2.1.7.1 Clinical Features

The patients are of a wide age range, from 4 to 80 years old with a peak incidence between the 3rd and 5th decades (Ghosh et al. 1973). The patients with von Recklinghausen's disease are younger than those without (D'Agostino et al. 1983; Sordillo et al. 1981). The sex ratio is equal in sporadic lesions, whereas men predominate in von Recklinghausen's disease (D'Agostino et al. 1963; Guccion and Enzinger 1979). Most often the patients seek medical advice for a painless mass. A small number of patients may complain of pain. The patients with vulval tumours are between 25 and 66 years of age (DiSaia et al. 1971; Lawrence and Shingleton 1978) and consult their gynaecologists for a rapidly growing vulval mass.

11.2.1.7.2 Gross Appearance

The size of these tumours varies from 2.5 to 45 cm (Guccion and Enzinger 1979). They are fusiform, oval or round in shape, and soft, firm and rubbery in consistency. The cut surfaces vary from greyish-white to yellowish in appearance. In the majority of cases, the tumours are seen in relation to the nerves.

The vulval tumours vary in size from 2.5 to 6 cm, appear encapsulated and are surrounded by fibro-fatty tissue. The cut surfaces are a homogeneous grey-white and vaguely whorled in appearance.

11.2.1.7.3 Microscopical Appearance

The tumours are composed essentially of spindle cells arranged in tight, wavy or interlacing bundles. They are often monomorphic with scanty to a moderate amount of cytoplasm and hyperchromatic, plump or spindle-shaped nuclei, which display one or more mitotic figures per high power field. In some areas, the nuclei are arranged in a palisading manner reminiscent of a benign schwannoma. Perivascular proliferation of the tumour cells with myxoid stroma in the intervening areas has also been noticed. Several other features such as focal necrosis of the tumour cells and hyalinisation of the stroma can be seen. In some tumours, the cells may be round to oval with epithelioid characteristics, possessing abundant cytoplasm, vesicular nuclei and prominent nucleoli (McCormack et al. 1954), or rhabdomyoblastic in the so-called triton tumours (Dewit et al. 1986). Foci of mesenchymal differentiation towards malignant osteoblasts and chondroblasts, epithelial differentiation forming acinar structures (Ducatman et al. 1984) and ganglion cells (Matsunou et al. 1985) have been noticed in some tumours.

Malignant schwannomas associated with plexiform neuroma and von Recklinghausen's disease tend to be more pleomorphic and more aggressive (Ghosh et al. 1973). The histological features of malignancy blend gradually with benign neurofibromatous areas. The co-existence of neurofibromatous components have been noticed in many tumours including those of the vulva (Davos and Abell 1976).

Ultrastructurally, the tumour cells display cytoplasmic processes covered by basal lamina (Taxy et al. 1981) and contain a moderate number of mitochondria, polyribosomes and scattered rough endoplasmic reticulum (Chen et al. 1980). Intercellular junctions and extracellular electron dense crystalline structures were also demonstrated (Chen et al. 1980). Lawrence and Shingleton (1978) noticed both Antoni A and Antoni B features of benign schwannoma except for cross-banded structures, as well as bizarre-shaped, indented nuclei, well-developed nucleoli, numerous mitochondria, endoplasmic reticulum surrounding a central lipid core and prominent Golgi complexes.

Immunohistochemically, the neoplastic cells react positively with at least one of three antibodies, namely S-100 protein, myelin basic protein and Leu 7 (Wick et al. 1987; Johnson et al. 1988). Also, 30% of all tumours show a positive reaction for neuron-specific enolase (Matsunou et al. 1985). While the sarcomatous areas are vimentin positive, the epithelial glandular component reacts positively to cytokeratin and CEA (Ducatman et al. 1986; Cross and Clarke 1988).

11.2.1.7.4 Behaviour

Malignant schwannomas tend to recur and metastasise. The incidence of recurrence and metastasis is higher in patients with von Recklinghausen's disease (Ducatman et al. 1986). Tumours arising at the site of previous irradiation also tend to be more aggressive than other malignant schwannomas (Sordillo et al. 1981).

11.2.1.7.5 Treatment

Ducatman et al. (1986) have recommended radical excision with removal of all tissues other than the most vital ones and including a wide margin of normal tissue. Excision and adjunctive radiotherapy should be used where radical surgery is not possible. Sordillo et al. (1981) achieved encouraging results with adjunctive chemotherapy and surgery. Vulval tumours have been treated by local excision, hemivulvectomy and radical vulvectomy. Radical vulvectomy with well-cleared surgical margins and inguinal lymphadenectomy should be undertaken as with other vulval sarcomas. While one patient treated by radical vulvectomy survived 9 years, another patient treated initially by local excision and subsequently by more radical surgery died of widespread metastases (DiSaia et al. 1971).

In general, the 5-year survival rate is much less (30%) with von Recklinghausen's disease than without (65%) (Ghosh et al. 1973). Tumours less than 5 cm in diameter have a better prognosis.

11.2.1.8 Rhabdomyosarcoma

Rhabdomyosarcomas are more common in the vagina than in the vulva (see Vaginal rhabdomyosarcoma). While the vaginal rhabdomyosarcomas occur commonly in infants and young girls (James et al. 1969; Copeland et al. 1985), they are also seen in adult women over 30 years of age (Ober et al. 1953; Priore et al. 1966; Witt 1967; DiSaia et al. 1971). The three patients reported in a large series on vulval sarcomas (DiSaia et al. 1971) were 18, 28 and 44 years old, respectively. Vulval rhabdomyosarcomas are commonly seen on the labium, vestibule and perineal region. They grow rapidly and produce symptoms of local discomfort, irritation and dyspareunia.

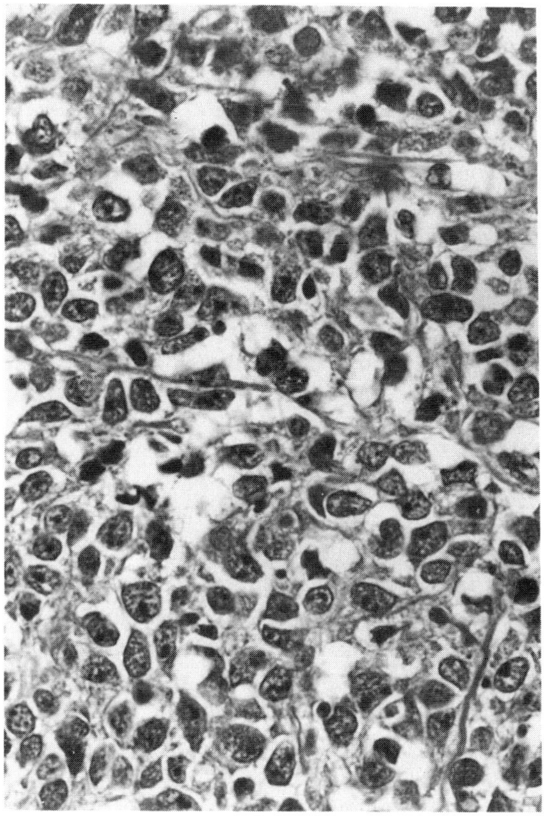

Fig. 11.17. Embryonal rhabdomyosarcoma: sheets of oval and round cells with hyperchromatic nuclei and scanty cytoplasm

11.2.1.8.1 Pathological Features

Gross and microscopical descriptions of vulval rhabdomyosarcomas are either scanty or altogether excluded from the literature. The gross anatomy of these tumours does not, however, seem to be significantly different from those of the vagina.

Rhabdomyosarcomas are usually classified according to the formulation by Horn and Enterline (1958). Of the four types – embryonal, alveolar, pleomorphic and botryoid – the botryoid and embryonal ones occur commonly in infants and children, while the pleomorphic variant, which is now considered to be a small group, occurs predominantly in adults.

Embryonal rhabdomyosarcoma is the most common type, occurring in children under 5 years of age. The head, neck and in particular orbits are frequently involved. Other areas affected include the urogenital tract and retroperitoneum. Except for the botryoid type, there is no significant difference among the rhabdomyosarcomas in their gross anatomy. They vary in consistency from soft to firm and are gelatinous, unencapsulated and deceptively circumscribed tumours of 2–20 cm in diameter. The cut surface is greyish to light tan in appearance.

Microscopically, these tumours are composed of spindle cells, round to ovoid cells with abundant eosinophilic cytoplasm and small round cells with scant cytoplasm (Fig. 11.17). The nuclei are hyperchromatic and elongated or ovoid in shape. Cytoplasmic longitudinal and cross-striations may be seen in occasional spindle cells.

Alveolar rhabdomyosarcoma, which is commonly seen in teenagers and young adults, occurs in the extremities. Its cells are arranged in an alveolar pattern lining the alveoli-like spaces, which are separated from their neighbours by delicate fibrovascular septae. The neoplastic cells are small and round to oval with small hyperchromatic nuclei resembling cells of the embryonal type. Some of the cells may be free floating within the alveolar spaces or may be arranged in small nests. Multinucleate giant cells and strap cells are also commonly seen in this type. Cross-striations can be seen in some of the strap cells.

The pleomorphic type occurs commonly in the extremities of adults and, as the name suggests, is composed of a pleomorphic cell population consisting of strap cells, tadpole-shaped cells, giant cells and small, round, anaplastic cells. Cross-striations can be seen in many of the strap and giant cells.

The botryoid type is commonly seen in the very young and occurs in the vagina. It can also occur in the cervix. This type differs from other types of rhabdomyosarcomas by its gross polypoid, soft, myxomatous, grape-like appearance. Occasionally, the tumour is a haemorrhagic, flesh-coloured, polypoid mass (see Sarcoma botryoides of the vagina).

Immunohistochemically, myoglobin has been found to be a reliable marker for rhabdomyosarcoma, and its staining correlates with the degree of cytoplasmic differentiation of the tumour cells (Brooks 1982). A high degree of specificity could be found with the battery of markers of myosin, myoglobin and isoenzymes of creatine kinase (Tsokos et al. 1983). According to Autio-Harmainen et al. (1986), staining for the basement membrane components, particularly type IV collagen and laminin, is very helpful in differentiating benign and malignant tumours of straited muscle origin. According to the stage of maturity, these components can be demonstrated both intra- and extra-cellularly. Skalli et al. (1988), after using various immunological methods, have concluded that alpha-sr actin is also a good marker.

Ultrastructurally, rhabdomyosarcomas contain complexes of thick and thin myofilaments and consistently glycogen (Bundtzen and Norback 1982; Weiss and Warhol 1984). The cytoplasm also contains swollen mitochondria and abundant rough endoplasmic reticulum. The nuclei are large, with a scalloped contour and prominent nucleoli (Horvat et al. 1970).

11.2.1.8.2 Treatment and Prognosis

Rhabdomyosarcoma of the vulva metastasises locally to the regional nodes as well as to distant sites, commonly to the lungs by the haematogenous route.

Two patients with vulval tumours were treated by local excision and subsequently by radiation and chemotherapy. Both patients died of widespread metastatic disease within 9 months. One patient who had undergone radical vulvectomy and inguinal lymphadenectomy was alive at 7 years (DiSaia et al. 1971). The outlook of rhabdomyosarcoma is much better than it was a decade and a half ago. The combined modality of pre-operative chemotherapy and post-operative radiotherapy has greatly reduced the necessity of mutilating surgery and improved the prognosis significantly (Bell et al. 1986). A well-planned and aggressive multidisciplinary programme (Bertholomew et al. 1979) has contributed greatly to the increasing survival rate of what used to be considered a fatal disease.

11.2.1.9 Angiosarcoma

Angiosarcomas or haemangiosarcomas are malignant tumours of vascular origin which occur at various sites of the body, namely, the head and neck region (Hodgkinson et al. 1979), particularly in the scalp and face (Wilson-Jones 1964), breast (McConnell and Haslam 1959; Masse et al. 1977), bones and muscles (Stout 1943) and lymphoedematous extremities (McConnell and Haslam 1959; Eby et al. 1967). They can also occur in the internal organs (Girard et al. 1970).

Clinically, the patients are usually elderly with an average age of 70 years (Wilson-Jones 1964). The cutaneous lesions are generally asymptomatic, but some patients may complain of a gradually increasing swelling which bleeds spontaneously or upon minor irritation (Girard et al. 1970). Angiosarcomas are rare on the vulva. Rosenzweig (1970) reported a haemangioendothelioma in a 57-year-old woman occurring at the site of Bartholin's gland. The other patient reported by Davos and Abell (1976) was an 83-year-old woman, who had the tumour on the left labium majus for 3 years. Another 66-year-old patient, who had previously had radiotherapy for vulval carcinoma developed angiosarcoma in the lymphoedematous thigh (Huey et al. 1985).

11.2.1.9.1 Gross Appearance

Angiosarcoma occurring in the dermis is a bluish or violaceous nodule (or nodules) while the deeper tumours tend to be colourless (Maddox and Evans 1981). In the early stage, they may be flat lesions with ill-defined borders (Rosai et al. 1976). Three gross types – diffusely infiltrative, papulonodular and ulcerated – have been described (Maddox and Evans 1981). In some patients, bullae or blood-filled vesicles may be seen on the skin.

11.2.1.9.2 Microscopical Appearance

The lesions are commonly located in the dermis, but deeper infiltrations are frequently noticed. Angiosarcomas vary in their degree of differentiation. The well-differentiated tumours consist of irregular vascular spaces lined by plump endothelial cells with slightly atypical hyperchromatic nuclei (Fig. 11.18). These cells can also be noticed in the stroma between the vascular spaces. Upon initial observation, the lesions may appear haemangiomatous, but close examination reveals intercommunicating blood vessels of irregular outline forming anastomosing channels. Fronds of endothelial cells projecting into the lumen and hyperchromasia of endothelial cells should raise a suspicion of low grade angiosarcoma. Mitoses are rarely seen. A variable number of lymphocytic infiltrations are common. The poorly differentiated tumour is markedly cellular and composed of diffuse sheets of atypical spindle cells and pleomorphic cells which line the blood vessels (Fig. 11.19) as well as infiltrate the stroma. Papillary fronds are infrequently seen in the undifferentiated tumours. Mitoses are usually numerous. Occasional tumours designated as epithelioid haemangioendothelioma (Weiss and Enzinger 1982) are composed of nests and cords of plump round and polygonal cells which fill the lumen of vascular channels and expand them. They often infiltrate the vessel wall, mimicking a carcinoma. McWilliam and Harris (1985) described a granular cell variant of the tumour in which the granular cells were positive for factor VIII-related antigen.

Immunohistochemically, well-differentiated tumours show a positive reaction for factor VIII-related antigen, whereas the undifferentiated tumours are only weakly positive (Guarda et al. 1982). Using monoclonal antibody BMA 120 against the endothelial cells, Alles and Bosslet (1988) demonstrated consistent positive results in all angiosarcomas.

Ultrastructurally, the well-differentiated tumour cells display many characteristics of normal endothelial cells. They contain numerous junctional complexes, a moderate number of pinocytic vesicles and a large number of cytoplasmic processes into the lumen and are surrounded by basal lamina (Rosai et al. 1976).

The aetiology of angiosarcoma is not known. It is known to complicate chronic lymphoedema (Eby et al. 1967; Woodard et al. 1972) and develop at the site of therapeutic radiation (Paik and Komorowski 1976; Chen et al. 1979). Although trauma has been mentioned in some reports (Girard et al. 1970), its role seems to be insignificant in the causation of angiosarcoma. Two angiosarcomas, one in a 14-year-old boy and another in a 61-year-old man with stigmata of von Recklinghausen's disease, have been reported (Chaudhuri et al. 1980; Millstein et al. 1981). It was suggested that the angiosarcoma represents an expression of an abnormal genome in the vascular tissue (Millstein et al. 1981).

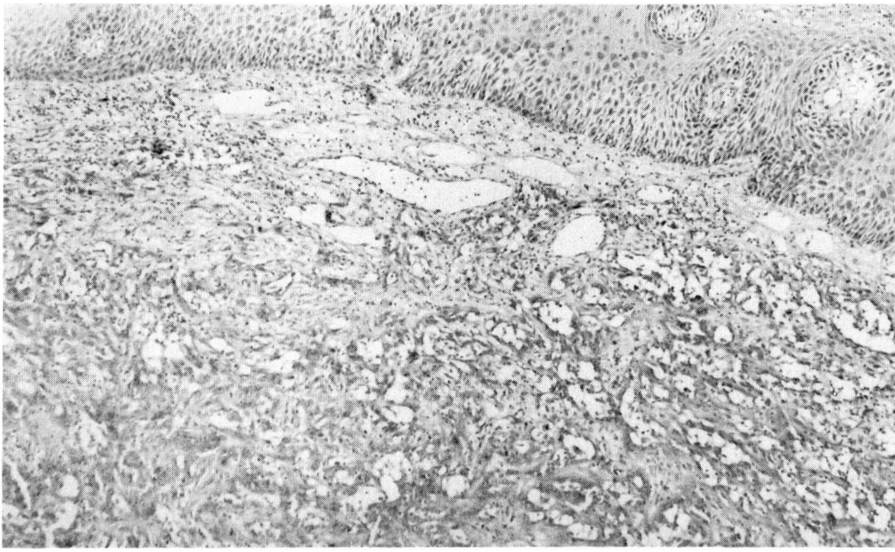

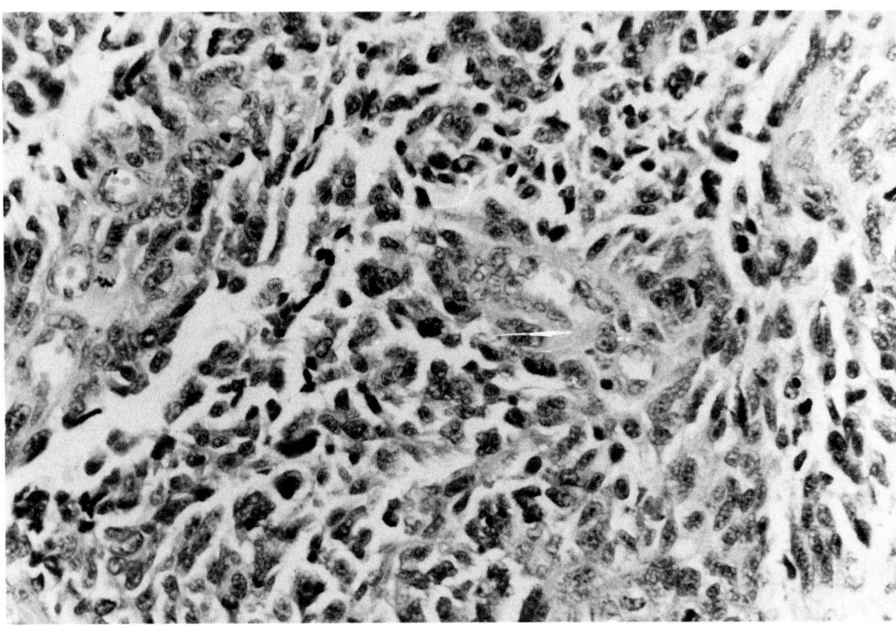

Fig. 11.18. Angiosarcoma: irregular vascular spaces lined by malignant endothelial cells beneath the epidermis

Fig. 11.19. Angiosarcoma: poorly differentiated tumour cells. Area of spindle-shaped cells

11.2.1.9.3 Behaviour

Angiosarcomas tend to recur and metastasise early and widely (Maddox and Evans 1981). They are considered highly malignant (Hodgkinson et al. 1979) with a poor outlook and median survival of only about 20 months (Maddox and Evans 1981). Although documentation of vulval angiosarcomas is inadequate, their behaviour does not seem to differ from these tumours at other sites.

11.2.1.9.4 Treatment

Wide surgical excision of the circumscribed and solitary lesions and radiation of multiple or ill-defined tumours have been advocated (Rosai et al. 1976). As these tumours also metastasise to the lymph nodes (Girard et al. 1970), radical surgical removal of the primary tumour with lymph node dissection followed by high dose radiation has also been recommended (Hodgkinson et al. 1979).

11.2.1.10 Kaposi's Sarcoma

These uncommon lesions, originally described by Kaposi as multiple idiopathic haemangiosarcoma of the skin (Kaposi 1872), have been known to occur with a higher frequency in some parts of Africa. They can appear sporadic or endemic and in immunosuppressed patients. They show a distinct preponderance for men. Immunocompromised homosexual men and intravenous drug users are particularly at high risk in non-African countries (Masur et al. 1981).

Clinically, these lesions present as violaceous papules or plaque-like lesions commonly on the lower distal extremities, which may ultimately ulcerate. While the older lesions progress, new lesions develop. The patients in non-African countries are over 50 years of age, but in African countries they are between the 2nd and 4th decades (Reynolds et al. 1965). Symptoms may be slight, altogether absent or simply a burning sensation and pruritus. A higher frequency of other malignancies, particularly lymphomas, has been noticed in association (Cox and Helwig 1959). The one documented patient with vulval Kaposi's sarcoma was a 64-year-old woman who presented with an indurated, raised, yellow-grey, scaling lesion involving the entire labium majora and satellite lesions on the buttock. The patient died of renal failure 1 year after the onset of symptoms (Hall et al. 1979).

11.2.1.10.1 Pathological Features

Taylor et al. (1971) classified Kaposi's sarcoma into nodular (nodules less than 2 cm in size), lymphadenopathic (with painless lymphadenopathy), florid or fungating and infiltrating (infiltrates deeper structures) types.

Microscopically, Kaposi's sacoma is characterised by proliferations of small and irregular vascular channels with jagged outlines which are lined by plump endothelial cells. They are surrounded by supporting spindle cells, inflammatory cells and extravasated red cells and may mimic granulation tissue. The spindle cells are generally uniform in size, with scanty cytoplasm and hyperchromatic nuclei with inconspicuous nucleoli. Characteristic cytoplasmic eosinophilic bodies

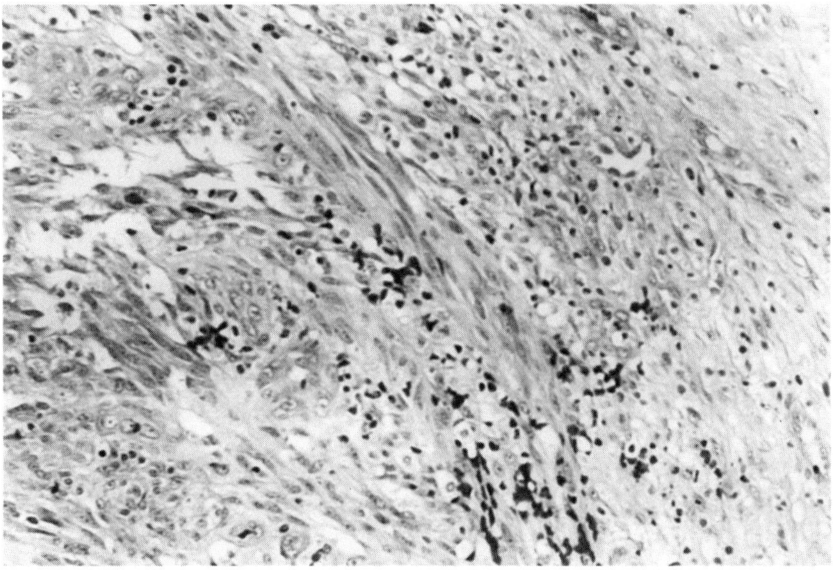

Fig. 11.20. Kaposi's sarcoma: spindle-shaped cells with interlacing fascicles

have been reported in the lesions of 92% of Malawi patients (O'Connell 1977). Kaposi's sarcomas may also masquerade as angiomas when vascular proliferation is abundant. Haemosiderin pigments from the extravasated red cells can often be seen in the lesion. The extravasation of red cells has been attributed to weak and imperfectly closed vascular channels (Dutz and Stout 1960). Dictor (1986) demonstrated aberrant lymphatico-venous connections in which lymphatic channels selectively penetrated the veins. In the later stage of the disease, the spindle cells predominate with obliteration of many vascular channels (Fig. 11.20), and the lesions may mimic a fibrosarcoma. In the poorly differentiated lesions, mitotic figures become frequent, and the cells become pleomorphic with loss of the spindle cell character.

The origin of neoplastic spindle cells is not clear. A relationship to the reticuloendothelial system has been suggested but not proven. Guarda et al. (1981) and Nadji et al. (1981) demonstrated factor VIII-related antigen (rag) in these cells by immunohistochemical methods. These findings, however, could not be confirmed in other studies (Mukai et al. 1980). Beckstead et al. (1985), using several markers for endothelial cells, concluded that neoplastic cells closely resemble cells of the lymphatic endothelium and that Kaposi's sarcoma could originate from the lymphatic channels. Ultrastructural studies (Hashimoto and Lever 1964; Mottaz and Zelickson 1966) demonstrated fibroblasts, endothelial cells, perithelial cells and other mesenchymal cells in Kaposi's sarcoma. McNutty et al. (1983) observed a lack of pericytic investment around the small blood vessels. The endothelial cells have small dilated endoplasmic reticulum and a few mitochondria and lack basal lamina. Necrosis of individual endothelial cells and prominent cytoplasmic processes trapping collagen fibres in some aggressive lesions were seen.

The nature of Kaposi's sarcoma is not clear. A relationship to reticulo-endothelial neoplasm has been suggested but not proven. The histogenesis of neoplastic spindle cells has remained the centre point of controversy. Immunohistochemical demonstration of factor VIII-related antigen (Guarda et al. 1981; Nadji et al. 1981) in both normal and neoplastic endothelial cells (Mukai et al. 1980) points toward endothelial cell origin. It was suggested that the tumour cells arise from undifferentiated mesenchymal cells which could differentiate toward several types of mesenchymal cells (Harrison et al. 1978). According to Akhtar et al. (1984), Kaposi's sarcoma arises from the vasoformative mesenchyme, and the spindle cells arise from endothelium of blood vessels (Fachetti et al. 1988).

11.2.1.10.2 Prognosis

Kaposi's sarcoma in general bears a good prognosis (Templeton and Bhana 1975). The disease pursues a prolonged course. O'Brien and Brasfield (1966) mentioned eight patients who were still alive after 16 years. Lesions with pleomorphic histological features tend to be aggressive. With locally aggressive disease, 64% of patients survives 3 years (Templeton and Bhana 1975). Generalised lymph node involvement indicates a poor prognosis. The outlook seems to be poor also in immunosuppressed patients.

11.2.1.10.3 Treatment

Surgery was advocated for localised disease (McCarthy and Pack 1950). The disease is often multicentric and treated by chemotherapy and radiotherapy. A multiagent chemotherapeutic regimen with actinomycin D, vincristine and dacarbazine (DTIC) has been found encouraging in vulval lesions (Hall et al. 1979).

11.2.1.11 Alveolar Soft Part Sarcoma

Alveolar soft part sarcoma, first described by Christopherson et al. (1952), is a soft tissue tumour of uncertain histogenesis (also see Vagina). It constitutes about 1% of all soft tissue sarcomas (Morton 1974).

Clinically, alveolar soft part sarcoma is a slow-growing, painless tumour in the deep tissue of one of the extremities. The patient is usually a young adult and more often female with an average age of 20 years. Both adolescents and adults can be affected (Lieberman et al. 1966). A patient with a vulval tumour was a 62-year-old woman who presented after 1 year with an asymptomatic mobile mass on the right labia majora (Shen et al. 1982). The tumour was about 4 cm in size, smooth surfaced and rubbery in consistency, with the cut surface homogeneous yellow to tan in appearance.

Microscopically, the tumour presents an organoid pattern with characteristic irregular alveolar compartments supporting large, round or polygonal cells which possess abundant eosinophilic, sometimes granular or clear cytoplasm, vesicular nuclei and prominent small nucleoli. Lieberman et al. (1966) noticed diastase-resistant, PAS-positive crystalline material in the cell cytoplasm in 11 of 50 tumours. The alveolar compartments are separated from their neighbours by thin strands of vascular connective tissue which are well demonstrated by reticulin stain. The tumours are usually very vascular, and dilated vascular channels can often be seen at the peripheral zone.

Various theories on the histogenesis of these tumours have been forwarded. A relationship to paraganglioma (Smetena and Scott 1951; Welsh et al. 1972), rhabdomyosarcoma (Fisher and Reidbord 1971) and granular cell myoblastoma (Stout and Lattes 1967) have all been suggested.

Immunohistochemical investigations have yielded variable results. Mukai et al. (1986) noted positive reactions in the tumour cells with desmin. This could not be confirmed by Auerbach and Brooks (1987), who found only a weakly positive vimentin reaction. These authors concluded that alveolar soft part sarcoma was neither myogenic nor paraganglionic in origin, because the tumour cells did not react to myoglobin, S-100 protein, non-specific enolase or factor VII-related antibodies.

Ultrastructurally, the round and polygonal tumour cells resting on the basement membrane contain numerous mitochondria of various sizes, sparse endoplasmic reticulum and well-developed Golgi apparatus (Shipkey et al. 1964). The mitochondria are collected near the basal part of the cell. A few granules with dense cores and limited by a single membrane are seen close to the Golgi zone in some cells (Unni and Soule 1975; Ekfors et al. 1979). The crystals are rhomboid or sharp spicules consisting of light and dark lines with a periodicity of 10 nm.

11.2.1.11.1 Behaviour

These tumours are highly malignant but often pursue a prolonged course with a tendency to late metastases (Asvall et al. 1969). Local recurrences are common. They metastasise via the blood stream to the lungs, bones and brain. Metastases to the lymph nodes occur infrequently. The survival rate in the series of Lieberman et al. (1966) was 82.8% at 2 years, 59% at 5 years and 47.1% at 10 years. One of their patients died of disseminated disease at the 20th year of the follow-up period. Deaths are most often due to metastatic disease (Baum et al. 1981.

11.2.1.11.2 Treatment

Surgical management has been the mainstay of treatment. Aggressive local excision or even amputation when localised in the extremities may be necessary (Wobbes 1978). The tumour has been reported to be insensitive to radiation (Rubenfeld 1971). Chemotherapy with vincristine, adriamycin and cyclophosphamide has not been encouraging (Blumberg and Chang 1976). A patient with a vulval tumour was treated by radical vulvectomy with right groin node dissection and superficial dissection of the left groin. She was free of disease during the 2 years of the follow-up period (Shen et al. 1982).

11.2.1.12 Dermatofibrosarcoma Protuberans

Dermatofibrosarcoma protuberans (DDSP) is an uncommon tumour of the skin, accounting for 1% of all skin tumours (Bonnaebeau et al. 1974). Its histogenesis has been variably argued to be histiocytic (Ozzello and Hamels 1976), fibroblastic (Hertzler 1926) or neurogenic (Bednar 1957).

11.2.1.12.1 Clinical Features

About 50% of the patients are between 20 and 40 years old (McPeak et al. 1967). The trunk is a common site, but the proximal extremities are also frequently affected (Taylor and Helwig 1962). The tumour, in fact, can arise in any part of the body except palm and sole (Brenner et al. 1975). The main complaint is the discovery of a slowly growing nodule. Some patients may notice discoloration of the skin preceding the appearance of the tumour. They may also notice new nodules appearing close to the original one after a latent period of months or years, which coalesce to form a larger nodule. There is an occasional history of trauma at the tumour site. On examination, the nodule is found to be fixed to the skin but freely mobile over the deeper tissue. Mannual pressure causes the nodule to blanch.

The age of patients with vulval tumours ranges between the 3rd and 9th decades (Davos and Abell 1976; Soltan 1981; Agress et al. 1983; Boek 1985). The main complaints are a long-standing, asymptomatic, slowly or rapidly growing, ulcerated mass either on the labia majora, mons pubis or upper part of the vulva.

11.2.1.12.2 Gross Appearance

The tumour appears as a firm and well-circumscribed, raised nodule or multinodular mass. Its size varies from 1 to 25 cm in greatest diameter (Burkhardt et al. 1966) with an average diameter of 5 cm (Taylor and Helwig 1962). Cut surfaces are firm, homogeneous, glistening and greyish in appearance but may also be partly myxomatous. Areas of haemorrhage may be scattered on the cut surface. The superficial skin may be stretched and discoloured.

11.2.1.12.3 Microscopical Appearance

At its cellular portion, the tumour is composed of spindle cells arranged in whorls or a cartwheel pattern around an inconspicuous blood vessel or a collagenous focus (Fig. 11.21). The spindle cells are uniform and plump, containing scanty cytoplasm and round to oval nuclei. Mitotic figures may be seen but are infrequent. A high mitotic count is an ominous sign, although a low count does not preclude the metastatic potential of the tumour (Brenner et al. 1975). Giant cells may be present sparsely but are never conspicuous. Haemosiderin pigments are quite common. Some tumours, particularly the recurrent ones, show focal myxoid changes due to accumulation of hyaluronic acid (Frierson and Cooper 1983). In these areas, a storiform pattern may be absent, the cells tending to be stellate. A characteristic feature is the presence of scattered, trapped, fat cells within the tumour. The tumour

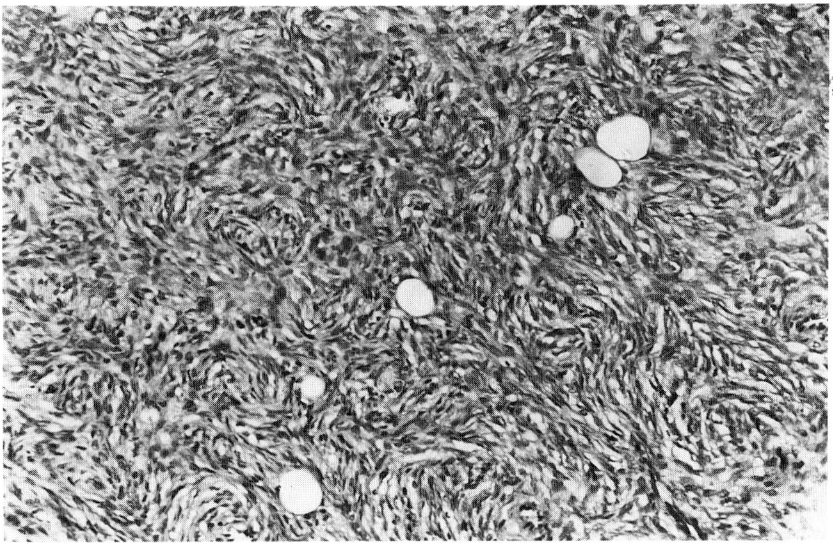

Fig. 11.21. Dermatofibrosarcoma protuberans: cartwheel pattern and trapped fat cells

involves the corium, extends into the subcutaneous fat in a web-like fashion and may infiltrate the underlying striated muscles (Burkhardt et al. 1866).

Occasional tumours show melanin pigment in the multipolar dendritic cells. These tumours are known as Bednar's tumours, coined after Bednar who originally noticed these features and thought these tumours to be neurofibromas (Bednar 1957).

Ultrastructural studies reveal cytoplasmic processes, rough endoplasmic reticulum, Golgi lamellae, spotty basal lamellae-like material and conspicuous absence of intracellular lysosomes and lipid. These features were suggestive of a perineural or endoneural cell origin (Hashimoto et al. 1974). A similar inference was made in the studies of Alguacil-Garcia et al. (1978), who suggested that the tumour originated from primitive fibroblastic cells with a sheath-forming cell differentiation. The immunohistochemical investigations, however, failed to demonstrate S-100 protein in these cells (Dupree et al. 1985). Positive reactions with the marker enzymes for histiocytic cells such as α-antitrypsin, lysozymes and ferritin in 75% of cases, on the other hand, lent support to the fibrohistiocytic character of the cells (Kindblom et al. 1982).

11.2.1.12.4 Behaviour

Transformation of the dermatofibrosarcoma protuberans to fibrosarcoma occurs generally after repeated recurrences (Wrotnowski et al. 1988). The sarcomatous area displays pleomorphism with loss of the storiform pattern, frequent mitoses and an absence of trapped fat cells. Dermatofibrosarcoma protuberans recurs in almost 50% of cases (Taylor and Helwig 1962), and recurrences are due to unintentional and unsuspected incomplete initial removal (Pack and Tabah 1951). Metastases, although rare, may occur after recurrences to the regional lymph nodes (Brenner et al. 1975), lungs and other sites (Penner 1951).

11.2.1.12.5 Treatment

Wide local excision including a border of 2.5–3 cm from the palpable visible periphery of the tumour is agreed upon as the treatment of choice (Brenner et al. 1975). Vulval lesions have been treated by local excision with a 1-cm healthy margin (Soltan 1981), wide local excision (Davos and Abell 1976), with a 3–4-cm free margin (Bock et al. 1985) and radical vulvectomy (Agress et al. 1983). None recurred during a follow-up period ranging from 6 months to 20 years.

11.2.1.13 Aggressive Angiomyxoma

Although there are sporadic reports of myxoid neoplasm occurring in the female genitalia and pelvis, Steeper and Rosai (1983) recognised a distinctive myxoid neoplasm which they termed aggressive angiomyxoma of the female pelvis and perineum. Subsequently, these neoplasms were also found to occur in the perineum and perianal region of the male (Begin et al. 1985).

11.2.1.13.1 Clinical Features

The patients are of a wide age range, but the majority are in their 3rd and 4th decades. The tumour grows slowly as an ill-defined or polypoid lump on the vulva, vagina, perineum and pelvic floor and perianal region. The majority of the patients consult their gynaecologists for vulval tumours or its pressure effects.

11.2.1.13.2 Gross Appearance

The size of the tumour varies widely from 3 to 60 cm (Steeper and Rosai 1983). The external surface may appear partially encapsulated but is generally irregular due to lobulations and finger-like projections. The cut surface may be soft or rubbery with grey-white to a glistening gelatinous appearance. Peticheal haemorrhages may be noticed in some tumours.

11.2.1.13.3 Microscopical Appearance

The tumour is composed of a loosely structured population of small spindle and stellate cells with one or more slender cytoplasmic processes. The cytoplasm contains occasional or a few vacuoles and is amphophilic and ill-defined. The nuclei are small, uniform in shape and bland in appearance. Mitoses are not seen. The cells are set in a myxoid background made of delicate collagen fibrils. Scattered within the tumour are occasional areas of increased cellularity merging imperceptibly with hypercellular areas. An important component of the tumour is the prominent, thick-walled, various-sized blood vessels which are distributed within the mesenchymal cell population. There are also scattered foci of microhaemorrhages, but cystic spaces are not seen. Mast cells are almost always seen. The tumour often displays, at its periphery, advancing columns of cells which infiltrate into the neighbouring fat or muscle tissue. The neoplasm is unencapsulated.

An aggressive angiomyxoma needs to be differentiated from myxoma which lacks blood vessels and microhaemorrhages, from the myxoid variant of malignant fibrous histiocytoma which involves the extremities and displays many pleomorphic giant cells and a vague storiform pattern. It is also to be differentiated from myxoid liposarcoma, which contains lipoblasts, arborising and thin-walled blood vessels, and lipid droplets ultrastructurally. The nerve sheath myxoma is superficial in location, contains nerve sheath cells and shows Schwann cells and fibroblasts.

Immunohistochemical investigations have demonstrated positive reactions for actin and negative for CEA, factor VIII-related antigen, S-100 protein and keratin (Begin et al. 1985). These findings have been interpreted as suggesting a fibroblastic origin.

11.2.1.13.4 Treatment

The tumour is locally aggressive and recurs if incompletely excised (Hilgers et al. 1986). Complete excision with wide tumour-free margin is the recommended treatment.

11.2.1.14 Haemangiopericytoma

Haemangiopericytoma is an uncommon vascular tumour which was first described by Stout and Murray (1942). These authors thought them to be of pericytic origin. The lesion occurs in patients of all age groups, from infancy to the 9th decade.

The common sites are the lower extremities, affecting predominantly the anterior part of the thigh and groin (McMaster et al. 1975). Although the musculo-skeletal system is involved in 50% of cases, the tumour can arise in any part of the body in which capillaries are found (Backwinkel and Diddams 1970). The usual symptom is a painless, slowly growing mass (Gerner et al. 1974). Some tumours may produce pressure effects when occurring in the deeper tissues. Rarely, hypoglycaemia (Crocker and Veith 1965) or hypertension (Robertson et al. 1967) may occur as paraneoplastic syndrome. Haemangiopericytomas are uncommon tumours of the female genital tract, occurring sporadically in the uterine wall (Greene et al. 1970) and rarely on the vulva (De Sousa and Lash 1959). Slattery et al. (1956) mentioned three vulval tumours in a series of 207 haemangiopericytomas collected by Stout. The patient reported by Reymond et al. (1972) developed metastasis in the bone 14 years after the removal of the vulval tumour.

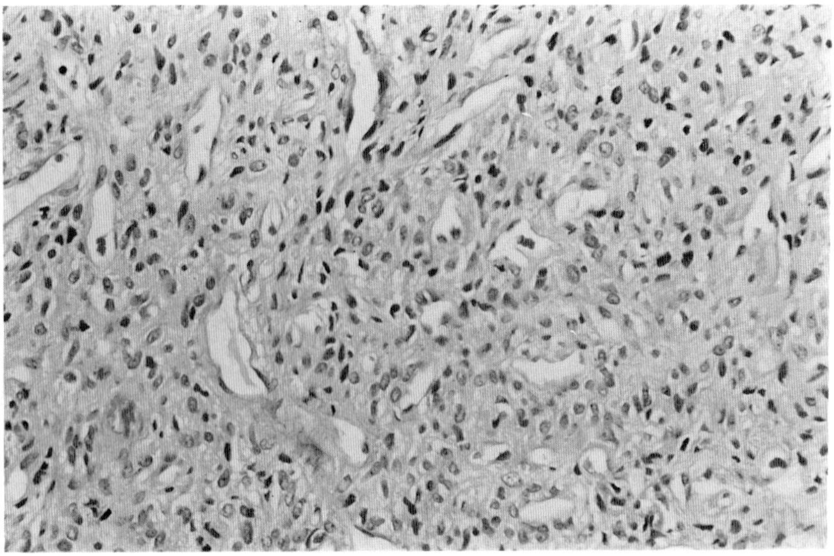

Fig. 11.22. Haemangiopericytoma: tightly packed tumour cells around vascular spaces

11.2.1.14.1 Gross Appearance

The tumour is generally well-circumscribed with a somewhat bosselated external surface and round and oval in shape. Its size varies from 5 to 15 cm (Angervall et al. 1978). The cut surface is greyish-white to reddish-brown in colour and may contain areas of haemorrhage and necrosis.

11.2.1.14.2 Microscopical Appearance

The tumour is richly vascular and composed of tightly packed elongated cells with pale to eosinophilic cytoplasm, indistinct cell outlines and round to oval nuclei rich in chromatin (Fig. 11.22). The ramifying and anastomosing thin-walled vascular channels, a prominent component of the tumour are lined by a single layer of endothelial cells. The tumour cells are in intimate contact with these vascular channels and surround them. Reticulin stain demonstrates this perivascular arrangement of cells; reticulin fibres are often seen around the individual or group of tumour cells. Mitotic figures may vary from none to 5 or more per 10 high power fields. Areas of haemorrhage may be noticed.

The classification of haemangiopericytomas into benign and malignant variants on histological criteria has been attempted and considered arbitrary (Backwinkel and Diddams 1970). It is, however, thought that the large, deep-seated tumour compared with superficial ones (McMaster et al. 1975), showing few mitotic figures and cellular anaplasia is likely to be malignant. An infiltrative growth pattern and the presence of haemorrhage and necrosis are also suggestive of malignancy (Angervall et al. 1978).

Ultrastructurally (Battifora 1973; Hahn et al. 1973; Nunnery et al. 1982), the neoplastic cells are enveloped completely or partly by basement membrane. The cells with their complex cytoplasmic processes interdigitate with the neighbouring cells. The cells contain numerous round to oval mitochondria, abundant free ribosomes, granular endoplasmic reticulum and inconspicuous Golgi apparatus. In the majority of cells, bundles of fibrillar material within the cytoplasm resembling those of smooth muscle could be seen. Battifora (1973) observed the transition between the pericytes and endothelial cells and suggested a close relationship between haemangiopericytoma and haemangioendothelioma. In the immunohistochemical studies (Hultberg et al. 1988), the cells of haemangiopericytoma reacted weakly for factor VIII rag and laminin. The reactions with *Ulex europaeus* antigen-1 (UEA-1) were negative. The cells showed, however, positive reaction for actin. Haemangioendothelioma cells, on the other hand, showed positive reactions for factor VIII rag, UEA-1, laminin and actin.

11.2.1.14.3 Treatment

Removal of the tumour with a wide normal surgical excision margin is the treatment of choice (Backwinkel and Diddams 1970). Radiation has been used with some improvent of prognosis (Stout 1949; Slattery et al. 1956). The patients with haemangiopericytoma should be followed much longer than 5 years, as these tumours are known to recur several years after the original surgery. The patient with a vulval tumour was treated by vaginal hysterectomy, repair of the perineum and rectocele, excision of labial haemangiopericytoma and Bartholin's gland (De Sousa and Lash 1959). One patient had radical hysterectomy but developed metastasis 14 years later (Reymond et al. 1972).

11.2.1.15 Desmoid Tumour of the Vulva

Desmoid tumour is a non-metastasising, locally invasive, fibroblastic mass arising from the musculo-aponeurotic tissue of the body. About half (Reitamo et al. 1982) to two-thirds of these tumours occur in the abdominal wall (Caldwell 1976), but they can appear in any part of the body. Extra-abdominal desmoids show a predilection for the shoulder girdle, upper arm, buttock and thigh (McDougall and McGarrity 1979). Although commonly unicentric, multicentric extra-abdominal desmoids have occasionally been reported as sporadic (Barber et al. 1973; McDougall and McGarrity 1979) and familial (Zayid and Dihmis 1969; Gaches and Burke 1971).

Individuals of any age may be affected; two-thirds of the patients are between 20 and 40 years old (Brasfield and Das Gupta 1969). Although desmoid tumours occur predominantly among women (Pearman and Mayo 1941; Das Gupta et al. 1969), they are uncommon in the female genitalia. Kfuri et al. (1981) reported a desmoid tumour in the right vulva of a 19-year-old woman who sought medical advice for intermittent vulval pain for 3 years. An irregular mass about 6 cm in diameter was discovered in her right labia majora which was incompletely removed and found histologically to infiltrate the skin and round ligament.

The aetiology of the condition is not known. Pregnancy, trauma and hormones have all been suggested. Desmoid tumour is a well-known component of Gardner's syndrome, which is characterised by familial polyposis, desmoid tumour, osteoma and sebaceous cysts (Smith 1958).

There is considerable variation in the presentation of the condition. The majority of patients complain of an asymptomatic, firm mass of months or years' duration. Occasionally, a rapidly growing mass causing discomfort may be noticed. Pain and pressure symptoms may prompt the patient to see her physician.

11.2.1.15.1 Gross Appearance

The lesions are circumscribed but unencapsulated and located within the musculo-aponeurotic spaces with their long axis disposed along the direction of the muscle bundles. The tumour is usually hard, tough and greyish-white to pinkish in appearance. The cut surface is grey and fibrous with mucoid and cystic changes.

11.2.1.15.2 Microscopical Appearance

The tumour is composed of interlacing bundles and fascicles of spindle-shaped fibrous tissue (Fig. 11.23) with abundant collagenous stroma, often trapping attenuated bundles of striated muscle fibres. The spindle-shaped tumour cells contain a moderate amount of cytoplasm, spindle-shaped nuclei and inconspicuous nucleoli. Mitotic figures are not seen or are very rare. Cellularity varies in different areas of the tumour; the actively growing area tends to be somewhat more cellular. Myxoid changes may be seen scatteredly and may be prominent in some areas. The peripheral margins of the tumour are irregular due to infiltrations into the adjacent muscle bundles, which become atrophied and ultimately are engulfed. The tumour appears hypovascular, but mature blood vessels can be seen scattered in the tumour. Involvement of the skin and subcutaneous tissue by the desmoid is usually rare.

The tumour is differentiated from fibrosarcoma by its uniform growth pattern and lack of pleomorphism and mitotic figures. Differentiation from keloids is sometimes difficult. Keloids are composed of mature, hyalinised, fibrous tissue and are relatively acellular, with a paucity of blood vessels.

In ultrastructural studies (Stiller and Katenkamp 1975; Goelner and Soule 1980), the constituent cells appear as essentially elongated fibroblasts with slender processes. The cytoplasm often contains dilated endoplasmic reticulum with fibrillar content, smooth endoplasmic reticulum containing collagen fibrils and myofilaments with dense bodies. The nuclei are irregular and convoluted in outlines with condensed peripheral chromatins and contain large nucleoli.

11.2.1.15.3 Behaviour

Whether the desmoid tumour should be called a benign, malignant or low grade fibrosarcoma is still undecided. The tumour is unencapsulated and infiltrates locally but does not metastasise. The recurrence rate is high and has varied in different series from 19% (Das Gupta et al. 1969) to 57% (Enzinger and Shiraki 1967) and has been attributed to incomplete excision of the lesion (Hunt et al. 1960). The tumour has been noted to recur up to five times in some patients (Hunt et al. 1960).

11.2.1.15.4 Treatment

The treatment is surgical. Microscopic infiltrations into the surrounding tissues cannot often be detected macroscopically (Cole and Guiss 1969). Resectable desmoid should therefore be excised with generous normal tissue margins around the tumour (Berardi and Canlas 1973; Einola et al. 1979). Radiotherapy has been claimed to control the recurrences and virtually cause complete regression of the tumour (Wara et al. 1977). Radiation has also been advocated in non-resectable desmoids (Hill et al. 1973). Others have not found this modality of treatment to be useful (Dahn et al. 1963; Brewster and Ivins 1975). The role of hormones in treatment has not been clearly established (McAdam and Goligher 1970).

11.3 Tumour-like Conditions

11.3.1 Benign Enlargement of Labia Majora

Enlargement of the labia due to varicosities can occur during pregnancy (Kearns 1940) and as a developmental disorder (Jeffcoate 1975). The labia majora can attain the size of a hen's egg with tortuous large varicose veins on the surface as well as beneath the skin. The whole mass appears purplish-blue (Warner and Bancroft 1950) and fleshy. This is to be differentiated from Bartholin's cyst, endometriosis, labial hernia and neurofibroma. A developmental disorder of accessory growth of the labia majora involving the posterior commissure was reported in a 26-year-old woman whose main complaint was vaginal growth and dyspareunia (De Beer 1948).

Microscopically, the dermis and subcutaneous tissue are thickened due to a bulky increase of connective tissue. The veins are dilated and tortuous with an increase of the intervening supporting tissue (Fig. 11.24).

11.3.1.1 Treatment

Excision may be necessary for cosmetic reasons. Excessive local haemorrhage may be a surgical complication.

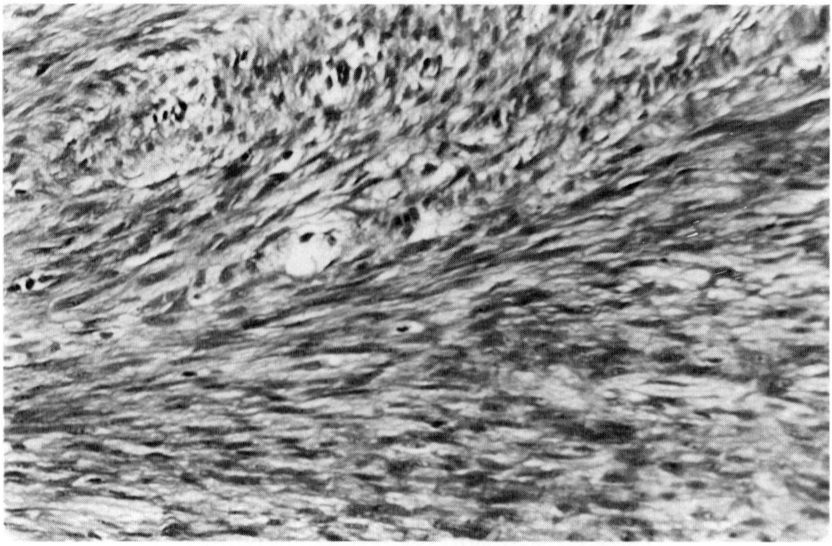

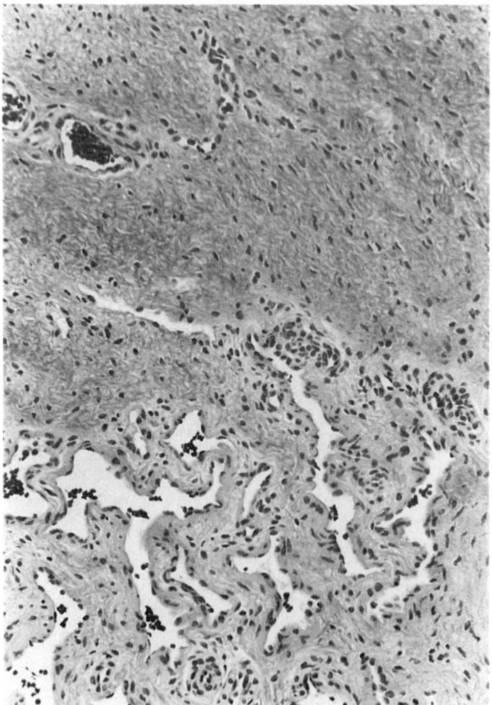

Fig. 11.23. Desmoid tumour: bundles of interlacing fibrocollagenous tissue

Fig. 11.24. Labial hypertrophy: hyperplastic connective tissue containing vascular spaces

11.3.2 Benign Enlargement of Labia Minora

Labial enlargement may occasionally be seen in young girls without any obvious cause. This has been variously thought to be due to a developmental defect (Jeffcoate 1975), excessive masturbation (Janovski and Doublas 1972) and post-filarial infections (Radman 1976). Taussig (1931) mentioned Hottentot's apron caused by the practice of manipulations of the parts by weight or manual stretching. The two young women with labial enlargement reported by Honore and O'Hara (1978) presented with labial discomfort and tenderness, and one 49-year-old woman reported by Gowen and Martin (1988) complained of pain, discomfort and difficulty in maintaining hygiene during menstruation. A developmental defect has been attributed as the main aetiological factor.

Microscopically, the labial tissue shows diffuse hyperplasia and hypertrophy of non-hair-bearing sebaceous glands which extend deep into the erectile fibromuscular tissue. The paillary and reticular dermis contains an excessive amount of collagen and reticulin. The superficial epidermis is acanthotic with hyperpigmentation (Honore and O'Hara 1978).

11.3.3 Clitoral Enlargement

Enlargment of the clitoris may be congenital due to idiopathic female intersex (Huben et al. 1981), true and pseudohermaphroditism and tumours like lipoma, neurofibroma and haemangioendothelioma (Haddad and Jones 1960).

11.3.4 Tumoral Calcinosis of the Vulva

Tumoral calcinosis is a large nodular mass of calcareous material in the subcutaneous tissue around the vicinity of the major joints. The disease tends to be familial and associated with hyperphosphatemia (Mazaffarian et al. 1972). The exact aetiology, however, is not known.

Clinically, the lesion is usually asymptomatic and slow growing over the years but may grow rapidly, attaining a large size in a few months (McClatchie and Bremner 1969). The majority of patients are young; only a few are 50 years old or older (Hacihanefioglu 1978).

The female genitalia is a rare site for these lesions. Clair and Majumdar (1980) reported two lesions, one occurring as a painful swelling on the left labia majora of a 53-year-old woman and the other as a swelling in the right inguinal area in a 67-year-old patient who also had endometrial carcinoma. In both patients, the lesion was suspected to be metastatic carcinoma. The sub-cutaneous masses were 4 cm in maximum diameter, circumscribed and hard.

Microscopically, the lesions are composed of amorphous calcific granular material (Fig. 11.25) with collections of multinucleate giant cells.

11.3.4.1 Treatment

Complete excision is the treatment of choice. Partial excision may be complicated by recurrence (Clair and Majumdar 1980).

11.3.5 Nodular Fasciitis of the Vulva

Nodular fasciitis, also known as pseudosarcomatous fibromatosis (Konwaler et al. 1955), is an uncommon lesion of the genital tract. This benign condition is characterised by nodular, tumour-like proliferations of fibrous tissue occurring commonly in the subcutaneous fascia of the extremities, trunk and neck.

The peak incidence occurs between 20 and 29 years of age (Allen 1972), although the lesions have been noticed in patients of a wide range of age, from 1 to 76 years old (Shimizu et al. 1984). Clinically, the lesion has a sudden onset and grows rapidly within a few weeks or months, raising suspicion of a malignant tumour. The patients with a vulval tumour were teenagers and had a short history of an asymptomatic tumour located on the labia majora and adjacent labia minora (LiVolsi and Brooks 1987).

11.3.5.1 Gross Appearance

The size of the lesion varies from less than 1 cm to 3 cm, with a mean of 1.5 cm. The lesion is a single, unencapsulated, round to ovoid nodule, firm rubbery to hard in consistency. The cut surface may be solid, gelatinous or myxoid and presents a grey-tan to flesh-pink appearance.

11.3.5.2 Microscopical Appearance

Nodular fasciitis presents a few diagnostic features which include (i) proliferations of spinde-shaped and plump fibroblasts in interlacing bundles and whorled curved fascicles (Fig. 11.26) – the fibroblasts contain abundant cytoplasm, oval and round nuclei with small nucleoli and may be bipolar or multipolar; (ii) cleft or slit-like spaces between the fibroblasts, which are not lined by endothelial cells and contain extravasated red blood cells and mucoid material (Fig. 11.27); (iii) mucoid ground substance which may be abundant. Price et al. (1961) divided these lesions into myxoid, cellular and fibrous types, while Bernstein and Lattes (1982) recognised four histological subtypes – reactive, densely cellular, those with osteoid or collagenous metaplasia and proliferative fasciitis. In a single lesion, cellular, hypocellular and storiform patterns may be seen. Mitoses are common, and according to Allen (1972), the diagnosis of nodular fasciitis should not be made in the absence of mitoses unless the lesion is hypocellular, hyalinised or fibrosed or there are cystic changes. Although bizarre cells are not seen, multinucleate giant cells are not uncommon. Lymphocytes, plasma cells and macrophages are frequently seen.

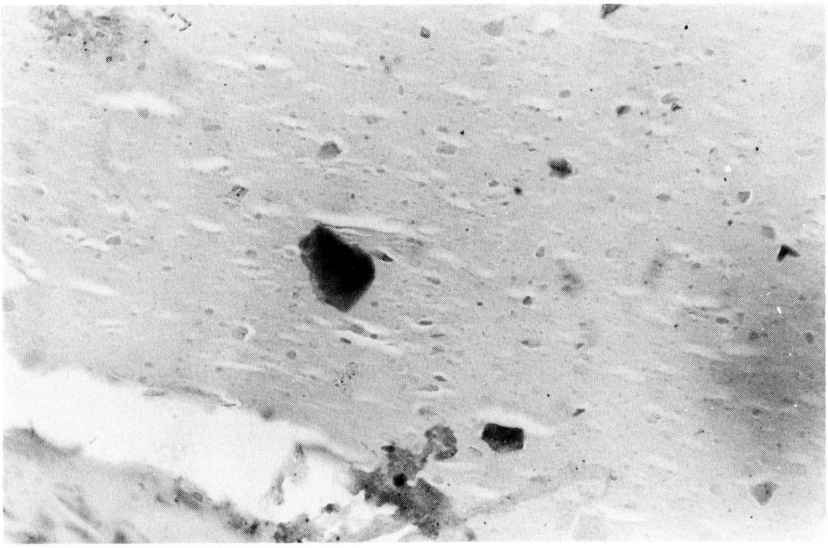

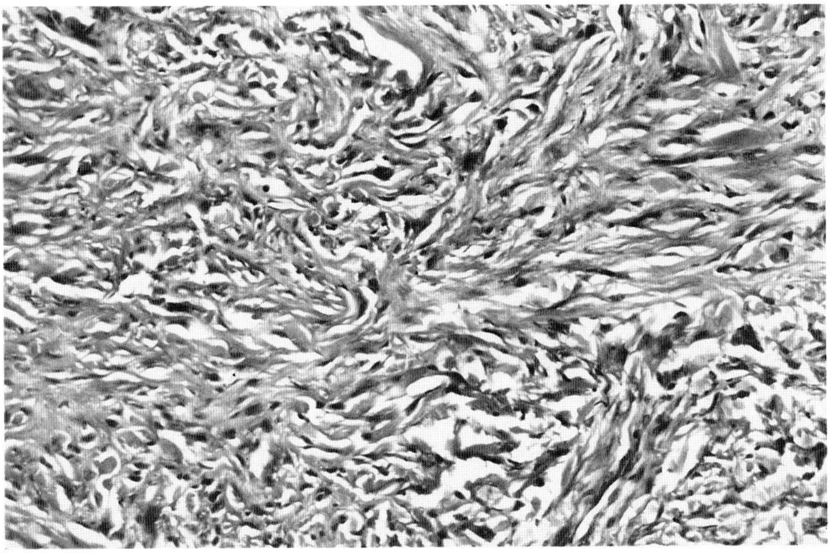

Fig. 11.25. Tumoral calcinosis. Calcium deposits in an amorphous background

Fig. 11.26. Nodular fasciitis: bundles and whorled fascicles of fibroblastic cells

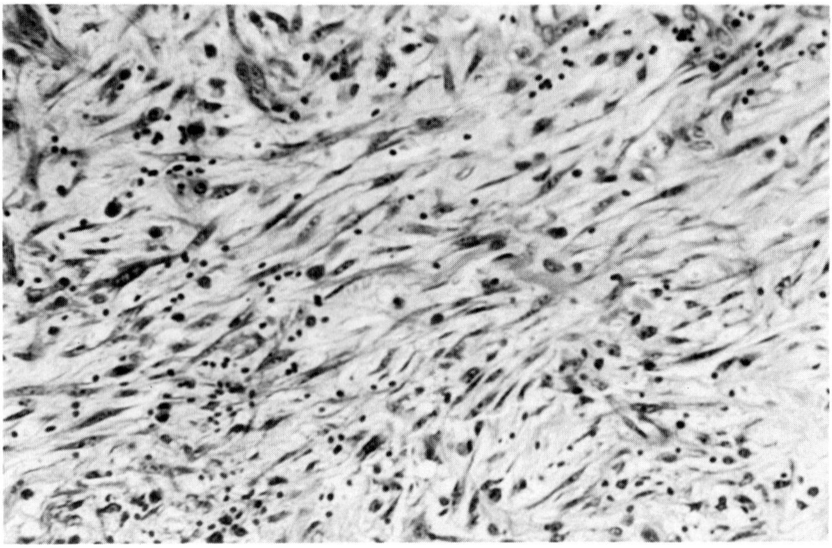

Fig. 11.27. Nodular fasciitis extravasated red blood cells and abundant mucoid material

The stroma is made of dense reticulin fibres and scanty collagen. Newly formed blood vessels, some of which are also dilated, are noticed scattered in the lesion.

The aetiology of this condition is unknown.

11.3.5.3 Treatment

Local excision is adequate, and recurrence is rare.

11.3.6 Traumatic Neuroma

Traumatic neuroma develops following trauma or severence of nerve fibres, where the proximal ends of the nerve fibres fail to meet the distal ends. This results in the formation of a tangled mass of neural tissue consisting of axons, Schwann cells and nerve sheath fibrous tissue.

Traumatic neuroma occurs commonly in the extremities and infrequently in the internal organs. Its appearance in the female genitalia is rare. I have seen only one case of vulval neuroma, which occurred after radical vulvectomy for vulval carcinoma.

11.3.6.1 Treatment

The lesion is to be excised.

11.3.7 Lymph Node Hyperplasia

Originally described as benign mediastinal lymph node hyperplasia (Castleman et al. 1956), this condition occurs less frequently in the lymph nodes of other sites (Dorfman and Warnke 1974). It is also uncommon in the soft tissues. In the female genital tract the lesion has been reported from the vulva of a 20-year-old woman who presented with a cystic mass of left labium majus of 8 years' duration (Kernen and Morgan 1970). The lesions have also been reported from the soft tissues of the female pelvis (Giaretta et al. 1971; Tsukamoto et al. 1980).

The two morphological types – hyaline vascular and plasma cell types – have been correlated with the clinical manifestations of the condition. The majority of patients with this type of lymphoid hyperplasia show a hyaline vascular type of lesion. They are usually asymptomatic. The lesions are detected incidentally during chest X-ray for other reasons. A few patients may present with pressure symptoms or rarely with pleural effusions. The plasma cell type commonly occurs in the mediastinum but may be multifocal (Gaba et al. 1978). The patients with this type of lesion tend to develop haematological abnormalities such as hypergammaglobinaemia, refractory anaemia, leucocytosis, thrombocytosis, splenomegaly (Kahn et al. 1973) and peripheral neuropathy (Yu and Carson 1976). Patients of both groups may complain of pyrexia.

The patients are of a wide age range, from childhood to octogenerian.

The nature of the condition is uncertain. An infectious process, hamartoma (Lattes and Pachter 1962) and neoplasia (Zettergren 1961) have been suggested. Immunosuppressed patients have been observed to develop the plasma cell type lesion which has been suggested to be a response to viral infections (Francis et al. 1988).

11.3.7.1 Gross Appearance

The lesion is an irregular, firm mass several centimeters in diameter. The vulval lesion is a sub-cutaneous mass about 3 cm in size with uniform, tan-coloured cut surfaces (Kernen and Morgan 1970).

11.3.7.2 Microscopical Appearance

In the hyaline vascular type, the nodal features are characterised by an increase in the number of lymphoid follicles which replace the whole node. The follicles are small, with their germinal centres transfixed by the radially penetrating capillaries which are ensheathed by hyalinised collagen. The germinal centres, as a result, look like Hassall's corpuscles (Keller et al. 1972). Around many of these germinal centres, there are concentric layers of mature lymphocytes arranged in onion-skin fashion. The interfollicular areas are vascular and contain many blood vessels lined by swollen endothelium. Plasma cells and eosinophils in variable number are also seen in these areas. In the plasma cell type lesions, the germinal centres are large and contain reactive lymphocytes with mitoses and histiocytes. Vascularisation of the germinal centres has not been noticed. Diffuse sheets of plasma cells are prominent features in the interfollicular areas. The soft tissue lesions also display a similar histological appearance. The reported vulval lesion was of the hyaline vascular type (Kernen and Morgan 1970).

11.3.7.3 Treatment

Complete surgical excision has been advocated (Keller et al. 1972).

11.3.8 Reactive Fibrohistiocytic Proliferation Simulating Histiocytoma

Occasionally, fibrohistiocytic proliferations may assume regular organoid or bizarre appearances which may simulate benign or malignant tumours. Many of these lesions are reactive in response to foreign material like silica or even to surgical manoeuvres. Some occur spontaneously. They can appear at different parts of the body but are very infrequent in the female genital tract.

The fibrohistiocytic lesion occurring at the site of previous surgery grows as an ill-defined nodule of average 1–3 cm in diameter. Histologically, it consists of bundles of spindle-shaped cells arranged in storiform pattern or intersecting fascicles of spindle cells (Snover et al. 1981; Proppe et al. 1984). A mild degree of cellular pleomorphism and mitotic figures may occasionally be noticed and lead to a mistaken diagnosis of malignancy. The overall bland appearance of the cells and the presence of acute or chronic inflammatory cells which are always noticed should point towards the benign nature of the lesion. The foreign body type of giant cells may also be seen.

References

General

Bernstein P (1939) Sarcoma of the vulva. Am J Surg 45:591–593

Cramer DW, Cutler SJ (1974) Incidence and histopathology of malignancies of the female genital organs in the United States. Am J Obstet Gynecol 118:443–460

Davos I, Abell MR (1976) Soft tissue sarcomas of the vulva. Gynecol Oncol 4:70–86

DiSaia PJ, Rutledge F, Smith JP (1971) Sarcoma of the vulva: report of 12 patients. Obstet Gynecol 38:180–184

Gallup DG, Abell MR, Morley GW (1974) Epitheliod sarcoma of the vulva. Obstet Gynacol 48 [Suppl]:14–17

Lundwall F (1961) Cancer of the vulva: a clinical review. Acta Radiol [Suppl] 208:1–326

Nolan RP (1957) Primary non pigmented sarcoma of the vulva with a report of a case complicating pregnancy. Am J Obstet Gynecol 73:134–140

Priore R, Patton GD, Conti EA (1966) Pregnancy complicated by non pigmented sarcoma of the vulva: report of a case and review of literature. Obstet Gynecol 27:420–427

Leiomyosarcoma
Audet-Lapointe P, Paquin F, Guerarad M-J et al. (1980) Leiomyosarcoma of the vulva. Gynecol Oncol 10:350–355
Berlin O, Stenner B, Kindblom L-G et al. (1984) Leiomyosarcoma of venous origin in the extremities. Cancer 54:2147–2159
Dahl I, Angervall L (1974) Cutaneous and subcutaneous leiomyosarcoma: a clinicopathologic study of 47 patients. Pathol Eur 9:307–315
Davos I, Abell MR (1976) Soft tissue sarcomas of vulva. Gynecol Oncol 4:70–86
Denk H, Krepler R, Artileb D et al. (1983) Proteins of intermediate filaments: an immunohistochemical and biochemical approach to the classification of soft tissue tumours. Am J Pathol 110:93–208
DiSaia PJ, Rutledge F, Smith JP (1971) Sarcoma of vulva: report of 12 patients. Obstet Gynecol 38:180–184
Fields JP, Helwig EB (1981) Leiomyosarcoma of the skin and subcutaneous tissue. Cancer 47:156–169
Gompel C, Silverberg SG (1977) Pathology in gynecology and obstetrics, 2nd edn. Lippicott, Philadelphia, p 37
Hashimoto H, Daimaru Y, Tsuneyoshi M et al. (1986) Leimyosarcoma of the external soft tissue. Cancer 57:2077–2088
Knapp RH, Wick MR, Goelner JR (1984) Leiomyoblastomas and their relationship to other smooth muscle tumors of gastrointestinal tract: an electronmicroscopic study. Am J Surg Pathol 8:449–461
Miettinen M (1988) Immunoreactivity for cytokeratin and epithelial membrane antigen in leiomyosarcoma. Arch Pathol Lab Med 112:637–640
Stout AP, Hill WT (1958) Leimyosarcoma of the superficial soft tissues. Cancer 11:844–854
Swanson PE, Stanley MW, Scheithauer BW et al. (1988) Primary cutaneous leiomyosarcoma: an electron and immunohistochemical study of 9 cases with ultrastructural correlation. J Cutan Pathol 15:129–141
Tavassoli FA, Norris HJ (1979) Smooth muscle tumors of the vulva. Obstet Gynecol 53:213–217
Varela-Duran JV, Oliva H, Rosai J (1979) Vascular leimyosarcoma, the malignant counterpart of vascular leiomyoma. Cancer 44:1684–1691
Witt MJ (1967) Sarcoma of the vulva. Proc R Soc Med 60:40–41

Malignant Fibrous Histiocytoma
Bertoni F, Capanna R, Biazini R et al. (1985) Malignant fibrous histiocytoma of soft tissue: an analysis of 78 cases located and deeply seated in the extremities. Cancer 56:356–367
Davos I, Abell MR (1976) Soft tissue sarcomas of the vulva. Gynecol Oncol 4:70–86
DiSaia PJ, Rutledge F, Smith JP (1971) Sarcoma of the vulva. Obstet Gynecol 38:180–184
Enzinger FM, Weiss SW (1983) Soft tissue tumors. Mosby, St Louis, pp 166–198
Fu Y-S, Gabbiani G, Kaye GI et al. (1975) Malignant soft tissue tumors of probable histiocytic origin (malignant fibrous histiocytomas): general considerations and electron microscopic and tissue culture studies. Cancer 35:176–198
Halpern J, Kopolvic J, Catane R (1984) Malignant fibrous histiocytomas developing in irradiated sacral chordoma. Cancer 53:2661–2662
Hensley GT, Friedrich EG Jr (1973) Malignant fibroxanthoma: a sarcoma of the vulva. Am J Obstet Gynecol 116:289–291
Hoffman MA, Dickersin GR (1983) Malignant fibrous histiocytomas: an ultrastructural study of eleven cases. Hum Pathol 14:913–922
Inoshita T, Youngberg GA (1984) Malignant fibrous histiocytoma arising in previous surgical sites: report of two cases. Cancer 53:176–183

Kearney MM, Soule EH, Ivins JC (1980) Malignant fibrous histiocytoma: a retrospective study of 167 cases. Cancer 45:167–178

Kempson RL, Kyriakos M (1972) Fibroxanthosarcoma of the soft tissues: a type of malignant fibrous histiocytoma. Cancer 29:961–976

Kindblom L-G, Jacobsoen GK, Jacobsen M (1982) Immunohistochemical investigation of tumors of supposed fibroblastic histiocytic origin. Hum Pathol 13:834–840

Kyriakos M, Kempson RL (1976) Inflammatory fibrous histiocytoma: an aggressive and lethal lesion. Cancer 37:1584–1606

Lawson CW, Fisher C, Gatter KC (1987) An immunohistochemical study of differentiation in malignant fibrous histiocytoma. Histopathology 11:375–383

Lee Y-S, Phoo RWH, Nather A (1984) Malignant fibrous histiocytoma of previous metal implant. Cancer 54:2286–2289

Malfetano JH, Dick AB, Hussain M (1986) Vulvar fibrous histiocytoma of low grade malignancy: case report. Br J Obstet Gynaecol 93:642–645

Markhede G, Angervall L, Stener B (1982) A multivirate analysis of surgical treatment of malignant soft tissue tumors. Cancer 49:1721–1733

Merkow LP, Frich JC, Silekin M et al. (1971) Ultrastructure of a fibroxanthoma (malignant fibroxanthoma). Cancer 28:372–383

O'Brien JE, Stout AP (1964) Malignant fibrous xanthomas. Cancer 17:1445–1458

Rydholm A, Syk I (1986) Malignant fibrous histiocytoma of soft tissue: correlation between clinical variables and histologic malignancy grade. Cancer 57:2323–2324

Sakamoto K (1986) Malignant fibrous histiocytoma induced by intraarticular injection of 9, 10- dimethyl-1,2-benzathracene in the rat. Cancer 57:2313–2322

Santa Cruz DJ, Kyriakos M (1981) Aneurysmal (angiomatoid) fibrous histiocytoma of the skin. Cancer 47:2053–2061

Santala M, Suino S, Syrjanaen K et al. (1987) Malignant fibrous histiocytoma of the vulva. Gynecol Oncol 27:121–126

Taylor RN, Bottles K, Miller TR (1985) Malignant fibrous histiocytoma of the vulva. Obstet Gynecol 66:145–148

Weiss SW, Enzinger FM (1978) Malignant fibrous histiocytoma: an analysis of 200 cases. Cancer 41:2250–2266

Fibrosarcoma

Bizer LS (1971) Fibrosarcoma: report of sixty four cases. Am J Surg 121:586–587

Burns WA, Kanhouwa S, Tillman L et al. (1972) Fibrosarcoma occurring at the site of plastic vascular graft. Cancer 29:66–72

Davos I, Abell MR (1976) Soft tissue sarcoma of vulva. Gynecol Oncol 4:70–86

DiSaia PJ, Rutledge F, Smith JP (1971) Sarcoma of the vulva. Obstet Gynecol 38:180–184

Gonzalez-Crussi F (1970) Ultrastructure of congenital fibrosarcoma. Cancer 26:1289–1299

Heller EL, Sieber WK (1950) Fibrosarcoma: a clinical and pathological study of sixty cases. Surgery 27:539–545

Keller J (1951) Fibrosarcoma labium vulvae. Can Med Assoc J 64:534–536

Mackenzie DH (1964) Fibroma a dangerous diagnosis: a review of 205 cases of fibrosarcoma of soft tissues. Br J Surg 51:607–612

Morris JM, Lucas DB (1964) Fibrosarcoma within a sinus tract of chronic draining osteomyelitis. J Bone Joint Surg [Am] 46:853–857

Oberman HA, Oneal RM (1970) Fibrosarcoma of the chest wall following resection and irradiation of cancer of the breast. Am J Clin Pathol 53:407–412

Priore RM, Patton GD, Conti EA (1966) Pregnancy complicated by nonpigmented sarcoma of the vulva, report of a case and review of the ltierature. Obstet Gynecol 27:420–427

Pritchard DJ, Soule EH, Taylor WF et al. (1974) Fibrosarcoma – a clinicopathologic and statistical study of 199 tumours of the soft tissues of the extremities and trunk. Cancer 33:888–897

Schwartz EE, Rothstein JD (1968) Fibrosarcoma following radiation therapy. JAMA 203: 296–298
Soule EH, Pritchard DJ (1977) Fibrosarcoma in infants and children: a review of 110 cases. Cancer 40:1711–1721
Stout AP (1948) The malignant tumor of fibroblasts. Cancer 1:30–63
Van der Werf-Messing B, van Unnik JAM (1965) Fibrosarcoma of the soft tissue: a clinicopathologic study. Cancer 18:1113–1123
Woodruff JD, Brack CB (1958) Unusual malignancies of vulvourethral region. Report of twelve cases. Obstet Gynecol 12:677–686

Liposarcoma

Battifora H, Nunez-Alonso C (1980) Myxoid liposarcoma: a study of ten cases. Ultrastruct Pathol 1:157–169
Bolen JW, Thorning D (1984) Liposarcoma: a histogenetic approach to the classification of adipose tissue neoplasms. Am J Surg Pathol 8:3–17
Brooks JJ, LiVolsi VA (1987) Liposarcoma presenting on the vulva. Am J Obstet Gynecol 156:73–75
Castleberry RP, Kelly DR, Wilson ER et al. (1984) Childhood liposarcoma: a report of a case and review of the literature. Cancer 54:579–584
Davos I, Abell MR (1976) Soft tissue sarcoma of the vulva: report of 12 patients. Obstet Gynecol 38:180–184
DiSaia PJ, Rutledge F, Smith JP (1971) Sarcoma of the vulva. Obstet Gynecol 38:180–184
Enterline HT, Culberson JD, Rochlin DB et al. (1960) Liposarcoma: a clinical and pathological study of 53 cases. Cancer 13:932–950
Enzinger FM, Weiss SW (1982) Liposarcoma. In: Soft tissue tumors. Mosby, St. Louis, pp 242–280
Enzinger FM, Winslow DJ (1962) Liposarcoma: a study of 103 cases. Virchows Arch [A] 335:367–388
Evans HL (1979) Liposarcoma: a study of 55 cases with re-assessment of its classification. Am J Surg Pathol 3:507–523
Genton CY, Maroni ES (1987) Vulval liposarcoma. Arch Gynecol 240:63–66
Gompel C, Silverberg SG (1977) Pathology in gynecology and obstetrics, 2nd edn. Lippincott, Philadelphia, p 37
Gondos B, Casey B (1982) Liposarcoma of the vulva. Am J Obstet Gynecol 33:1017–1026
Hashimoto H, Enjoji M (1982) Liposarcoma: a clinicopathologic subtyping of 52 cases. Acta Pathol Jpn 32:933–948
Kindblom L-G, Angervall L, Svendsen P (1975) Liposarcoma: a clinicopathologic, radiographic and prognostic study. Acta Pathol Microbiol Scand A [Suppl] 253:1–69
Krall RA, Kostianavsky M, Patchefsky AS (1981) Synovial sarcoma: a clinical, pathological and ultrastructural study of 26 cases supporting recognition of a monophasic variant. Am J Surg Pathol 5:137–151
Legace R, Jacob S, Seemayer TA (1979) Myxoid liposarcoma: an electron microscopic study. Biologic and histologic considerations. Virchows Arch [A] 384:159–172
Pack GT, Pierson JC (1954) Liposarcoma: study of 105 cases. Surgery 36:687–712
Reitan JB, Kaalhus O, Brennhovd IO et al. (1985) Prognostic factors in liposarcoma. Cancer 55:2482–2490
Reszel PA, Soule EH, Coventry MB (1966) Liposarcoma of the extremities and limb girdles. J Bone Joint Surg [Am] 48:229–244
Rossouw D, Cinti S, Dickrersin GR (1986) Liposarcoma: an ultrastructural study of 15 cases. Am J Clin Pathol 85:f649–667
Spittle MF, Newton KA, Mackenzie DH (1971) Liposarcoma: a review of 60 cases. Br J Cancer 24:696–704
Taussig FJ (1937) Sarcoma of the vulva. Am J Obstet Gynecol 33:1017–1026

Epithelioid Sarcoma

Blewitt RW, Aparacio SGR, Bird CC (1983) Epithelioid sarcoma: a tumor of myofibroblasts. Histopathology 7:573–584

Bloustein PA, Silverberg SG, Waddell WR (1976) Epithelioid sarcoma: a case results with ultrastructural review, histogenetic discussion and chemotherapeutic data. Cancer 38:2390–2400

Enzinger FM (1970) Epithelioid sarcoma simulating granuloma or carcinoma. Cancer 26:1029–1041

Fisher ER, Horwat B (1972) The fibrocytic derivation of the so-called epithelioid sarcoma. Cancer 30:1074–1081

Frable WJ, Kay S, Lawrence W et al. (1973) Epithelioid sarcoma: an electron microscopic study. Arch Pathol Lab Med 75:8–12

Gabbiani G, Fu Y-S, Kaye GI et al. (1972) Epithelioid sarcoma: a light and electron microscopic study suggesting a synovial origin. Cancer 30:486–499

Gallup PG, Abell MR, Morley GW (1976) Epithelioid sarcoma of the vulva. Obstet Gynecol 48 [Suppl]:14–17

Hall DG, Grimes MM, Goplerud DR (1980) Epithelioid sarcoma of the vulva. Gynecol Oncol 9:237–246

Manivel JC, Wick MR, Dehner LP (1987) Epithelioid sarcoma: an electron microscopic study. Am J Clin Pathol 87:319–326

Meis JM, Mackay B, Ordonez NG (1988) Epithelioid sarcoma: an immunohistochemical and ultrastructural study. Surg Pathol 1:13–31

Miettinen M, Lehto V-P, Vartio T et al. (1982) Epithelioid sarcoma: ultrastructural and immunohistological features. Arch Pathol Lab Med 106:620–623

Piver MS, Tsukada Y, Barlow J (1972) Epithelioid sarcoma of the vulva. Obstet Gynecol 40:839–842

Prat J, Woodruff JM, Marcove RC (1978) Epithelioid sarcoma: an analysis of 22 cases indicating prognostic significance of vascular invasion and regional lymph node metastasis. Cancer 41:1472–1487

Santiago H, Feinerman LK, Lattes R (1972) Epithelioid sarcoma: a clinical and pathologic study of 9 cases. Human Pathol 3:133–147

Shimm DS, Suit H (1983) Radiation therapy of epithelioid sarcoma. Cancer 52:1022–1025

Soule EH, Enriquez P (1972) Atypical fibrous histiocytoma, malignant fibrous histiocytoma, malignant histiocytoma and epithelioid sarcoma. Cancer 30:128–143

Malignant Schwannoma

Chandrasoma P, Shibata D, Radin R et al. (1986) Malignant peripheral nerve sheath tumor arising in an adrenal ganglioneuroma in an adult homosexual. Cancer 51:2022–2025

Chen KTK, Latorraca R, Fabrich D et al. (1980) Malignant Schwannoma: a light microscopic and ultrastructural study. Cancer 45:1585–1593

Cross PA, Clarke NW (1988) Malignant nerve sheath tumour with epithelial elements. Histopathology 12:547–561

D'Agostino AN, Soule EH, Miller RH (1963) Sarcomas of the peripheral nerves and somatic tissues associated with multiple neurofibromatosis (von Recklinghausen's disease). Cancer 16:1015–1027

Davos I, Abell MR (1976) Soft tissue tumours of the vulva. Gynecol Oncol 4:70–86

Dewit L, Albus-Lutter CE, Jong ASH, Voute PA (1986) Malignant Schwannoma with rhabdomyoblastic component: a so-called triton tumor: a clinicopathologic study. Cancer 58:1350–1356

DiSaia PJ, Rutledge F, Smith JP (1971) Sarcoma of the vulva: report of 12 patients. Obstet Gynecol 38:180–184

Ducatman BS, Scheithauer BW (1983) Postirradiation neurofibrosarcoma. Cancer 51:1028–1033

Ducatman BS, Scheithauer BW (1984) Malignant peripheral nerve sheath tumors with divergent differentiation. Cancer 54:1049–1057

Ducatman BS, Scheithauer BW, Piepgras DG et al. (1986) Malignant nerve sheath tumors: a clinicopathologic study of 120 cases. Cancer 57:2006–2021

Erlandson RA, Woodruff JM (1982) Peripheral nerve sheath tumours: an electron microscopic study of 43 cases. Cancer 49:273–287

Fletcher CDM, Fernando IN, Braimbridge MV et al. (1988) Malignant nerve sheath tumour arising in a ganglioneuroma. Histopathology 12:449–454

Ghosh BC, Ghosh L, Huvos AG et al. (1973) Malignant Schwannoma: a clinicopathologic study. Cancer 31:184–190

Guccion JG, Enzinger FM (1979) Malignant Schwannoma associated with von Recklinghausen's neurofibromatosis. Virchows Arch [A] 383:43–54

Johnson MD, Glick AD, Davis BW (1988) Immunohistochemical evaluation of Leu 7, myelin basic protein, S-100 protein, glial fibrillary acidic protein and LN3 immunoreactivity in nerve sheath tumors and sarcomas. Arch Pathol Lab Med 112:155–160

Lawrence WD, Shingleton HM (1978) Malignant Schwannoma of the vulva: a light and electron microscopic study. Gynecol Oncol 6:527–537

Matsunou H, Shimoda T, Kakimoto S et al. (1985) Histopathologic and immunocytochemical study of malignant tumours of peripheral nerve sheath (malignant Schwannoma). Cancer 56:2269–2279

McCormack LJ, Hazard JB, Dickson JA (1954) Malignant epithelioid neurilemmoma (Schwannoma). Cancer 7:725–728

Sordillo PP, Helson L, Hajdu SI et al. (1981) Malignant Schwannoma – a clinical characteristic, survival and response to therapy. Cancer 47:2503–2509

Storm FK, Eilber FR, Mirra J et al. (1980) Neurofibrosarcoma. Cancer 45:126–129

Taxy JB, Battifora H, Trujillo Y et al. (1981) Electron microscopy in the diagnosis of malignant Schwannoma. Cancer 48:1381–1391

Vieta JO, Pack T (1951) Malignant neurilemmomas of peripheral nerves. Am J Surg 82:416–431

Wick MR, Swanson PE, Scheithauer BW et al. (1987) Malignant peripheral nerve sheath tumor. Am J Clin Pathol 87:1425–433

Rhabdomyosarcoma

Autio-Harmainon H, Apaja-Sarkkinen M, Martikainen J et al. (1986) Production of basement membrane laminin and type IV collagen by tumors of striated muscle: an immunohistochemical study of rhabdomyosarcomas of different histological types and a benign rhabdomyoma. Hum Pathol 17:1218–1224

Bell J, Averette H, Davos J et al. (1986) Genital rhabdomyosarcoma: current management and review of the literature. Obstet Gynecol 41:257–263

Bertholomew TH, Conzales ET Jr, Starling KA et al. (1979) Changing concepts in management of pelvic rhabdomyosarcoma in children. Urology 13:613–616

Brooks JJ (1982) Immunohistochemistry of soft tissue tumors; myoglobin as a tumor marker for rhabdomyosarcoma. Cancer 50:1757–1763

Bundtzen LJ, Norback DH (1982) The ultrastructure of poorly differentiated rhabdomyosarcomas: a case report and literature review. Hum Pathol 13:301–313

Copeland LJ, Gershenson DM, Saul PB et al. (1985) Sarcoma botryoides of the female genital tract. Obstet Gynecol 262–266

DiSaia PJ, Rutledge F, Smith JP (1971) Sarcoma of the vulva: report of 12 patients. Obstet Gynecol 38:180–184

Horn RC Jr, Enterline HT (1958) Rhabdomyosarcoma: a clinicopathological study and classification of 39 cases. Cancer 11:181–199

Horvat BL, Caines M, Fisher ER (1970) The ultrastructure of rhabdomyosarcoma. Am J Clin Pathol 53:555–564

James GB, Guthrie W, Buchan A (1969) Embryonic sarcoma of the vulva in an infant. J Obstet Gynecol Br Commonw 76:458–461

Ober WB, Palmer RE, Glassy FJ (1953) Rhabdomyosarcoma of the vulva and vagina. Arch Pathol 56:364–373

Priore RM, Patton GD, Conti EA (1966) Pregnancy complicated by non pigmented sarcoma of the vulva. Report of a case and review of the literature. Obstet Gynecol 27:420–427

Skalli O, Gabbiani G, Babai F et al. (1988) Intermediate filament proteins and actin isoforms as markers for soft tissue tumor differentiation and origin. II Rhabdomyoma. Am J Pathol 130:515–531

Tsokos M, Howard R, Costa J (1983) Immunohistochemical study of alveolar and embryonal rhabdomyosarcoma. Lab Invest 48:148–155

Weiss LM, Warhol M (1984) Ultrastructural distinctions between adult pleomorphic rhabdomyosarcomas, pleomorphic liposarcomas and pleomorphic malignant fibrous histiocytomas. Hum Pathol 15:1025–1033

Witt MJ (1967) Sarcoma of the vulva. Proc R Soc Med 60:40–41

Angiosarcoma

Alles JU, Bosslet K (1988) Immunochemistry of angiosarcomas: a study of 19 cases with special emphasis on the applicability of endothelial cell specific markers to routinely prepared tissues. Am J Clin Pathol 89:463–471

Chaudhuri B, Ronan SG, Manaligod JR (1980) Angiosarcoma arising in aplexiform neurofibroma: a case report. Cancer 46:605–610

Chen RTK, Hoffman KD, Hendricks EJ (1979) Angiosarcoma folliowing therapeutic irradiation. Cancer 44:2044–2048

Davos I, Abell MR (1976) Soft tissue sarcomas of vulva. Gynecol Oncol 4:70–86

Eby CS, Brennan MJ, Fine G (1967) Lymphangiosarcoma: a lethal complication of chronic lymphoedema. Arch Surg 94:223–230

Girard C, Johnson WC, Graham JH (1970) Cutaneous angiosarcoma. Cancer 26:868–883

Guarda LA, Ordonez NG, Smith L Jr et al. (1982) Immunoperoxidase localisation of factor VIII in angiosarcoma. Arch Pathol Lab Med 106:515–516

Hodgkinson DJ, Soule EH, Woods JE (1979) Cutaneous angiosarcoma of the head and neck. Cancer 44:1106–1113

Huey GR, Stehman F, Roth RM et al. (1985) Lymphangiosarcoma of the edematous thigh after radiation therapy for carcinoma of the vulva. Gynecol Oncol 20:394–401

Maddox JC, Evans HL (1981) Angiosarcoma of skin and soft tissue: a study of forty four cases. Cancer 48:1907–1921

Masse SR, Mongeau CJ, Rioux A (1977) Angiosarcoma of the breast. Can J Surg 20:341–343

McConnell EM, Haslam P (1959) Angiosarcoma in postmastectomy lymphoedema: a report of 5 cases and review of the literature. Br J Surg 46:322–332

McWilliam LJ, Harris M (1985) Granular cell angiosarcoma of the skin: histology, electron microscopy and immunochemistry of a newly recognised tumor. Histopathology 9:1205–1216

Millstein DI, Tang C-K, Campbell EW Jr (1981) Angiosarcoma developing in a patient with neurofibromatosis (von Recklinghausen's disease). Cancer 47:950–954

Paik HH, Komorowski R (1976) Hemangiosarcoma of the abdominal wall following irradiation therapy of endometrial carcinoma. Am J Clin Pathol 66:810–814

Rosai J, Sumner HW, Kostianovsky M et al. (1976) Angisoarcoma of the skin: a clinicopathologic and fine structural study. Hum Pathol 7:83–109

Rosenzweig E (1960) A rare case of vulvar sarcoma in the region of the Bartholin's gland. Gynecologia (Basel) 149:329–337

Stout AP (1943) Haemangioendothelioma: a tumor of blood vessels featuring vascular endothelial cells. Ann Surg 118:445–464

Weiss S, Enzinger FM (1982) Epithelioid hemangioendothelioma: a vascular tumor often mistaken for carcinoma. Cancer 50:970–981

Wilson-Jones E (1964) Malignant angioendothelioma of the skin. Br J Dermatol 76:21–39
Woodard AH, Ivins JC, Soule EH (1972) Lymphangiosarcoma arising in chronic lymphedematous extremities. Cancer 30:562–572

Kaposi's Sarcoma

Akhtar M, Bunuan H, Ashraf M et al. (1984) Kaposi's sarcoma in renal transplant receipients: ultrastructural and immunoperoxidase study of four cases. Cancer 53:258–266
Beckstead JH, Wood GS, Fletcher V (1985) Evidence for the origin of Kaposi's sarcoma from lymphatic endothelium. Am J Pathol 119:294–300
Cox FH, Helwig EB (1959) Kaposis's sarcoma. Cancer 12:289–298
Dictor M (1986) Kaposi's sarcoma. Virchows Arch [A] 409:23–35
Dutz W, Stout AP (1960) Kaposis's sarcoma in infants and children. Cancer 13:684–694
Facchetti F, Lucini L, Gavazzoni R et al. (1988) Immunohistochemical analysis of the role of blood vessel endothelium in the morphogenesis of cutaneous Kaposi's sarcoma. A study of 57 cases. Histopathology 12:581–593
Guarda LG, Silva EG, Ordonez NG et al. (1981) Factor VIII in Kaposis's sarcoma. Am J Clin Pathol 76:197–200
Hall DJ, Burns JC, Copelrud DR (1979) Kaposis's sarcoma of the vulva: a case report and brief review. Obstet Gynecol 54:478–482
Harrison AC, Kahn LB (1978) Myogenic cells in Kaposi's sarcoma: an ultrastructural study. J Pathol 124:151–160
Hashimoto K, Lever WF (1964) Kaposi's sarcoma: histochemical and electron microscopic studies. J Invest Dermatol 43:539–549
Kaposi M (1872) Idiopathisches multiples Pigmentsarkom der Haut. Arch Dermatol Syphilol 4:265–273
Masur H, Michelis MA, Greene JB et al. 1981) An outbreak of community acquired pneumocystis carinii pneumonia. N Engl J Med 305:1431–1438
McCarthy WD, Pack GT (1950) Malignant blood vessel tumors: report of 56 cases of angiosarcoma and Kaposi's sarcoma. Surg Gynecol Obstet 91:465–482
Mottaz JH, Zelickson AS (1966) Electron microscopic observatiosn of Kaposi's sarcoma. Acta Derm Venereol (Stockh) 46:195–200
McNutty NS, Fletcher V, Conant MA (1983) Early lesion of Kaposi's sarcoma in homosexual man. Am J Pathol 111:62–77
Mukai K, Rosai J, Burgdorf WHC (1980) Localization of factor VIII-related antigen in vascular endothelial cells using an immunoperoxidase method. Am J Surg Pathol 4:273–276
Nadji M, Morales AR, Zeigles-Weissmen J et al. (1981) Kaposis's sarcoma: immunohistochemical evidence for an endothelial origin. Arch Pathol Lab Med 105:274–275
O'Brien PH, Brasfield RD (1966) Kaposis's sarcoma. Cancer 19:1497–1502
O'Connell KM (1977) Kaposi's sarcoma histopathological study of 159 cases from Malawi. J Clin Pathol 30:687–695
O'Connell M (1977) Kaposi's sarcoma: histological study of 159 cases from Malawi. J Clin Pathol 30:687–695
Reynolds WA, Winklemann RK, Soule EH (1965) Kaposis's sarcoma: a clinicopathologic study with particular reference its relationship to the reticuloendothelial system. Medicine 44:419–443
Taylor JF, Templeton AC, Vogel CL et al. (1971) Kaposi's sarcoma in Uganda: a clinicopathological study. Int J Cancer 8:122–135
Templeton AC, Bhana D (1975) Prognosis in Kaposi's sarcoma. J NCI 55:1301–1304

Alveolar Soft Part Sarcoma

Asvall J, Hoeg K, Kleppe K et al. (1969) Alveolar soft part sarcoma. Clin Radiol 20:426–432
Auerbach HE, Brooks JJ (1987) Alveolar soft part sarcoma: a clinicopathologic and immunohistologic study. Cancer 60:66–73

Baum ES, Fickenscher L, Nackman JB et al. (1981) Pulmonary resection and chemotherapy for metastatic alveolar soft part sarcoma. Cancer 47:1946–1948

Blumberg MB, Chang CHJ (1976) Alveolar soft part sarcoma. South Med J 69:282–285

Christopherson WM, Foote FW Jr, Stewart F (1952) Alveolar soft part sarcomas: structurally characteristic tumors of uncertain histogenesis. Cancer 5:100–111

Ekfors TO, Kalimo H, Rantakokko V et al. (1979) Alveolar soft part sarcoma: a report of two cases with some histochemical and ultrastructural observations. Cancer 43:1672–1677

Fisher ER, Reidbord H (1971) Electron microscopic evidence suggesting the myogenous origin of the so-called alveolar soft part sarcoma. Cancer 27:150–159

Lieberman PH, Foote FW Jr, Stewart FW et al. (1966) Alveolar soft part sarcoma. JAMA 198:1047–1051

Morton DL (1974) Soft tissue sarcomas. In: Holland JF, Frei E III (eds) Cancer medicine. Lea and Febiger, Philadelphia, p 1845

Mukai M, Torikata C, Iri H et al. (1986) Histogenesis of alveolar soft part sarcoma: an immunochemical and biological study. Cancer 60:66–73

Rubenfeld S (1971) Radiatiaon therapy in alveolar soft part sarcoma. Cancer 28:577–580

Shen J-T, D'Ablaing G, Morrow P (1982) Alveolar soft part sarcoma of the vulva: report of first case and review of literature. Gynecol Oncol 13:120–128

Shipkey FH, Lieberman PH, Foote FW Jr et al. (1964) Ultrastructure of alveolar soft part sarcoma. Cancer 17:821–830

Smetena HF, Scott WF (1951) Malignant tumors of non chromaffin paraganglioma. Mil Surg 109:330–349

Stout AP, Lattes R (1967) Tumors of soft tissues. In: Atlas of tumor pathology; fasc 1, 2nd ser. A.F.I.P., Washington, p 180

Unni KK, Soule EH (1975) Alveolar soft part sarcoma: an electron microscopic study. Mayo Clin Proc 50:591–598

Welsh RA, Bray DM, Shipkey FH et al. (1972) Histogenesis of alveolar soft part sarcoma. Cancer 29:191–204

Wobbes T (1978) Alveolar soft part sarcoma. J Surg Oncol 10:201–204

Dermatofibrosarcoma Protuberans

Agress R, Figge DC, Tamini H et al. (1983) Dermatofibrosarcoma protuberans of the vulva. Gynecol Oncol 16:288–291

Alguacil-Garcia A, Unni K, Goellner JR (1978) Histogenesis of dermatofibrtosarcoma protuberans: an ultrastructural study. Am J Clin Pathol 69:427–434

Bednar B (1957) Storiform neurofibromas of the skin – pigmented and non pigmented. Cancer 10:368–376

Bock JE, Andreasson B, Thorn A et al. (1985) Dermatofibrosarcoma protuberans of the vulva. Gynecol Oncol 20:129–135

Bonnaebeau RC Jr, Soughton WB, Armanios AW et al. (1974) Dermatofibrosarcoma protuberans. Report of a case with pulmonary metastases and multiple intrathoracic reccurrences. Oncology 29:1–12

Brenner W, Schaeffer K, Chhabra H et al. (1975) Dermatofibrosarcoma protuberans metastatic to a regional lymphnode: report of a case and review. Cancer 36:1897–1902

Burkhardt BR, Soule EH, Winkelmann RK et al. (1966) Dermatofibrosarcoma protuberans: study of fifty six cases. Am J Surg 111:638–644

Davos I, Abell MR (1976) Soft tissue sarcomas of vulva. Gynecol Oncol 4:70–86

Dupree WB, Langloss JM, Weiss SW (1985) Pigmented dermatofibrosarcoma protuberans (Bednar tumor): a pathologic, ultrastructural and immunohistochemical study. Am J Surg Pathol 9:630–639

Frierson HF, Cooper PH (1983) Myxoid variant of dermatofibrosarcoma protuberans. Am J Surg Pathol 7:445–450

Hashimoto K, Brownstein MH, Jacobiec FA (1974) Dermatofibrosarcoma protuberans: a tumour with perineural and endoneural cell features. Arch Dermatol 110:874–885

Hertzler AE (1926) Fibrosarcomatous tumors of skin and trunk characterised by attenuated dermal surfaces. Ann Surg 84:489–496

Kindblom L-G, Jacobsen GK, Jacobsen M (1982) Immunohistochemical investigations of tumors of supposed fibroblastic histiocytic origin. Hum Pathol 13:834–840

McPeak CJ, Cruz T, Nicastri AD et al. (1967) Dermatofibrosarcoma protuberans: an analysis of 86 cases. Ann Surg 166 [Suppl] 12:803–1816

Ozzello L, Hamels J (1976) Histiocytic nature of dermatofibrosarcoma protuberans: tissue culture and electron microscopic study. Am J Clin Pathol 65:136–148

Pack GT, Tabah EJ (1951) Dermatofibrosarcoma protuberans: a report of nine cases. Arch Surg 62:391–411

Penner DW (1951) Metastasising dermatofibrosarcoma protuberans: a case report. Cancer 4:1083–1085

Soltan MH (1981) Dermatofibrosarcoma protuberans of the vulva: case report. Br J Obstet Gynaecol 88:203–205

Taylor HB, Helwig EB (1962) Dermatofibrosarcoma protuberans: a study of 115 cases. Cancer 18:712–725

Wrotnowski U, Cooper PH, Schmookler BM (1988) Fibrosarcomatous changes in dermatofibrosarcoma protuberans. Am J Surg Pathol 12:287–293

Aggressive Angiomyxoma

Begin LR, Clement PB, Kirk ME et al. (1985) Aggressive angiomyxoma of pelvic soft parts: a clinicopathologic study of nine cases. Hum Pathol 16:621–628

Hilgers RD, Pai R, Bartow SA et al. (1986) Aggressive angiomyxoma of the vulva. Obstet Gynecol 68 [Suppl]:60–62

Steeper TA, Rosai J (1983) Aggressive angiomyxoma of the female pelvis and perineum: report of nine cases of distinctive type of gynecologic soft tissue neoplasm. Am J Surg Pathol 7:463–475

Haemangiopericytoma

Angervall L, Kindblom L-G, Nielson JM et al. (1978) Hemangiopricytoma: a clinicopathologic, angiographic and microangiographic study. Cancer 42:2412–2427

Backwinkel KD, Diddams JA (1970) Hemangiopericytoma: report of a case and comprehensive review of the literature. Cancer 25:896–901

Battifora H (1973) Hemangiopericytoma: ultrastructural study of five cases. Cancer 31:1418–1432

Crocker DW, Veith FJ (1965) Mesodermal tumors associated with hypoglycemia; review of the literature and report of a case. Ann Surg 161:418–427

DeSousa LM, Lash AE (1959) Haemangiopericytoma of the vulva. Am J Obstet Gynecol 78:295–298

Gerner RE, Moore GE, Pickern JW (1974) Hemangiopericytoma. Ann Surg 179:128–132

Greene RR, Gerbie AB, Gerbie MV et al. (1970) Haemangiopericytoma of the vulva. Am J Obstet Gynecol 106:1020–1028

Hahn MJ, Dawson R, Esterly JA et al. (1973) Hemangiopericytoma: an ultrastructural study. Cancer 31:253–261

Hultberg BM, Duagaard S, Johansen HF et al. (1988) Malignant hemangiopericytomas and haemangioendotheliosarcomas: an immunohistochemical study. Histopathology 12:405–414

McMaster MJ, Soule EH, Ivins JG (1975) Hemangiopericytoma: a clinicopathologic study and long term follow up of 60 patients. Cancer 36:2232–2244

Nunnery EW, Kahn LB, Reddick RL et al. (1982) Hemangiopericytoma: a light microscopic and ultrastructural study. Cancer 47:906–914

Reymond RD, Hazra TA, Edlow DW et al. (1972) Haemangiopericytoma of the vulva with metastasis to bone 14 years later. Br J Radiol 45:765–768

Robertson PW, Klidjian A, Harding LK et al. (1967) Hypertension due to renin secreting renal tumor. Am J Med 43:963–976

Slattery LR, Aronson SG, Lowman EW et al. (1956) Hemangiopericytoma: review of abdominal cases. Am J Surg 91:985–900

Stout AP (1949) Hemangiopericytoma: a study of twenty-five new cases. Cancer 2:1027–1054

Stout AP, Murray MR (1942) Hemangiopericytoma. A vascular tumor featuring Zimmerman's pericytes. Ann Surg 116:26–33

Desmoid Tumour

Barber HM, Galasko CSB, Woods CG (1973) Multicentric extraabdominal desmoid tumours: report of two cases. J Bone Joint Surg [Br] 55:858–863

Berardi RS, Canlas M (1973) Desmoid tumour and laparotomy scar. Int Surg 58:254–256

Brasfield RD, Das Gupta TK (1969) Desmoid tumors of the anterior abdominal wall. Surgery 65:241–246

Brewster RC, Ivins JC (1975) Extra abdominal desmoid tumors: a clinicopathologic study. J Bone Joint Surg [Am] 57:1026

Caldwell EH (1976) Desmoid tumor: musculoaponeurotic fibrosis of the anterior abdominal wall. Surgery 79:104–106

Cole MN, Guiss LW (1969) Extra abdominal desmoid tumors. Arch Surg 98:530–533

Dahn I, Jonsson N, Lundh G (1963) Desmoid tumors, a series of 33 cases. Acta Chir Scand 126:305–314

Das Gupta TK, Brasfield RD, O'Hara J (1969) Extra abdominal desmoid: a clinicopathological study. Ann Surg 170:109–121

Einola S, Aho AJ, Lauren P et al. (1979) Extra abdominal desmoid tumour: report of three cases. Acta Chir Scand 145:563–569

Enzinger FM, Shiraki M (1967) Musculo-aponeurotic fibromatosis of the shoulder girdle (extraabdominal desmoid): analysis of thirty cases followed up for 10 or more years. Cancer 20:1131–1140

Gaches C, Burke J (1971) Desmoid tumour (fibroma of the abdominal wall) occurring in siblings. Br J Surg 58:495–498

Goelner JR, Soule EH (1980) Desmoid tumors: an ultrastructural study of eight cases. Hum Pathol 11:43–50

Hill DR, Newman H, Phillips TL (1973) Radiation therapy of desmoid tumors. Am J Roentgenol Radium Ther Nucl Med 117:84–89

Hunt RTN, Morgan HC, Ackerman LV (1960) Principles in the treatment of extra abdominal desmoids. Cancer 13:825–835

Kfuri A, Rosenstein N, Dorfman H et al. (1981) Desmoid tumor of the vulva. J Reprod Med 26:272–273

McAdam WAF, Goligher JC (1970) The occurrence of desmoids in patients with familial polyposis coli. Br J Surg 57:618–631

McDougall A, McGarrity G (1979) Extra abdominal desmoid tumours. J Bone Joint Surg [Br] 61:373–377

Pearman RO, Mayo CW (1942) Desmoid tumors: a clinical and pathologic study. Ann Surg 115:114–125

Reitamo JJ, Hayry P, Nykuri E et al. (1982) The desmoid tumor 1. Am J Clin Pathol 77:665–673

Smith WG (1958) Multiple polyposis, Gardner's syndrome and desmoid tumors. Dis Colon Rectum 1:323–332

Stiller D, Katenkamp D (1975) Cellular features in desmoid fibromatosis and well differentiated fibrosarcomas: an electron microscopic study. Virchows Arch [A] 369:155–164

Wara WM, Phillips TL, Hill DR et al. (1977) Desmoid tumors – treatment and prognosis. Radiology 124:225–226

Zayid I, Dihmis C (1969) Familial multicentric fibromatosis-desmoids: a report of three cases in a Jordanian family. Cancer 24:786–795

Tumour-like Conditions of Mesenchymal and Neural Origin

Benign Enlargement of Labia and Clitoris

De Beer GR (1948) An accessory growth on the posterior commissure of the labia majora. J Obstet Gynaecol Br Emp 65:36–40
Gowen RM, Martin VL (1988) Labia minora reduction in an iron lung disabled woman. Obstet Gynecol 71:488–489
Haddad HM, Jones HW Jr (1960) Clitoral enlargement simulating pseudohermaphroditism. Am Dis Child 99:282–287
Honore LH, O'Hara KE (1978) Benign enlargement of the labia minora: report of two cases. Eur J Obstet Gynecol Reprod Biol 8:61–64
Huben RP, Devine PC, Harkins GA et al. (1981) Clitoromegaly and megalourethra in idiopathic female intersex. J Urol 126:849–851
Janovski NA, Douglas CP (1972) Diseases of the vulva. Harper and Row, Hagerstown NY, p 54
Jeffcoate N (1975) Principles of gynaecology, 4th edn. Butterworth, London, p 151
Kearns PJ (1940) Some clinical lesion of the vulva. Can Med Assoc J 42:361–363
Radman H (1976) Hypertrophy of the labia minora. Obstet Gynecol 48 [Suppl]:78–80
Taussig FJ (1931) Diseases of the vulva. Gynecol Obstet Monogr 13:104–106
Warner MP, Bancroft FW (1950) Unilateral massive varicosities of the vulva in a twenty one year old virgin. NY State Med J 50:2571–2572

Tumorous Calcinosis

Clair JTS, Majumdar B (1980) Tumoral calcinosis masquerading as metastatic carcinoma. Gynecol Oncol 10:69–74
Hacihanefioglu U (1978) Tumoral calcinosis: a clinical and pathological study of eleven unreported cases in Turkey. J Bone Joint Surg [Am] 60:1131–1135
Mazaffarian G, Lafferty FW, Pearson OH (1972) Treatment of tumoral calcinosis with phosphorous derivation. Ann Intern Med 77:741–745
McClatchie S, Bremner AD (1969) Tumoral calcinosis – an unrecognised disease. Br Med J 1:153–155

Nodular Fasciitis

Allen PW (1972) Nodular fasciitis. Pathology 4:9–26
Bernstein KE, Lattes P (1982) Nodular (pseudosarcomatous) fasciitis, a nonrecurrent lesion: clinicopathologic study of 134 cases. Cancer 49:1668–1678
Konwaler BE, Keasbey L, Kaplan L (1955) Subcutaneous pseudosarcomatous fibromatosis (fasciitis): report of 8 caseds. Am J Clin Pathol 25:241–252
LiVolsi VA, Brooks JJ (1987) Nodular fasciitis of the vulva: a report of two cases. Obstet Gynecol 69:513
Price EB Jr, Silliphant WM, Shuman R (1961) Nodular fasciitis: a clinicopathologic analysis of 65 cases. Am J Clin Pathol 35:122–136
Shimizu S, Hashimoto H, Enjoji M (1984) Nodular fasciitis: an analysis of 250 patients. Pathology 16:161–166

Lymphnode Hyperplasia

Castleman B, Iverson L, Menendez V (1956) Localised mediastinal lymphnode hyperplasia resembling thymoma. Cancer 9:822–830
Dorfman RF, Warnke R (1974) Lymphadenopathy simulating the malignant lymphoma. Hum Pathol 5:519–550
Francis ND, Hollowood K, Gabriel R (1988) Angiofollicular lymphnode hyperplasia. J Clin Pathol 41:353–356

Gaba AR, Stein RS, Sweet DL et al. (1978) Multicentric giant lymphnode hyperplasia. Am J Clin Pathol 69:86–90
Giaretta MI, Hyun J, Gibson JM Jr (1971) Angiomatous lymphoid hyperplasia as pelvic mass. Obstet Gynecol 38:391–394
Kahn LB, Ranchod M, Stables DP et al. (1973) Giant lymphnode hyperplasia with haematological abnormalities. S Afr Med J 47:811–816
Keller AR, Hochholzer L, Castleman B (1972) Hyaline vascular and plasma cell types of giant lymphnode hyperplasia of the mediastinum and other locations. Cancer 29:670–683
Kerner JA, Morgan ML (1970) Benign lymphoid hamartoma of the vulva: report of a case. Obstet Gynecol 35:290–292
Lattes R, Pachter MR (1962) Benign lymphoid masses of probable hamartomatous nature: analysis of 12 cases. Cancer 15:197–214
Tsukamoto N, Iraha H, Matsuyama T et al. (1980) Giant lymph node hyperolasia: report of two interesting caes. Gynecol Oncol 9:394–404
Yu GSM, Carson JW (1976) Giant lymphnode hyperplasis, plasma cell type of the mediastinum, with peripheral neuropathy. Am J Clin Pathol 66:46–53
Zettergren L (1961) Probable neoplastic prliferation of lymphoid tissue follicular (lymphoreticuloma). Acta Pathol Microbiol Scand A 51:113–126

Reactive Fibrohistiocytic Proliferation

Proppe KH, Scully RE, Rosai J (1984) Post operative spindle cell nodules of genitourinary tract resembling sarcomas. Am J Surg Pathol 8:101–108
Snover DC, Phillips G, Dehner LP (1981) Reactive fibrohistiocytic proliferation simulating fibrous histiocytoma. Am J Clin Pathol 76:232–235

12 Lymphomas

Although lymphomas with first manifestation in the vulva have been reported, vulval lymphomas primary or secondary are, indeed, rare (also see Part II on the vagina). Buckingham and McLure (1955) reported in a 33-year-old patient a rapidly growing labial mass which had been causing interference with walking and intercourse. The tumour ($12 \times 7 \times 5$ cm) was removed and found to consist of non-epithelial moderately pleomorphic cells with scanty cytoplasm, round to oval vasicular nuclei and prominent nucleoli. Reticulin stains showed branched reticulin fibres in intimate association with malignant cells. The tumour was vascular and contained scattered areas of necrosis. It was diagnosed to be a reticulum cell sarcoma. A lymphoma reported by Taussig (1937) was an ulcerated, firm, nodular, 2-cm clitoral mass in a 63-year-old woman. It was composed of dense aggregates of round cells with sparse pale cytoplasm, slightly irregular cell outlines, well-defined nuclear membranes and nucleoli. The femoral node of the patient showed similar features.

References

Buckingham JC, McLure JH (1955) Reticulum cell sarcoma of the vulva: report of a case. Obstet Gynecol 6:138–143

Taussig FJ (1937) Sarcoma of the vulva. Am J Obstet Gynecol 33:1017–1026

13 Neuroendocrine Carcinoma (Merkel Cell Tumour) and Amphicrine Tumours

Merkel cell was named after Friedrich Sigmund Merkel, who in 1875 described a special sensory cell ("tastzell") in the epidermis of vertebrates. These cells are also present in the hair follicles of mammals and have ultrastructural similarities to APUD cells containing neurosecretory granules. The tumours originating in these cells have been variously labelled as trabecular carcinoma of the skin (Toker 1972), neuroendocrine carcinoma of the skin (Sibley et al. 1980), small cell neuroepithelial tumour of the skin (Silva and Mackay 1980), primary small cell carcinoma of the skin (Taxy et al. 1980) and cutaneous APUDOMA (Wolf-Peters et al. 1980). They occur commonly in the head and neck region and extremities (Frigerio et al. 1982; Raaf et al. 1986) but have also been reported from the face, ear, cheek, leg, buttock and forearm. The vulval tumour reported by Bottles et al. (1984) occurred on the left labium majus of a 73-year-old woman who also had in situ squamous cell carcinoma adjacent to the Merkel cell tumour. She had nodal and bony metastases. The patient reported by Copeland et al. (1985) was 59 years old and presented with a painful lump in the left Bartholin's gland area. She was treated by left hemivulvectomy and left superficial lymph node dissection followed by radiation. There was local recurrence and pulmonary metastases, and she died 4 months later (Copeland et al. 1985). Husseinzadeh et al. (1988) reported a lesion in a 47-year-old woman who presented with vaginal discharge and right labial and groin swelling for 3 months and was treated by radical vulvectomy and inguinal node dissection followed by post-operative radiation. She died of metastatic disease.

Merkel cell tumours are sub-cutaneous nodules of 1–7 cm in size, firm in consistency and display a greyish-tan cut surface.

Microscopically, they are composed of uniform, undifferentiated, round cells with very scanty, ill-defined cytoplasm and uniform, round nuclei with evenly stippled, fine chromatin, a well-defined nuclear border and several small inconspicuous nucleoli (Fig. 13.1). Mitoses are often frequent. The cells are arranged in compact masses, organoid or trasbecular pattern, and anastomosing nests of cords. The tumour cells are PAS-positive and may be argyrophilic.

Immunohistochemical studies by van Muijen et al. (1985) demonstrated cytokeratin in all of their ten patients and neurofilaments in two. Neuron-specific enolase, which is thought to be a marker of neuroendocrine carcinoma of the lung, could not be demonstrated by Warner et al. (1983) in any of their six patients. Husseinzadeh et al. (1988) have demonstrated ACTH in vulval tumours.

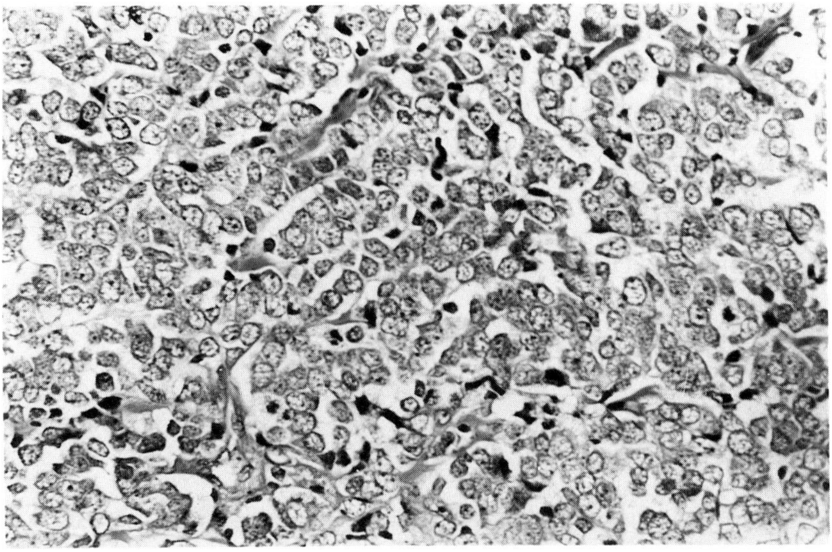

Fig. 13.1. Neuroendocrine carcinoma: uniform, undifferentiated, round cells with well-defined nuclear border and vague trabecular arrangement

Some patients with Merkel cell tumour show elevated levels of plasma ACTH and the presence of ACTH (Iwasaki et al. 1981) and calcitonin in the tumour tissue (Johannessen and Gould 1980).

Ultrastructurally, the cells contain neurosecretory-type membrane-bound granules of 130 nm average diameter in the cytoplasm of most cells (Tang and Toker 1978; Pajor et al. 1986). While desmosomes are seen in all cases, tonofilaments are not constant features (van Muijen et al. 1985). The cells are rich in polyribosomes and display a prominent Golgi zone, scant endoplasmic reticulum and loose aggregates of microfilaments (Sidhu et al. 1980).

In differential diagnosis, secondary deposits from primary undifferentiated carcinoma at some other site, lymphoma and amelanotic melanoma should be excluded. The neuroendocrine cells contain an isoenzyme neuron-specific enolase which can be used as a diagnostic marker (Gu et al. 1983). Ultrastructural demonstration of dense core granules forms an additional diagnostic feature.

The histogenesis of Merkel cell tumours has not been clearly established. Neuroectodermal, neuroendocrine and APUD systems have all been suggested. Sidhu et al. (1980) noticed keratinocytic differentiation and transition from Merkel to squamous cell. They concluded that Merkel cell tumours were not neuroectodermal in origin.

These tumours are more aggressive than squamous cell carcinoma (Bottles et al. 1984). Metastases to the lymphatics are common and occur also to other distant sites. The prognosis seems to be disappointing.

13.1 Treatment

Before establishing the primary malignancy in the skin, other primary sites, particularly the lungs, should be excluded. The common modality of treatment is local excision. Local excision, radiotherapy and combined chemotherapy have been used, but the ultimate outcome is poor (Taxy et al. 1980).

13.2 Amphicrine Tumour

Recently, Hidvegi et al. (1988) described an adenocarcinoid tumour in a 75-year-old woman who had presented with an ulcerated vulval tumour 12 cm in diameter which had been growing for 5 years. The tumour was grey-white on its cut surface. Microscopically, it was composed of pleomorphic, undifferentiated, malignant cells with a trabecular arrangement and myxoid stroma. The tumour cells and stroma were PAS- and alcian blue-positive.

The tumour was labelled as an amphicrine tumour because of its dual composition of both exocrine and endocrine cells. Such tumours occur commonly in the gastrointestinal tract. The histogenesis of this tumour is uncertain. Multidirectional differentiation of neoplastic cells derived either from the Merkel cell proper or epithelial cells is possible.

References

Bottles K, Lacey CG, Goldberg J et al. (1984) Merkel cell carcinoma of the vulva. Obstet Gynecol 63 [Suppl]:61–65

Copeland LJ, Cleary K, Sneige N et al. (1985) Neuroendocrine (Merkel cell) carcinoma of the vulva: a case report and review of the literature. Gynecol Oncol 22:367–378

Frigerio R, Carella C, Euseri V et al. (1982) Merkel cell carcinoma of the skin. Histopathology 7:229–249

Gu J, Polak JM, Noorden SV et al. (1983) Immunostaining of neuron specific enolase as a diagnostic tool for Merkel cell tumors. Cancer 52:1039–1043

Hidvegi J, Zsolnai B, Szinay G (1988) Amphicrine tumor of the vulva. Pathol Res Pract 183:505–508

Husseinzadeh N, Wesseler T, Newman N et al. (1988) Neuroendocrine (Merkel cell) carcinoma of the vulva. Gynecol Oncol 29:105–112

Iwasaki H, Mitsui T, Kikuchi M et al. (1981) Neuroendocrine carcinoma (trabecular carcinoma) of the skin with ectopic ACTH production. Cancer 48:735–756

Johannessen JV, Gould VE (1980) Neuroendocrine skin carcinoma associated with calcitonin production: a Merkel cell carcinoma? Hum Pathol 11:586–589

Merkel F (1875) Tastzellen und Tastkörperchen bei den Haustieren und beim Menschen. Arch Mikr Anat 11:636–652

Pajor L, Balazs M, Balogh J et al. (1986) Ultrastructural, lectin histochemical and immunohistological observations on Merkel cell tumors. Path Res Pract 181:45–49

Raaf JH, Urmacher C, Knapper WK et al. (1986) Trabecular (Merkel cell) carcinoma of the skin. Cancer 57:178–182

Sibley RK, Rosai J, Foucar E et al. (1980) Neuroendocrine (Merkel cell) carcinoma of the skin: a histologic and ultrastructural study of two cases. Am J Surg Pathol 4:211–221

Sidhu GS, Mullins JD, Feiner H et al. (1980) Merkel cell neoplasms. Am J Dermatopathol 2:101–119

Silva EG, Mackay B (1980) Small cell neuroepithelial tumor of the skin. Lab Invest 42:151

Tang C-K, Toker C (1978) Trabecular carcinoma of the skin: an ultrastructural study. Cancer 42:2311–2321

Taxy JB, Ettinger DS, Wharam MD (1980) Primary small cell carcinoma of the skin. Cancer 46:2308–2311

Toker C (1972) Trabecular carcinoma of the skin. Arch Dermatol 105:107–110

van Muijen GNP, Rutter DJ, Warnaar SO (1985) Intermediate filaments in Merkel cell tumors. Hum Pathol 16:590–595

Warner TFCS, Uno H, Hafez GR et al. (1983) Merkel cells and Merkel cell tumors: ultrastructure, immunochemistry, and review of the literature. Cancer 52:238–245

Wolf-Peters CD, Marien K, Mebis J et al. (1980) A cutaneous APUDOMA or Merkel cell tumor. Cancer 46:1810–1816

14 Germ Cell Tumour

14.1 Endodermal Sinus Tumour

Teilum (1959) first drew attention to the histological features of a tumour originally described by Schiller in 1939 as mesonephroma, which had a close structural resemblance to the rat placenta. He thought this structural display was an attempt at extra-embryonic differentiation; the tumour was therefore of germ cell origin. He designated the tumour as an endodermal sinus tumour.

In women, the most common site of endodermal sinus tumours, which can occur either as a pure form or admixed with other germ cell tumours, particularly immature teratomas, is the gonads. Rarely, the tumours are noticed at extra-gonadal sites and believed to arise from germ cells misplaced or arrested during their migration from the yolk sac. Vulval endodermal sinus tumours have occasionally been reported (Ungerleider et al. 1978; Castaldo et al. 1980; Krishnamurthy and Sampat 1981; Dudley et al. 1983).

Clinically, patients with vulval tumours are young with an age range from 22 months to 26 years. One patient (Krishnamurthy and Sampat 1981) was pregnant at the time of diagnosis. The main symptom was the vulval mass.

14.1.1 Gross Appearance

The tumours of the vulva vary in size from 1.5 to 7 cm in diameter and occur either as an indurated area or a tan nodule with no preferential site on the vulva.

14.1.2 Microscopical Appearance

The gonadal tumours generally display several histological patterns. The most common is reticular, which may also be the predominant pattern in vulval tumours. It consists of irregular, interlacing cords of vacuolated and immature cells forming a loose reticular network often enclosing small cystic spaces (Fig. 14.1). In some areas, the tumour cells may also be arranged in ill-defined, loose nests and sheets separated by incomplete, thin, fibrous septae. Many PAS-positive, intra- and extracellular hyaline bodies which have the composition of basement membrane (No-

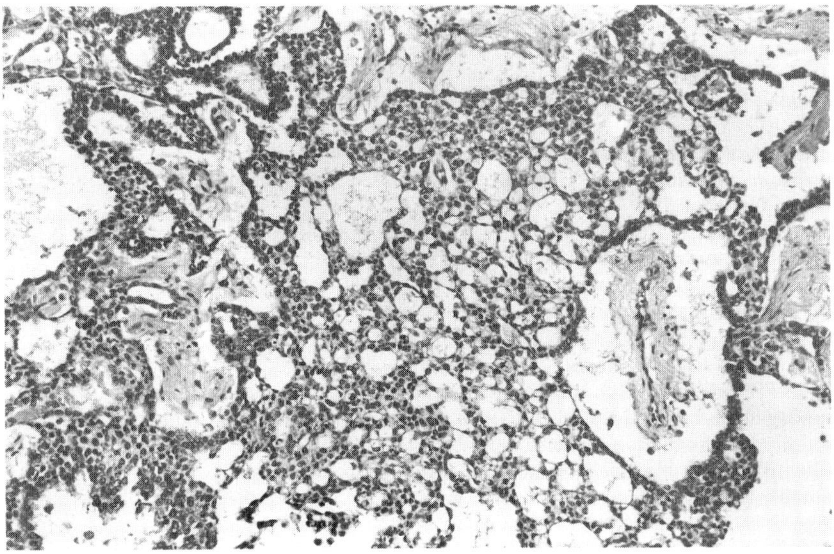

Fig. 14.1. Endodermal sinus tumour: irregular, interlacing cords of immature cells

gales et al. 1977) can often be seen. The tumour cells elaborate alpha-fetoprotein, which is used as a marker for the endodermal sinus tumour. Other patterns of the gonadal tumours such as solid, cystic and microcystic are also reflected in the vulval tumours.

These tumours recur invariably and show a strong tendency to spread by the lymphatics and blood stream. The overall prognosis is poor, with a median survival of only 10 months (Huntington and Bullock 1971). The prognosis appears to depend not so much on the stage but on complete resectibility of the tumour mass (Ungerleider et al. 1978). Three of the four patients with vulval neoplasms died within 1 year of diagnosis.

14.1.3 Treatment

Radical vulvectomy with bilateral node dissection should be the treatment of choice (Dudley et al. 1983). Radiotherapy to control local and pelvic disease (Dudley et al. 1983) and post-operative multiagent chemotherapy to sterilise microscopical local and metastatic disease (Ungerleider et al. 1978) have been advocated. Improved survival has been reported by using vincristine, actinomycin D and cyclophosphamide (VAC) in ovarian yolk sac tumours (Kurman and Norris 1976; Gerhenson et al. 1983). Others (Tsukamoto et al. 1985; Swada et al. 1985) have used different combinations of chemotherapeutic agents and achieved good results. At present chemotherapy seems to offer the brightest hope for this condition (Ungerleider et al. 1978).

References

Castaldo TW, Petrilli ES, Ballon SC et al. (1980) Endodermal sinus tumor of the clitoris. Gynecol Oncol 9:376–380

Dudley AG, Young RH, Lawrence WD et al. (1983) Endodermal sinus tumor of the vulva in an infant. Obstet Gynecol 61 [Suppl]:76–79

Gerhenson DM, Junco GD, Herson J et al. (1983) Endodermal sinus tumor of the ovary. Obstet Gynecol 61:194–202

Huntington RH Jr, Bullock WK (1971) Endodermal sinus and other yolk sac tumours, a re-apprisal. Acta Pathol Microbiol Scand [A] 80 [Suppl 233]:26–31

Krishnamurthy SC, Sampat MB (1981) Endodermal sinus (yolk sac) tumor of the vulva in a pregnant female. Gynecol Oncol 11:379–382

Kurman RJ, Norris HJ (1976) Endodermal sinus tumor of the ovary: a clinical and pathological analysis of 71 cases. Cancer 38:2404–2419

Nogales FF, Silverberg SG, Blaustein PA et al. (1977) Yolk sac carcinoma (endodermal sinus tumor): ultrastructural and histogenesis of gonadal and extragonadal tumors in comparison with normal human yolk sac. Cancer 39:1452–1472

Schiller W (1939) Mesonephroma ovarii. Am J Cancer 35:1–21

Swada M, Okudaira Y, Matsui Y et al. (1985) Cisplatin, vinblastin and bleomycin therapy of yolk sac tumors of the ovary. Gynecol Oncol 20:162–169

Teilum G (1959) Endodermal sinus tumors of the ovary and testis: comparative morphogenesis of the so-called mesonephroma ovarii (Schiller) and extraembryonic (Yolk-allantoic) structures of the rat placenta. Cancer 12:1092–1105

Tsukamoto N, Imachi M, Ucheno H et al. (1985) Modified VAB-3 combination chemotherapy of advanced and recurrent endodermal sinus tumors of the ovary. Gynecol Oncol 20:336–345

Ungerleider RS, Donaldson SS, Warnke RA et al. (1978) Endodermal sinus tumor: the Stanford experience and first reported case arising in the vulva. Cancer 41:1627–1634

15 Histiocytosis X

The non-commital term histiocytosis X comprises three clinical conditions, namely, Letterer-Siwe disease, Hand-Schüller-Christian disease and eosinophilic granuloma. Each condition used to be regarded as a distinct clinical entity, but all of them are now believed to be inter-related conditions. The basic characteristic of these lesions is proliferation of histiocytes, the aetiology of which is unknown. The most fatal of the conditions is Letterer-Siwe disease, which occurs in infancy and involves the major internal organs particularly the spleen, bone marrow, lymph nodes, liver, lungs, intestinal mucosa and skin. Hand-Schüller-Christian disease occurs in early childhood and affects predominantly bones, particularly of the skull, producing exophthalmos, diabetes insipidus and loosening of the teeth from the mandible. The visceral involvement is minor. This type pursues a prolonged course, and if not treated, about half of the patients die of other diseases. Eosinophilic granuloma is the least severe of the conditions, generally localised in the bone and occasionally involving the skin and oral mucosa. Older children and young adults are affected. This condition has a chronic course and responds well to treatment.

The female genital tract is infrequently involved in histiocytosis X. Several reports indicate that the vulva is more commonly affected than any other part of the genital system (Curtis and Cawley 1947; McKay et al. 1953; Kierland et al. 1957; Borglin et al. 1966; Miodovnik et al. 1979; Issa et al. 1980; Lechner et al. 1983). The vulval lesion is either the sole manifestation of the disease (Rose et al. 1984) or occurs as part of widespread lesions (Thomas et al. 1986). The lesion may present as local induration, bullae or ulcer. The common symptoms are itching, pain, polyuria and vaginal bleeding. Diabetes insipidus is present in 75% of patients (Issa et al. 1980) with generalised disease.

Microscopically, there are pronounced histiocytic proliferations in the dermis. The histiocytes are large, round and ovoid in shape, with pink granular cytoplasm and round or reniform nuclei which may be multilobulated and folded (McKay et al. 1953). A varying number of eosinophils, a few polymorphs, occasional lymphocytes and plasma cells can be seen in the lesion. The histiocytes, which constitute the main cellular component, together with other types of inflammatory cells infiltrate the epidermis, which becomes eroded or ulcerated. In some lesions, multinucleate giant cells are also present, and the pathological features simulate giant cell granulomas.

Ultrastructural studies have demonstrated Langerhans' granules (x-bodies) in the histiocytes (Gianotti and Caputo 1969; Nezelof et al. 1973). These granules can also be seen in the Langerhans' cells of the normal epidermis. Both the histiocytes of histiocytosis X and epidermal Langerhans' cells share many immunochemical and ultrastructural characteristics (Rowden et al. 1983; Beckstead et al. 1984; Ide et al. 1984). Both types of cell contain S-100 protein and OKT6 antigens, and both are positive for adenosine triphosphate, alphanaphthyl acetate and acid phosphatase enzymes. These observations have led to the suggestion that histiocytosis X is the proliferative disorder of the Langerhans' cells. The epidermal Langerhans' cells are thought to originate in the bone marrow.

15.1 Treatment and Prognosis

Nezelof et al. (1979) identified two prognostic groups, one severe with combined symptoms of thrombocytopenia, spontaneous anaemia, hepatosplenomegaly, respiratory insufficiency and absence of osteolytic lesions, and the other which has a more favourable prognosis, with skin lesions, diabetes insipidus, multiple bone lesions and radiological lung lesions.

The treatment has varied and has included surgery, steroids, chemotherapy and radiotherapy with variable results (Nezolof et al. 1979; Jonese et al. 1974; Lechner et al 1983). No particular modality of treatment has, however, shown a better result (Rose et al. 1984). Depending on the extent of the disease, individualisation of the treatment has been recommended (Lechner et al. 1983; Issa et al. 1980). A 90% 5-year survival rate can be achieved with excision and/or radiotherapy for the localised lesion and more aggressive chemotherapy in disseminated disease (Lechner et al. 1983). Follow-up of the patients with localised disease has been recommended to guard against systemic development (Wolfson et al. 1981).

References

Beckstead JH, Wood GS, Turner RR (1984) Histiocytosis X-cells and Langerhans' cells: enzyme histochemical and immunologic similarities. Hum Pathol 15:826–833

Borglin NE, Soderstrom J, Wehlin L (1966) Eosinophilic granuloma (Histiocytosis-X) of the vulva. J Obstet Gynaecol Br Commonw 73:478–486

Curtis AC, Cawley EP (1947) Eosinophilic granuloma of bone with cutaneous manifestation. Arch Dermatol 55:810–818

Gianotti AC, Caputo R (1969) Skin ultrastructure in Hand-Schüller-Christian disease. Arch Dermatol 100:342–349

Ide F, Iwase T, Saito I et al. (1984) Immunological and ultrastructural analysis of the proliferating cells in histiocytosis-X. Cancer 53:917–921

Issa P-Y, Saleem PA, Brihi E et al. (1980) Eosinophilic granuloma with involvement of female genitalia. Am J Obstet Gynecol 608–612

Jones B, Kung F, Chevalier L et al. (1974) Chemotherapy of reticuloendotheliosis. Cancer 34:1011–1017

Kierland RB, Epstein JG, Weber WE (1957) Eosinophilic granuloma of skin and mucous membrane. Arch Dermatol 75:45–54

Lechner W, Ortner A, Thoni A et al. (1983) Histiocytosis-X in gynecology. Gynecol Oncol 15:253–260

McKay DG, Street RB, Benirschke K et al. (1953) Eosinophilic granuloma of the vulva: Surg Gynecol Obstet 96:437–447

Miodovnik M, Adatto R, Adoni A et al. (1979) Vulval eosinophilic granuloma: Acta Obstet Gynecol Scand 58:565–567

Nezelof C, Basset F, Rousseau MF (1973) Histiocytosis-X: histogenetic arguments for a Langerhans' cell origin. Biomedicine 18:365–371

Nezelof C, Frileux-Herbet F, Cronier-Sachat J (1979) Disseminated histiocytosis-X. Cancer 44:1824–1838

Rose PG, Johnston GC, O'Toole RV (1984) Cutaneous histiocytosis-X of the vulva. Obstet Gynecol 64:587–590

Rowden G, Connelly EM, Winkleman RK (1983) Cutaneous histiocytosis X: the presence of S-100 protein and its use in diagnosis. Arch Dermatol 119:553–559

Thomas R, Barnhill D, Bibro M et al. (1986) Histiocytosis-X in gynecology: a case presentation and review of the literature. Obstet Gynecol 67 [Suppl]:46–49

Wolfson SL, Botero F, Hurtwitz S et al. (1981) Pure cutaneous histiocytosis-X. Cancer 48:2236–2238

16 Some Inflammatory Conditions That May Simulate Tumours

Young et al. (1977) classified erosions and ulcers of the vulva into four groups. The first group comprises syphilis, hidradenitis suppuritiva, aphthosis, Behçet's syndrome and chancroid; the second group is vesicobulbous dermotoses; the third group is pruritic and factitial dermotoses; and the fourth group in situ and invasive carcinomas. Although the overwhelming majority of the first three groups of lesions has clinical and macroscopical features distinctive from neoplastic conditions, a few may occasionally pose diagnostic problems which can be resolved by histological examination.

16.1 Specific

16.1.1 Human Papillomavirus Infections of the Vulva

Since the recognition of a link between human papillomaviruses (HPV) and lower female genital tract cancers, numerous reports have vindicated that there is a strong argument in favour of their causative role in these neoplasias. It has become evident from the worldwide cervical cytological screening programme that the incidence of HPV infection can be noticed in 2%–4% of smears in any laboratory (Meisels et al. 1981; Nash et al. 1987). This is a manifold increase in recent times over what was thought to be a rarity a decade and a half ago. This increase and the association with genital neoplasia have generated added impetus to the investigation of these viruses. HPV belong to the group Papovaviruses, an abbreviation of papilloma, polyoma and simian vacuolating viruses (Melnick 1962), which are double-stranded DNA viruses with a molecular length of about 7900 base pairs and a molecular weight of about 5 200 000 daltons (Orth et al. 1977). With various restriction endonucleases, cleavage sites in the genome of different types of papillomavirus have been found (Gissmann and zur Hausen 1978). This information is employed in the nucleic acid hybridisation technique, and by this technique, a virus is considered to be a new type when there is less than 50% homology with the known types, that is, when the viruses share less than 50% of their base sequences under stringent conditions of hybridisation (Coggin and zur Hausen 1979). Up to now, more than 50 strains of HPV have been identified. Many of them have been associated with benign and malignant lesions in the human with preferential distribution in certain tissues. Types 6, 11, 16, 18, 33 and 35 have been particularly noticed in genital tract lesions. Of them, types 6, 11, 16, 18 and 31 constitute 75% of the infections (Wilbur et al. 1988). Types 16 and 18 have been consistently found in about 70% of pre-invasive and invasive squamous cell carcinoma of the cervix and types 6 and 11, in more than 90% of condylomata acuminata (Gissmann et al. 1984). While extensive investigations of the HPVs in relation to cervical lesions have been made, studies of the role of these viruses in relation to vulval lesions are relatively less intense. According to some data, HPV capsid antigen can be detected in 64% (Pilotti et al. 1984) and HPV DNA in 83% of vulval intra-epithelial neoplasia (Bornstein et al. 1988). HPV type 16 has been detected more frequently in patients with lesions limited to the vulva than in patients with multicentric lesions. Koilocytosis, which is thought to be the morphological expression of HPV infection, can be demonstrated in from 65.5% (Crum et al. 1984) to 70.7% cases. In some studies, type 16 is predominantly associated with vulval intra-epithelial neoplasia and types 6 and 11, with condylomata acuminata (Gupta et al. 1987; Buscema et al. 1988). In other studies, 78% of vulval carcinoma contained types 6 and 11 DNA, 33% type 16 DNA, and 28% type 18 DNA (Sutton et al. 1987). In bowenoid papulosis, which is an intra-epithelial neoplasia with a tendency to occur particularly in young patients and occasionally undergoes spontaneous regression, type 16 DNA has been identified (Ikenberg et al. 1983). Recently, a verrucous carcinoma has been reported to contain an unusual type of HPV 6 (Randoo et al. 1986) and a condylomatous carcinoma (carcinoma arising in the condylomata acuminata), types 6 and 16 (Downey et al. 1988).

At present it appears that HPV 16 is the predominant type in vulval intra-epithelial neoplasia and invasive carcinoma, and types 6 and 11 are common types found in condylomata acuminata. There are still a few problems to be resolved – the mechanism of oncogenesis, specificity of the viruses for particular lesions and predilection for anatomical sites – before their causative role is established beyond doubt.

16.1.2 Condylomata Acuminata

Condylomata acuminata, also known as venereal warts, are caused by HPV. As already mentioned, some strains of these viruses have been linked to warts, pre-invasive and invasive squamous cell carcinoma of the female lower genital tract. Types 1 (Staguet et al. 1981), 6 and 11 (Gissmann et al. 1983) and in occasional cases, 16 and 18 have been identified in condylomata acuminata (Vallejos et al. 1987).

Condylomata acuminata are transmitted mainly through sexual contact, although non-sexual transmission is known to occur. In the recent years, their incidence have increased in epidemic proportion. The affected individuals are usually sexually active. Women of child-bearing age are more susceptible. The incubation period varies from 4 to 6 weeks after exposure. On the vulva, warts occur in the posterior introitus in 73%, labia minora and clitoris in 32%, labia majora in 31%, perineum in 23%, anus in 18% and urethra in 8% of patients (Oriel 1971).

Patients with vulval condylomata have a high risk of cervical condylomata (Walker et al. 1984). In about one-third of all patients with vulval condylomata, cervical intra-epithelial neoplasia may co-exist (Campion et al. 1985).

Spontaneous regression of warts is noticed in a small number of patients and is said to depend on the immunological status of the individuals. Both humoral and cell-mediated immunity are thought to be responsible. In the early stage of infection, most patients develop IgM antibodies, and later IgG antibodies seem to play some role (Lynch 1985). The cell-mediated immunity, however, seems to be more important in resistance to initial infection and subsequent resolution of the lesion. In HPV infection, the cell-mediated immunity is impaired (Obalek et al. 1980). In cervical condylomata B lymphocytes are more important than the T lymphocytes (Syrjanen 1983). Although the significance of this finding is not clear, the ratio of T-helper and T-suppressor cells appears to be more important (Syrjanen et al. 1984). The ratio in favour of suppressor cells facilitates the progression of the lesion.

16.1.2.1 Gross Appearance

The genital warts are flat, expophytic and endophytic (Meisels and Roy 1977). The vulval condylomata are mostly exophytic. The warts are multiple, soft to rubbery, finger-like, verrucous growths one to several centimeters in diameter. These may coalesce to form larger masses or even bulky, cauliflower-like growths. The giant condyloma acuminatum of Löwenstein and Buschke and verrucous carcinoma appear to be the lesions at the other end of the spectrum which begins with the flat condyloma, as different strains of HPV have been identified in all of them. In condyloma acuminatum, type 6 can be demonstrated in 93% of patients (Gissmann et al. 1982).

When the condylomata are massive, they may complicate labour (Benschine 1941; Gorthey and Krems 1954), even necessitating Caesarean section (Wilson 1973).

It has been claimed that colposcopic examination (McCance and Singer 1986) can detect 52% of sub-clinical HPV-associated lesions. (i) Microwarts with villous projections are found frequently on the labia minora, introitus and posterior fourchette. Histologically, the microwart consists of a single villus with a central capillary loop. Koilocytes are seen in 80% of patients. (ii) Fused villi in estensive lesions are found commonly on the labia minora and posterior fourchette. Histologically, evidence of HPV and in 30% of patients associated intra-epithelial neoplasia grade 1 or 2 are noticed. (iii) Villi appear white after application of 5% acetic acid. Histologically, evidence of HPV infection and intra-epithelial neoplasia grade 1 or 2 can be seen.

16.1.2.2 Microscopical Appearance

The lesions are composed of thickened and multilayered squamous cells, parakeratosis and vacuolated cells (koilocytes) in the upper malpighian layer (Fig. 16.1). The hyperplastic squamous epithelium is thrown into complex papillary folds, often with fibrovascular cores. Bulky infolding of the thickened epithelium (Fig. 16.2) with atypia and mitoses should be carefully evaluated for malignant change which can supervene condylomata acuminata. Lymphocytes and plasma cells are almost always seen in the underlying connective tissue.

DNA analysis of the condylomata shows a diploid and polypoid distribution in contradistinction to the aneuploid DNA quantitation of intra-epithelial neoplasia (Shevchuk and Richart 1982).

Intranuclear viral particles were demonstrated in the warts by ultrastructural examination (Dunn and Ogilvie 1968; Oriel and Almedia 1970).

16.1.2.3 Treatment

Trichloracetic acid and podophyllin have been successfully used in the treatment of condylomata acuminata (Powell 1978). Podophyllin is used with caution because of its undesirable side effects (Gardner and Kaufman 1965) and is contraindicated in pregnancy. Cryosurgery has been used with a very high success rate (Ghosh 1978). For refractory and extensive lesions, the laser has been advocated (Ferenczy 1983; Reid 1985). Topical 5-fluorouracil (Sillman et al. 1985) has been found useful. Intramuscular injection of interferon (Schonfeld et al. 1984) and injection of interferon alpha-2b directly into the genital warts (Eron et al. 1986) have also been found to be effective.

16.1.3 Squamous Papilloma

So-called squamous papilloma is a non-specific term representing various conditions in which the hyperplastic epidermis is thrown into papillary folds. The pruritic vestibular papilloma (Growdon et al. 1985; Moncharan and Sommervill 1987) which causes pruritus, pain, burning sensation and dyspareunia has been thought to be due to HPV infections. The hirsutoid papilloma of the vulva (Grob et al. 1987) has been linked to the pearly papilloma of the penis (Ackerman and Kornberg 1973).

16.1.4 Herpes Virus Infection

Herpes simplex viruses (HSV) are members of the herpesvirus family, which includes many human and animal viruses. The common members causing human infections are cytomegalovirus, varicella (chicken pox) and Epstein-Barr virus (infectious mononucleosis).

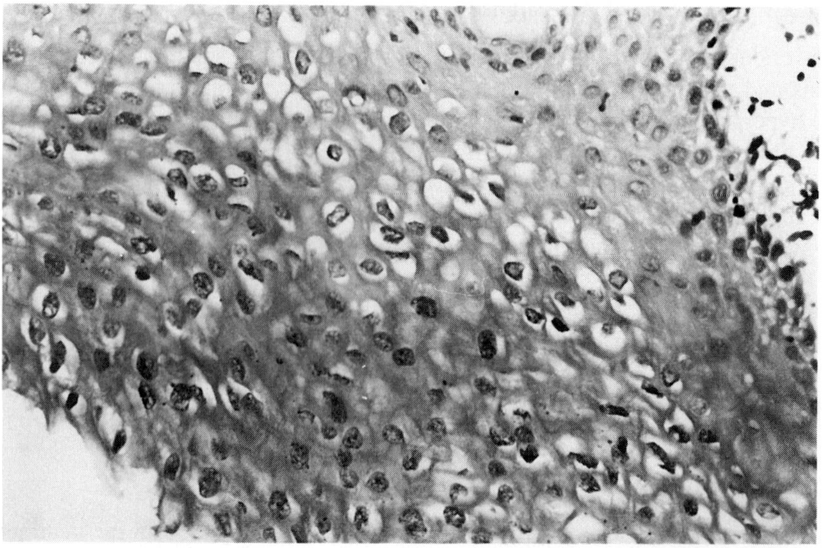

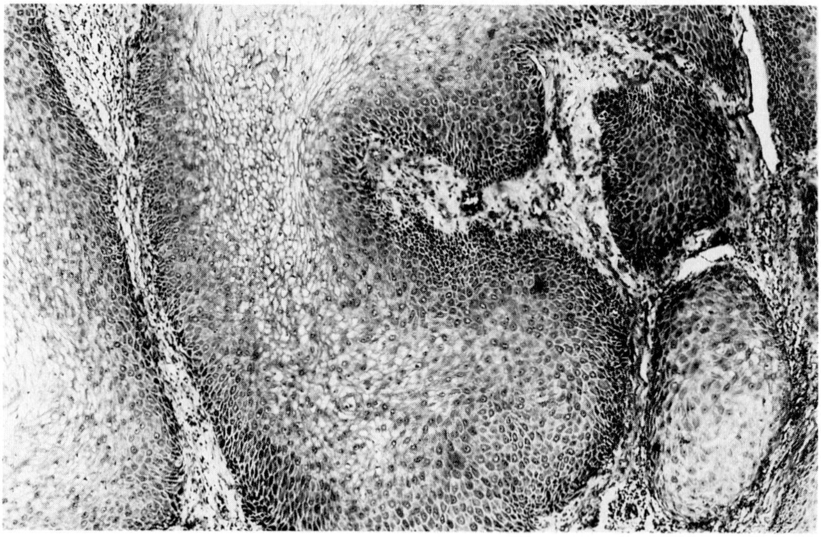

Fig. 16.1. Condylomata acuminata: koilocytic changes of epidermal cells

Fig. 16.2. Condylomata acuminata: bulky infolding of squamous cells. There is no cellular atypia

Two types of herpes simplex virus have been identified. Type 1 causes non-genital infections, and type 2, which is sexually transmitted, causes genital infections.

HSV are double-stranded DNA viruses. About 50% of the DNA of type 1 differs from that of type 2.

Clinically, herpes genitalis may be manifested as a primary lesion which is extensive, severe and painful and a focal recurrent lesion which is localised. The true primary infection occurs in patients who do not have circulating antibodies against either HSV type 1 or 2. If the patient has circulating antibodies, the lesion is localised and less severe. The third group of patients develops recurrent infections from the reactivation of the primary infection.

The typical vulval lesion appears as multiple vesicles that rupture with the formation of shallow ulcers. Similar ulcers may also develop on the vaginal and ectocervical mucosae. In the primary infections, the genital area becomes extremely painful. This is associated with inguinal lymphadenopathy, systemic symptoms and involvement of a wide ara of the perineum and buttocks. The ulcers may coalesce to form a large necrotic ulcer simulating a carcinoma.

After the primary infection, the viruses may remain dormant in the dorsal root ganglia and migrate to the territorial skin.

The recurrence of lesions commonly follows the primary infections by HSV-2 and depends on the presence of circulating neutralising antibodies in the patient's serum (Reeves et al. 1981). After the primary infection, the viruses remain dormant in the dorsal root ganglia and migrate to the territorial skin (Adams et al. 1976). They are thought to be reactivated by several conditions such as stress and ultraviolet light. Prostaglandins have been thought to be involved in some way in the process of reactivation of the virus and recurrence of the lesions (Hill and Blyth 1976).

Recurrent disease is usually mild and is manifested in a solitary ulcer which heals in about 1 week (Guinan et al. 1981).

The role of herpes genitalis in the genesis of cancer of the female lower genital tract has been discussed in an earlier chapter. Using immunological and in situ hybridisation techniques, herpesvirus DNA and herpesvirus antigens have been demonstrated in the lesions and patients' serum (Cabral et al. 1982; Kaufman et al. 1988). Although the oncogenic role of these viruses are yet not very clear, it has been suggested that they act synergistically with HPV in the oncogenesis of the cervix, vagina and vulva.

16.1.4.1 Microscopical Appearance

Wilbanks et al. (1970) and Ng et al. (1970) have described the cellular changes following the infections in detail. Within a few hours after infection, the nuclei display clumping and fragmentations of chromatin and small vacuoles which subsequently coalesce. The nuclei develop a basophilic ground glass appearance. The acidophilic intranuclear inclusion body, which is central in location, ultimately occupies most of the nuclear area and becomes surrounded by a clear halo. The individual infected cells coalesce to form multinucleate giant cells (Ng et al. 1970). The infected cells finally undergo necrosis. If a biopsy is taken at a later phase of infection, the inclusion bodies and cellular changes may not be evident. Under experimental conditions the whole process takes about 5 days (Munoz et al. 1969). The cells affected are keratinocytes of the middle zone and basal cells. A fully developed lesion is manifested in an intra-epidermal bulla containing floating cellular debris and a few leucocytes. The dermal papillae become oedematous, and both superficial and deep dermal plexuses become infiltrated by lymphocytes, histiocytes, eosinophils and a few neutrophils (Hertz et al. 1977).

Cytological investigation of the scrappings from fresh ulcers and tissue culture during the early phase yield a high percentage of positive results. Immunoperoxidase and immunofluorescent techniques are also used for the diagnosis with a high yield of accurate results. While serodiagnosis of antibodies is useful in detecting a primary lesion, it is of little help in differentiating perimary from reactivated lesions (Corey and Holmes 1983).

16.1.4.2 Treatment

Corey and Holmes (1983) outlined the goals of treatment, which should include increasing the rate of healing, resolving symptoms and lesions, decreasing complications and preventing subsequent recurrences. The anti-viral drug acyclovir is now widely used. The prevention of recurrence is not always achieved with the drugs available, but human leucocyte interferon has been found to decrease the frequency of reactivation (Pazin et al. 1978).

16.1.5 Tuberculous Ulcers

Tuberculous lesions of the vulva are rare and may occasionally present in ulcerative and hypertrophic forms, involving the labia, clitoris and vulval skin (Corbet 1953; Bhattacharya 1978). Both forms may be seen in one lesion. While the hypertrophic lesions appear as a firm nodular mass or irregular thickening of the area with ulcerations or discharging sinuses, the ulcerative lesions have well-defined, heaped up or punched out edges and a necrotic floor. The draining lymph nodes may also be involved.

Microscopically, the typical tuberculous granulomas consist of a central caseation necrosis which may be minimal or even absent, surrounded by epitheloid cells, Langerhans' type giant cells with a peripheral row of nuclei, monocytes and lymphocytes (Fig. 16.3). Acid-fast bacilli may be demonstrated by Ziehl-Neelsen stain and bacteriological culture of the infected tissue.

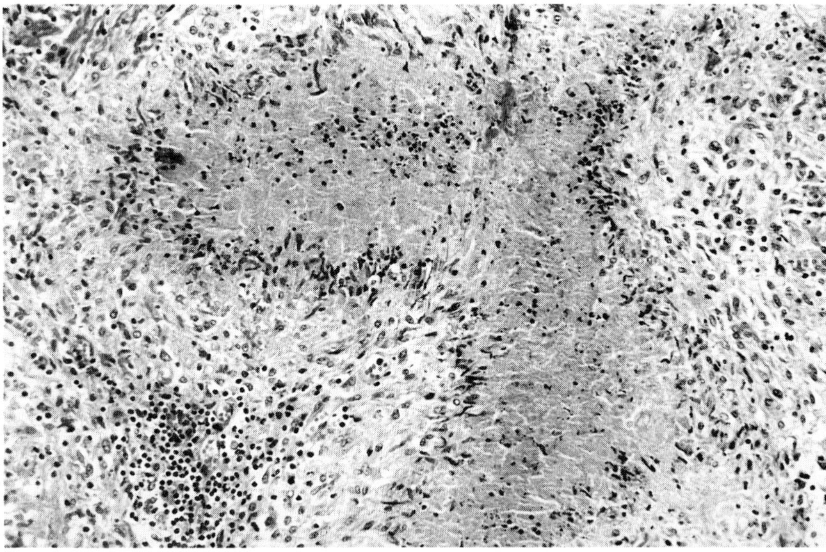

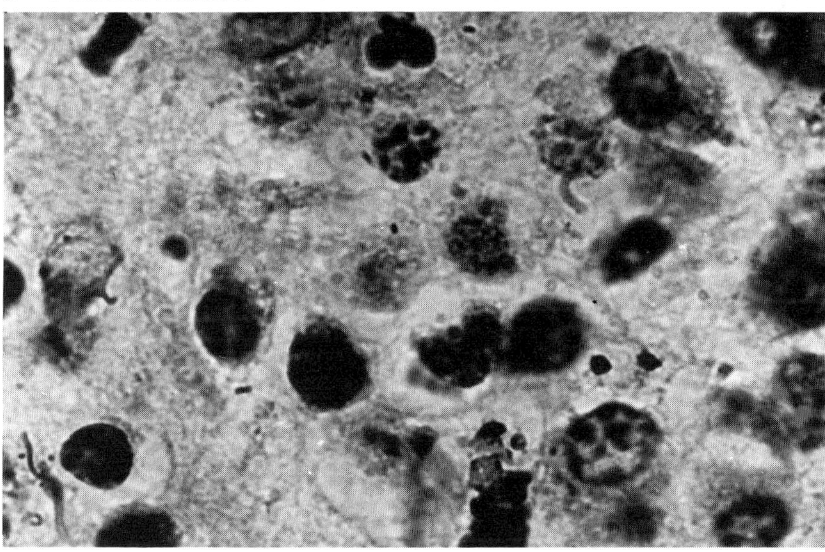

Fig. 16.3. Tuberculous lesion: central area of caseation surrounded by pale-staining epithelioid cells and other chronic inflammatory cells

Fig. 16.4. Granuloma inguinale: histiocytes containing Donovan bodies

16.1.5.1 Treatment

After establishing the diagnosis, an anti-tuberculous regimen is instituted. The hypertrophied tissues may be removed by surgery at a later date when the patient's condition improves.

16.1.6 Syphilis

With any ulcerative lesion of the vulva, the differential diagnosis of syphilitic ulcer should be kept in mind. The chancre of the primary stage is an indurated, smooth ulcer with a raised margin. This is associated with regional lymphadenopathy.

Microscopically, inflammatory cell infiltrations consisting of plasma cells, lymphocytes and histiocytes are pronounced in the area. These are associated with fibroblastic reactions and endarteritis obliterans.

Clinically, the history of exposure and demonstrations of spirochaetes differentiate this lesion from herpetic ulcer and chancroid. In secondary syphilis, the disseminated lesions are manifested as maculopapular rashes in all parts of the body. Perivascular plasma cell infiltrates, enarteritis obliterans and epidermal hyperplasia can be seen also in this stage. The late syphilitic lesion of the skin is characterised by the formation of gumma, which may at times become tumour-like masses. Microscopically, these consist of non-specific granulomas with a central necrosis surrounded by plasma cells, lymphocytes, epithelioid cells, multinucleate giant cells and fibrous tissue reactions. Serological tests including specific treponemal tests are used to confirm the diagnosis.

16.1.6.1 Treatment

Penicillin, tetracyclin and a few other antibiotics are quite effective in the treatment of syphilis.

16.1.7 Lymphogranuloma Venereum

The obligatory intracellular, bacteria-like *Chlamydia trachomatis* is now known to be the causative organism of the sexually transmitted disease lymphogranuloma venereum as well as of inclusion conjunctivitis, cervicitis, urethritis and psittacosis. Of the several serotypes, types 1, 2 and 3 are related to lymphogranuloma venereum. In women, the primary lesion may involve any part of the external genitalia, but it commonly affects the posterior vaginal wall and tissues adjacent to the fourchette (Holder and Duncan 1972). The initial lesion after exposure is a transient, vulval nodule which may become ulcerated. This is followed by inguinal and femoral lymphadenitis; constitutional symptoms like fever, malaise and sweating may develop in association with the lymphadenitis. The nodes are initially discrete but subsequently matted together to form a bubo. Stellate abscesses develop, which may coalesce and eventually rupture through multiple sinuses. In the later stage of the disease, fibrosis and destruction of the tissue are characteristic. Destruction of the labia minora and clitoris may disfigure the whole area. Sometimes extensive necrosis is associated with polypoid growths (Koteen 1945). The vulval surface becomes irregularly nodular and is covered with warty polypoid excrescences (Pund and Dick 1947). Rectal stricture and recto-vaginal fistula may also result (Douglas 1962).

16.1.7.1 Microscopical Appearance

The abscesses are initially surrounded by epithelioid histiocytes which often show a plaisading arrangement. With increasing size, the abscesses undergo central necrosis. Collections of numerous, polymorphonuclear cells and a varying number of other chronic inflammatory cells including multinucleate giant cells gradually become pronounced in the setting of granulation tissue. In the chronic stage, scarring with disfigurement of the vulva and cicatrical stricture of the rectum due to destructive infiltrations may occur. The marginal epidermis shows pseudoepitheliomatous hyperplasia with thickening of the malpighian layer and prolongation of rete pegs. This should be differentiated from invasive squamous cell carcinoma which is known to complicate lymphogranuloma venereum (Swink 1949).

Physical examination alone does not help establish the diagnosis (Schacter 1978). This is made by the isolation of the organism from the aspirates of bubos and the complement fixation test. A single titre of 1:64 or higher in the complement fixation test is highly suggestive. The microfluorescent test is now considered to be a more sensitive method.

16.1.7.2 Treatment

A syphilitic lesion should be excluded before instituting treatment. Fluctuant bubos should be aspirated through healthy skin. Tetracycline for 2 weeks has been recommended. Alternatively, other antibiotics like erythromycin or sulfamethoxazole can be used.

16.1.8 Granuloma Inguinale

Granuloma inguinale is also a sexually transmitted disease caused by *Calymmatobacterium granulomatis*, a gram-negative, encapsulated bacteria which can be grown only in medium containing yolk of fertilised chicken eggs. The condition is known to be mildly contagious and is seen in men and women between 20 and 40 years of age. Although the lesion occurs preponderantly in the genitalia, extra-genital lesions in the oral cavity (Garg 1978), axillae (Spagnolo et al. 1984), perianal region (Milton 1958), uterus, tubes and ovary (Pund and Gotcher 1948) and bone (Kirkpatrick 1970) have been reported.

Granuloma inguinale begins as a small nodule in the mons pubis or labia minora, which ulcerates. It becomes progressively larger by local infiltrations as well as by coalescence with adjacent ulcers, which are formed by auto-inoculation. The lesion can also extend by lymphatic permeation. Four clinical forms of the ulcer have been described: (i) the ulcero-granulomatous type is beefy-red and non-tender, (ii) the verrucous type has raised irregular edges, (iii) the necrotic type is a destructive and foul-smelling lesion, and (iv) the cicatrical variety is a band-like scar around the genitalia (Sehgal and Shyam-Prasad 1986).

The vulval ulcers are often mistaken for carcinoma, which may occasionally complicate the lesion. The incidence of vulval carcinoma in association with granuloma inguinale is stated to be high in some geographical areas (Stewart 1964).

Microscopically, the lesion is characterised by formation of granulation tissue with predominant plasma cells and histiocytic cell infiltrations (Fig. 16.4). The histiocytes have a foamy cytoplasm which contains Donovan bodies. The Donovan bodies are infrequently seen in formalin-fixed and wax-embedded tissues. Tissues fixed in glutaraldehyde and embedded in plastic give the best result (Dodson et al. 1974). Davis (1970) advocated Wright or Giemsa staining of the smear prepared from crushed fresh tissue for routine use.

The lesion shows scattered small microabscesses. Lymphocytes are usually fewer in number. Pseudoepitheliomatous hyperplasia of the epidermis mimicking invasive squamous cell carcinoma is common and should be differentiated from true carcinoma which can occasionally develop in these chronic lesions.

16.1.8.1 Treatment

Tetracyclines, chloramphenicol and erythromycin are all effective in this condition. Co-trimoxazole, a sulpha derivative, is considered to be the drug of choice (Lal and Garg 1980). Other infections which are often associated should also be looked for (Hart 1983).

16.1.9 Chancroid of the Vulva

Chancroid or soft chancre is a sexually transmitted disease caused by the gram-negative coccobacillus *Haemophilus ducreyi*. The median incubation period is about 7 days (Ronald 1986). The lesions consist of single or multiple, saucer-shaped ulcers which are tender and have irregular, undermined margins. The ulcers, generally deep with an excavated appearance and covered by purulent material, are commonly seen in the clitoris or vestibule. There is no induration either at the base or surrounding area. Inguinal lymphadenitis is common and seen in 33%–50% of all patients (Gaisin and Heaton 1975; Mohanty 1988). Extension to the surrounding area with eventual ulceration can occur.

Microscopically, three layers can be noticed in the lesion: the superficial layer consisting of necrotic debris, fibrin, polymorphonuclear cells and gram-negative coccobacilli; the wider middle layer containing many newly formed blood vessels oriented perpendicularly to the surface with peri- and endovasculitis, fibrinoid necrosis of the blood vessels and formation of intravascular thrombi; and the deepest layer showing chronic inflammatory cell infiltration comprising lymphocytes and plasma cells and fibroblastic proliferations (Sheldon and Heyman 1946).

Diagnosis is confirmed by isolation of the organisms in culture. Gram stain of the smears from the lesion and of the biopsied tissue may show gram-negative, rod-shaped organisms.

16.1.9.1 Treatment

Sulphonamide and tetracycline are used effectively in treating the condition.

16.1.10 Molluscum Contagiosum

Molluscum contagiosum is a disease caused by a virus related to the variola and paravaccinia group and is considered to spread by direct contact. The disease can spread also by sexual contact, which according to some authors is the common cause of transfer (Gudgel 1968). The genital lesions are considered to be venereal in origin. Trauma caused by coitus and supported by moisture and a dirty bed, furniture or fomites provides a favourable background for establishing the virus (Lynch and Minkin 1968). In children the distribution of the lesion is generalised or localised in the hands, forearm and face (Wilkin 1977). The lesions may increase during pregnancy. Spontaneous involution occurs in a few months or years.

The lesions appear as asymptomatic clusters of small, flesh-coloured, discrete papules 2–4 mm in size with a central umbilication.

16.1.10.1 Microscopical Appearance

Molluscum contagiosum consists of marked acanthosis with prolongation of the epidermis into the dermis. The epidermal cells show characteristic, numerous, large, intra-cytoplasmic inclusion bodies. These are acidophilic at deeper parts and gradually become basophilic towards the surface. It has been suggested that the mollusca bodies stimulate the basal portion of the epidermis and induce the formation of follicles (Reed and Parkinson 1977). The epidermis adjacent to the lesion is normal. A moderate number of chronic inflammatory cells with vascular proliferations can be seen in the dermis around the lesion.

16.1.10.2 Treatment

Small, discrete lesions can be treated by a sharp curette. Cryosurgery has also been applied successfully.

16.1.11 Amoebic Ulcer

Entamoeba histolytica, which is the causative organism of the amoebic lesions, is a protozoon belonging to the phylum protozoa. They commonly inhabit the large intestine. Their life cycle in humans begins with the ingestion of mature tetranucleate cysts which eventually become eight nucleate. From them develop eight amoebula, which become metacystic trophozoites invading the tissue, causing lesions. Trophozoites are non-infective. Some days after the establishment of lesions, the trophozoites can be transformed into cysts, which are excreted in the faeces.

Amoebic infection occurs worldwide but is more prevalent in tropical regions. A poor hygenic environment favours the propagation of infection, but the conditions which favour establishment of the lesions are unknown (Brandt and Tamayo 1970).

The skin around the anus, vulva and vaginal surfaces are affected by direct implantation of the trophozoites. Lesions in the cervix (Carter et al. 1954) can occur through a rectovaginal fistula or, as suggested by Veliath et al. (1987), sexual contact. Tubal (Bhaduri 1957), uterine (de Rivas 1944) and vaginal (Hingorani and Mahapatra 1964) lesions have also been reported.

The squamous epithelium is generally resistant to *E. histolytica*, but once the infection is established, it becomes chronic, causing proliferative lesions which mimic carcinoma.

Patients with genital tract lesions may present with various complaints such as ulcer, fetid and bloody vaginal discharge, leukorrhoea, menorrhagia, etc. Clinically, malignancy may be suspected in elderly patients. A mistaken diagnosis of cancer is often made with large ulcer of the vulva, perianal region and labia (Heinz 1973) or fungating lesion of the clitoris (Majumdar et al. 1976). Amoebic ulcers are described as flask shaped in the large bowel, but lesions of the vulva and vagina tend to be large, shallow, soft and friable. Diagnosis is made by taking a biopsy from the ulcer margin. Cytological examination of the smears from ulcers have yielded a high incidence of positive results in some series (Munguia et al. 1966; De Torres and Benitez-Bribiesca 1973).

Microscopically, the tissue taken from the biopsy shows pronounced necrosis, congestion and inflammatory cells consisting mainly of polymorphs. The vegetative form of amoeba (trophozoites) is seen usually at the periphery, adjacent to necrotic tissue and the base of the ulcer. The organisms can be identified by their large size of about 20–30 μm single inconspicuous nucleus and clear cytoplasm containing ingested red blood cells. Sometimes a clear zone can be seen around the parasite in tissue sections.

16.1.11.1 Treatment

As these patients also harbour the intestinal lesions, examination of the stool is essential. The anti-amoebic drugs chloroquin, emetine hydrochloride and metronidazole have been used successfully. The prevention of reinfection is important.

16.1.12 Schistosomiasis

Schistosomes, commonly known as flukes, belong to the class Trematodes. Of the three main species, *Schistosoma haematobium* and *S. mansoni* are prevalent in the tropical and subtropical regions of Africa, while *S. japonicum* is found in the Far East. The adult *S. haematobium* live in the rectal and vesical venous plexuses, *S. mansoni* in the veins of lower part of the large bowel and *S. japonicum* in the tributaries of the superior and inferior mesenteric veins. At these sites the adult females lay eggs which are passed through the faeces (*S. mansoni* and *S. japonicum*) and urine (*S. haematobium*). When the eggs come in contact with water, they develop into miracidia and enter the snail hosts in which they become cercariae. The cercariae come out of the snails into water and wait to infect humans. Humans are infected while bathing, wading in or drinking water. The young worms migrate to the portal and vesical venous systems, where they develop into adult worms. The eggs of *S. haematobium* are oval or spindle-shaped with a terminal spine, those of *S. mansoni* are oval with a lateral spine and those of *S. japonicum* are round with a lateral knob-like thickening.

Schistosoma can infect any organ of the body. Even the central nervous system is not spared (*S. japonicum*). The liver, to a variable degree, can be affected by all species, most particularly by *S. japonicum*. The urinary tract is the preferential site of affliction by *S. haematobium* and the gastrointestinal tract, by *S. mansoni* and *S. japonicum*. Tissue reactions are generally caused more by the dead adult worms and living ova than by living adult worms and dead ova (Berry 1966).

The basic pathological changes in the urinary bladder are formation of granulomas and pseudotubercles in the subepithelial tissue and muscular wall and hyperplastic changes in the epithelium. In the lungs, there may be pneumonitis during the migration of young flukes and granulomas, with necrotising arteriolitis due to lodgement of the flukes and allergic reactions to them or to their disintegration products. Granulomas may also occur as localised, para-arterial and interstitial lesions and are composed of epithelioid cells, lymphocytes, plasma cells, giant cells and eosinophils. Extensive peripheral fibrosis around the granulomas may convert them to discrete fibrous nodules.

Schistosomiasis of the female genital tract in endemic areas is not uncommon. The fallopian tubes and cervix are stated to be more frequently affected than other genital areas (Charlewood et al. 1949; Al-Adnani and Saleh 1982). According to Gelfand et al. (1971), *Schistosoma* eggs can be found in all areas of the female genital tract but more commonly in the cervix and vaginal wall. The tissue reactions such as hyperaemia, ulcerations and proliferative changes in all these areas may be mistaken for malignancies (Berry 1966). Cytological smears have been stated to be helpful in detecting the ova and establishing the diagnosis (Berry 1976). Oedema, hypertrophy and ulcers may also raise the possibilities of venereal warts, lymphogranuloma venereum, granuloma venereum and syphilis (Attili et al. 1983).

Detection of the ova in various stages of degeneration and tissue reactions are the basis of the histopathological diagnosis. The histopathological changes of the female genital tract lesions are not different from those at other locations. The collection of eosinophils in large numbers in the tissues forming eosinophilic abscesses, circumscribed granulomas and foreign body-type giant cell reactions can all be seen in the female genital tract (Wright et al. 1982). The vulval lesions can manifest like warts, warty nodules, vitiligo (McKee et al. 1983), ulcerated nodules on the clitoris and painless nodules on the labia (Attili et al. 1983).

16.1.13 Elephantiasis

Primary congenital lymphoedema of the vulva is very uncommon, but in tropical and temperate areas where filariasis is endemic, lymphoedema of the vulva and lower extremities can occasionally be seen. These lesions result from lymphatic blockage due to recurrent lymphangitis caused by *Wuchereria bancrofti* and *Brugia malayi*.

Microscopically, the blubbery tissue is composed of dilated lymphatic vessels, fibrosis, interstitial oedema, infiltrations of lymphocytes, plasma cells, eosinophils and occasional giant cells. The epidermis is thickened and shows hyperkeratosis.

16.1.14 Loxosceles reclusa Spider Bite

Magrina and Masterson (1981) reported a patient who developed a chronic necrotic ulcer on the vulva and systemic symptoms following *Loxoceles reclusa* spider bite. Biopsy revealed chronic inflammation, abscess and reactive inguinal lymphadenitis. Partial vulvectomy was curative (Magrina and Masterson (1981).

16.2 Non-specific

16.2.1 Granulation Tissue

Formation of granulation tissue following hysterectomy is not uncommon. Occasionally, it attains a large size and becomes a polypoid tumour-like mass. The main complaint of the patient is vaginal discharge or post-coital bleeding. Microscopically, the tissue consists of numerous young fibroblasts, capillaries, inflammatory cells including macrophages, lymphocytes, plasma cells and polymorphonuclear cells.

16.2.2 Granuloma Pyogenicum

The term granuloma pyogenicum is incorrect as no granuloma is seen in the lesion. The inflammatory cell infiltrations are so common in the lesion that it is believed to be a type of granulation tissue. Because of its very vascular character and close resemblance to a capillary haemangioma, the lesion is considered also to be a variant of the latter.

It is a polypoid mass of a few millimeters to a few centimeters in size, either sessile or projecting from the skin or mucous surface by a short stalk. It is a red-brown, granular and friable mass which bleeds easily. Granuloma pyogenicum has also been observed within the vein (Ulbright and Santa-Cruz 1980).

Microscopically, the lesion consists of lobules of compact clusters of bland endothelial cells and newly formed capillaries surrounded by loose, myxomatous stroma (Fig. 16.5). Some of the capillaries within the lobules may be dilated. Inflammatory cellular infiltrations, which may be absent in the early phase, can be extensive in the older lesions. The overlying epithelium may be thickened or thin and ulcerated. Invagination of the epidermis at the neck of the lesion may produce an epidermal collarette (Kaufman and Gardner 1961). The hallmark of the histological diagnosis of the condition is its lobular pattern. According to some authors, the lesion should be called lobular capillary haemangioma (Cooper and Mills 1982).

16.2.2.1 Treatment

Simple excision is adequate.

16.2.3 Hidradenitis Suppuritivum

Hidradenitis suppuritivum appears as chronic, progressive, unrelenting and recurrent abscesses of the skin and subcutaneous tissue of the perineum, axillae and groin. The lesion occurs initially as firm, tender, pea-sized nodules which rupture and form sinuses. Although the redness disappears, induration persists, and in 2–3 months, palpable cords with contracture of the area result from subcutaneous fibrosis (Vickeers 1975). The condition probably begins as obstructions of the apocrine ducts from inspissated secretions with eventual discharge into the dermis (Broadwater et al. 1982) which becomes secondarily infected (Masson 1969). The disease occurs after puberty, and the majority of patients are in their 2nd and 3rd decades (Thornton and Abcarian 1978). Hidradenitis suppuritivum has been noticed with a somewhat increasing frequency in women taking certain types of combined oestrogen-progesterone contraceptive pills (Stellon and Wakeling 1989). Because of the chronic pain and malodour of the discharge, the patients may avoid social contacts and suffer from depression (Shaughnessy et al. 1972).

Microscopically, the lesion is characterised by acute and chronic inflammations, dilatation of the apocrine glands with inspissated glandular secretions (Shaughnessy et al. 1972) and later destruction of pilosebaceous units and eventual scarring. The long-standing lesions can be complicated by squamous cell carcinoma (Thornton and Abcarian 1978; Donsky and Mendelson 1964) which occurs in about 3% of patients (Jackman 1959).

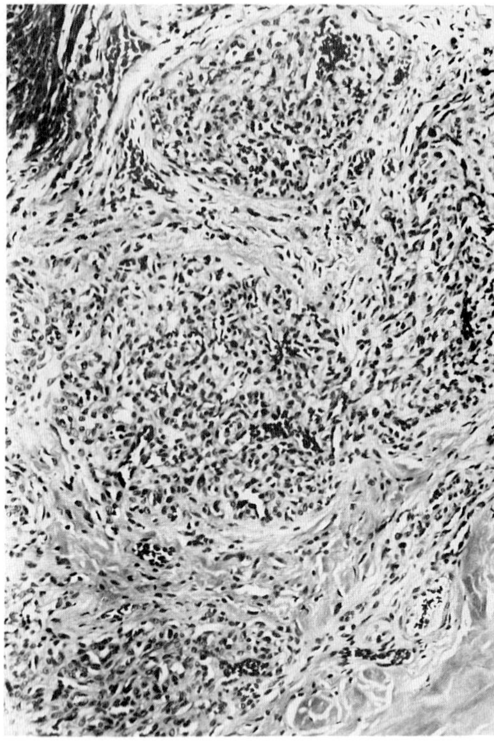

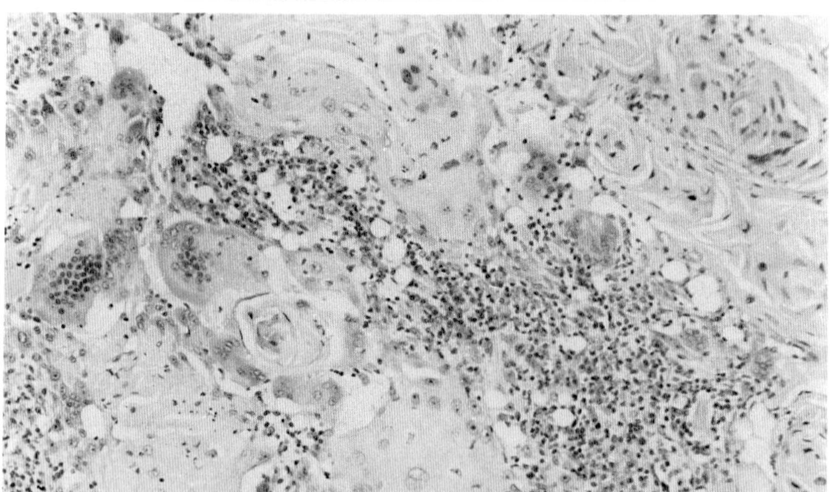

Fig. 16.5. Pyogenic granuloma: lobules of endothelial-lined spaces

Fig. 16.6. Pilonidal sinus: foreign body-type giant cells and other inflammatory cells. A hair shaft can be seen in many lesions

16.2.3.1 Treatment

Early treatment has been advocated by most authors (Shaughnessy et al. 1972; Vickeers 1975; Bhatia et al. 1984). Injections of steroid, incision and drainage, and topical and systemic antibiotics have not been found successful in the treatment of vulval lesions (Thomas et al. 1985). Wide excision of the apocrine gland followed by skin grafting has been recommended as the treatment of choice for advanced disease and to prevent recurrence (Broadwater et al. 1982). Although the results of treatment with isotretinoin in different series are not uniform, Brown et al. (1988) noticed a very good response with oral administration of this drug. The drug is contraindicated in pregnancy.

16.2.4 Pilonidal Sinus of the Vulva

The pilonidal sinus most commonly occurs at the base of the spine. It is a chronic abscess cavity containing hair follicles, hair shaft, granulation tissue, inflammatory cells and occasional giant cells (Fig. 16.6). The cavity communicates with the surface through a sinus which is lined by granulation tissue. Because of its location at the lower part of the back, the lesion was thought to be congenital in origin. Similar lesions can, however, be seen in the interdigital webs of the hands of barbers. It is now generally believed that these lesions occur as a result of penetration of hairs to the subcutaneous tissue which becomes secondarily infected.

In the vulva, pilonidal sinuses occur in the clitoris and labia minora (Betson et al. 1962; Palmer 1957; Smith 1951). The patients usually present with pain and swelling in the genitalia and occasionally with a discharging sinus.

16.2.4.1 Treatment

An acute abscess is treated by drainage, and the chronic abscess is removed by surgical excision.

16.2.5 Sclerosing Lipogranuloma

Sclerosing lipogranuloma is a granulomatous type of fat necrosis which occurs in the genitalia and other regions after the injection of foreign oil and sometimes without any known aetiological agent (Kempson and Sherman 1968). The lesion can present as a mass in the vulval region with lymphadenopathy and be mistaken for a malignant tumour.

Grossly, the lipogranulomatous mass is well-delineated with a firm to rubbery consistency.

Microscopically, the lesion consists of foam cells, small clear spaces formed by fat cells and larger cyst-like spaces lined by foreign body-type giant cells, set in dense and loose bands of hyalinised fibrocollagenous tissue.

16.2.5.1 Treatment

The treatment is surgical excision.

16.2.6 Crohn's Disease

The gynaecological importance of Crohn's disease lies in the fact that clinical manifestations of the disease may mimic other gynaecological problems, such as lower abdominal and pelvic pain and an abdominal mass which may be misdiagnosed as inflammatory pelvic disease or ovarian cysts. Also, the complications like abscess and fistula formation and its skin manifestation may directly affect the genital area (Parks et al. 1965; Kao et al. 1975). Although involvement of the vulva in Crohn's disease is infrequent, perianal manifestations are quite common (Gray et al. 1965), with an estimated incidence ranging between 11% and 93% of patients (Williams 1971). In some patients, the perianal lesion is the first manifestation of the disease (Spiro 1983). Dermatological manifestations occur in about 45% of patients (McCallum and Kinmont 1968) and consist of erythema nodosum, pyoderma gangrenosum, furunculosis and ulcerations. The ulcers may be perineal, parastomal and metastatic (Maountain 1970). The metastatic lesions develop remote from the gastrointestinal lesions and are separated from other ulcers by normal skin. The vulva can be affected both by metastatic and direct spread of the perineal lesions (Levine et al. 1982; Kao et al. 1975; Ansell and Hogbin 1973; Devroede et al. 1975).

Clinically, the patients are in their 20s and 30s and have a clinical history of Crohn's disease of the bowel. On rare occasions, the vulval lesion is the sole presenting feature (Holohan et al. 1988), which may consist of swelling, mass, abscess, ulceration and induration with discharging sinuses. The patient's initial complaints may be prutitus, vaginal discharge, bleeding and painful vulval ulcer. Anterior vulva, clitoris, labia majora and pernineum are the sites usually affected. Extensive destruction of the tissue by the sinus tracts may eventually lead to the formation of skin tags and bridges (Kao et al. 1975).

16.2.6.1 Microscopical Appearance

Before the ulcers develop, the earliest changes in the swollen area consist of oedema, collections of lymphocytes, plasma cells, histiocytes and neutrophils. The typical lesion is characterised by non-caseating granulomas composed of foreign body giant cells, epithelioid cells, and lymphocytes (Fig. 16.7). Abscesses, cleft fissures, granulation tissue and fibrosis are also frequent components of the lesions. In long-standing lesions, fibrosis may be extensive, causing disfigurement of the vulva. Crohn's disease can be differentiated from actinomycosis and tuberculosis without much difficulty. Lymphogranuloma venereum is associated with inguinal lymphadenitis.

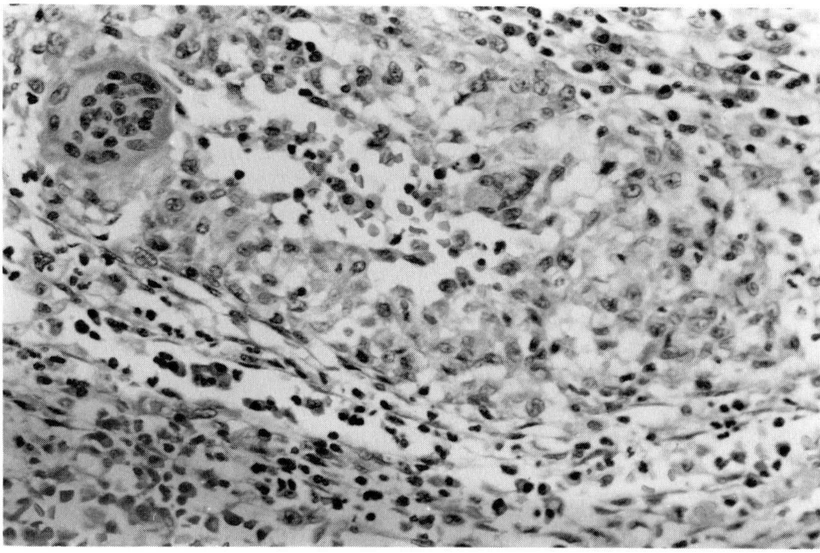

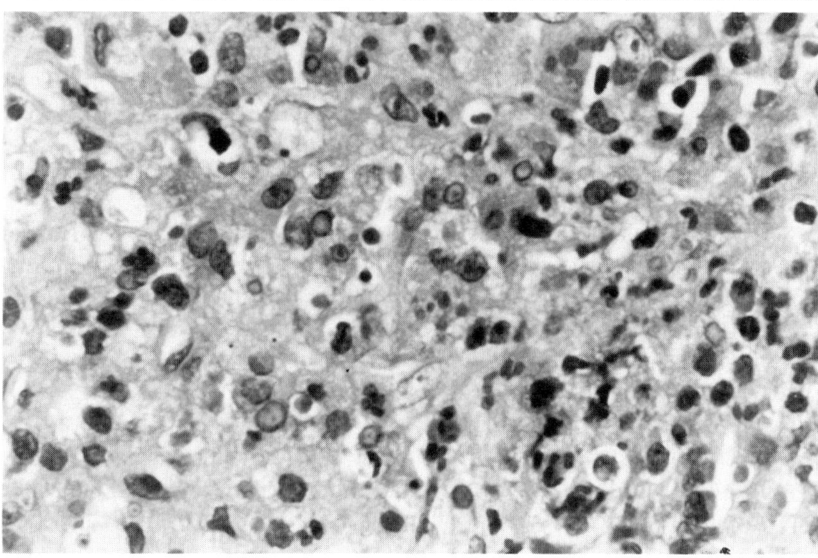

Fig. 16.7. Crohn's disease: non-caseating granuloma with giant cells and epithelioid cells

Fig. 16.8. Malakoplakia: scattered calcified (Michaelis Gutmann) bodies and chronic inflammatory cells

16.2.6.2 Treatment

Medical management with corticosteroids, sulphasalazine and azothiaprine has been advocated as the mainstay of therapy, as in the gastrointestinal disease (Holland and Greiss 1983). Surgery is generally reserved for complications (Donaldson 1976). The surgical management includes simple debridement, simple excision, myocutaneous skin graft and vulvectomy (Holland and Greiss 1983). Radical excision of the whole lesion may be necessary to offer a cure, particularly in those patients whose intestinal lesions are well controlled but whose mutating vulval lesions persist (Kao et al. 1975).

16.2.7 Malakoplakia of the Vulva

Malakoplakia is an unusual chronic inflammatory process which has been noticed in many organs including skin (Moore et al. 1973), eyes, tonsils, lungs, gastrointestinal and urinary systems, testes (Brown and Smith 1967) and female genital tract. Concerning the last, the vagina appears to be the most commonly afflicted site (McClure 1983). Lesions affecting the endometrium (Thomas et al. 1977; Molnar and Poliak 1983), broad ligament, inguinal region (Rao 1969), cervix (Wahl 1982; Willen et al. 1983; Chen and Hendricks 1985), Bartholin's gland (Pasquin et al. 1986) and vulva have been reported. The patients are mostly elderly, with a mean age of 61 years (McClure 1983). They may present with a cyst or mass in the Bartholin's gland area or an ulcer on the vulva (Arul and Emmerson 1977).

Microscopically, malakoplakia is characterised by the predominance of macrophages with pale eosinophilic, coarsely granular cytoplasm (von Hansemann cells). The presence of intra- and extra-cellular calcified bodies commonly known as Michaelis-Gutmann bodies is considered a hallmark of the diagnosis (Fig. 16.8). These bodies are round or oval, concentrically laminated structures stained for calcium and iron. They are commonly seen within the cytoplasm of macrophages. The other cellular infiltrates of the lesions comprise lymphocytes, plasma cells, neutrophils and occasionally giant cells.

The ultrastructural studies suggest that in the histiocytes, Michaelis-Gutmann bodies are formed within single membrane-bound cytoplasmic inclusions containing finely granular matrix material and concentric freagments in which hydroxyapatite crystals are laid (Price et al. 1973). Degradation of intra-cellular bacteria or incorporation and persistence of bacteria within the phagolysosomes as dense aggregates which later become calcified are also considered to be sources of Michaelis-Gutmann bodies (McClurg et al. 1973).

The aetiology is not known. The condition may be an infective process (Lewin et al. 1976). Infection with *Escherichia coli* has been commonly associated with this condition (Chalvardijan et al. 1980). It has been suggested that the macrophages are defective in their phagocytic function, leading to incomplete destruction of bacteria within the cytoplasm, which are ultimately calcified to form the Michaelis-Gutmann bodies.

Malakoplakia has been frequently reported in patients with immunological disorders such as lymphoma (Lewin et al. 1976), rheumatoid arthritis (Moore et al. 1973), carcinoma (Dockerty 1972), renal transplants (Sian et al. 1981) and familial immune deficiency syndrome (Almagro et al. 1981).

16.2.7.1 Treatment

The treatment is excision of the lesion. Abdou et al. (1979) using a cholinergic agonist raised the level of cyclic guanosine monophosphate in macrophages and achieved a dramatic improvement of the condition.

References

Human Pailloma Virus Infections

Bornstein J, Kaufman RH, Adam E et al. (1988) Multicentric intraepithelial neoplasia involving the vulva: clinical features and association with human pailloma virus and herpes simplex virus. Cancer 62:1601–1604

Buscema J, Naghashafar Z, Swadar E et al. (1988) Predominance of human papilloma virus type 16 in vulvar neoplasia. Obstet Gynecol 71:601–606

Coggin JR, zur Hausen H (1979) Workshop on papilloma virus and cancer. Cancer Res 39:545–546

Crum CP, Liskow A, Petras P et al. (1984) VIN (severe atypia and carcinoma in situ): a clinicopathologic study of 41 cases. Cancer 54:1429–1434

Downey GO, Okagaki T, Ostrow RS et al. (1988) Condylomatous carcinoma of the vulva with special reference to human papilloma virus DNA. Obstet Gynecol 72:68–73

Favre M, Orth G, Croissant O et al. (1975) Human Papilloma virus DNA: physical map. Proc Natl Acad Sci USA 72:4810–4814

Gissmann L, zur Hausen H (1978) Physical characterisatiaon of the deoxyribonucleic acids of different human papilloma viruses (HPV). Med Microbiol Immunol 166:3–11

Gissmann L, Boshart M, Durst M et al. (1984) Presence of human pailloma virus in genital tumors. J Invest Dermatol 83 [Suppl]:26–28

Gupta J, Pilotti S, Shah KV et al. (1987) Human papilloma virus associated with early vulvar neoplasms investigated by in situ hybridisatiaon. Am J Surg Pathol 11:430–434

Ikenberg H, Gissmann L, Gross G et al. (1983) Human papilloma virus type 16 related DNA in genital Bowen's disease and Bowenoid papullosis. Int J Cancer 32:563–565

Meisels A, Roy M, Fortier M et al. (1981) Human papilloma virus of the cervix: the atypical condyloma. Acta Cytol (Baltimore) 25:7–16

Melnick JL (1962) Papova virus group. Science 135:1178–1130

Nash JD, Burke TW, Hoskings WJ (1987) Biological course of cervical human papilloma virus infection. Obstet Gynecol 69:160–162

Orth G, Favre M, Croissant O (1977) Characterisation of a new type of a human papilloma virus that causes skin warts. J Virol 24:108–120

Pilotti S, Rilke F, Shah K et al. (1984) Immunohistochemical and ultrastructural evidence of HPV infection associated with in situ and microinvasive squamous cell carcinoma of the vulva: Am J Surg Pathol 8:751–761

Randoo RF, Sedlacek TV, Hunt J et al. (1986) Verrucous carcinoma of the vulva associated with an unusual type 6 human papilloma virus. Obstet Gynecol 67 [Suppl]:70–75

Sutton GP, Stehman FB, Ehrlich CE et al. (1987) Human papilloma virus deoxyribonucleic acid in lesions of the female genital tract: evidence for type 6/11 in squamous carcinoma of the vulva. Obstet Gynecol 70:564–568

Wilbur DC, Bonfiglio TA, Stoler MH (1988) Continuity of human pailloma virus (HPV) type between neoplastic precursors and invasive cervical carcinoma: an in situ hybridisatiaon study. Am J Surg Pathol 12:182–186

Codylomata Acuminata

Benschine FW Jr (1941) Massive condylomata acuminata of the vulva complicating labor. Am J Obstet Gynecol 42:338–340

Campion MJ, Clarkson P, McCance DJ (1985) Squamous neoplasia of the cervix in relation to other genital tract neoplasia. Clin Obstet Gynecol 12:265–280

Dunn AEG, Ogilvie MM (1968) Intranuclear virus particles in human genital wart tissue: observations on the ultrastructure of the epidermal layer. J Ultzrastruct Res 22:282–295

Eron LJ, Judson F, Tucker S et al. (1986) Interferon therapy for condylomata acuminata. N Engl J Med 315:1059–1064

Ferenczy A (1983) Using the laser to treat vulvar condylomata acuminata and intraepidermal neoplasia. Can Med Assoc J 128:135–137

Gardner HL, Kaufman RH (1965) Condylomata acuminata. Clin Obstet Gynecol 8:938–945

Ghosh AK (1978) Cryosurgery of genital warts in cases in which podophyllin treatment has failed or was contraindicated. Br J Vener Dis 54:352–353

Gissmann L, De-Villiers EM, zur Hausen H (1982) Analysis of human genital warts (condylomata acuminata) and other genital tumours for human papilloma virus type DNA. Int J Cancer 29:143–146

Gissmann L, Wolnik L, Ikenberg H et al. (1983) Human papilloma viruses type 6 and 11 DNA sequences in genital and laryngeal papillomas and in some cervical cancer. Proc Natl Acad Sci USA 80:560–563

Gorthey RL, Krembs MA (1954) Vulvar condylomata acuminata complicating labor. Obstet Gynecol 4:67–74

Lynch PJ (1985) Condyloma acuminata (Anogenital warts). Clin Obstet Gynecol 28:142–151

McCance D, Singer A (1986) The importance of HPV infections in the male and female genital tract and their relationship to cervical neoplasia. In: Poland A, Kimbrough RD (eds) Viral etiology of cervical cancer. Cold Spring Harbour Labnoratory, Cold Spring Harbor NY, pp 311–319 (Branbury report 21)

Meisels A, Roy M (1977) Condylomatous lesions of the cervix. II Cytologic, colposcopic and histilogic study. Acta Cytol (Baltimore) 21:379–390

Obalek S, Glinski W, Haftek M et al. (1980) Comparative studies on cell mediated immunity in patients with different warts. Dermatoalogica 161:73–83

Oriel JD (1971) Natural history of genital warts. Br J Vener Dis 47:1–13

Oriel JD, Almedia JD (1970) Demonstration of virus particles in human genital warts. Br J Vener Dis 46:37–42

Powell LC Jr (1978) Condyloma acuminata: recent advances in development, carcinogenesis and treatment. Clin Obstet Gynecol 21:1061–1078

Reid R (1985) Superficial laser vulvectomy: efficacy of extended superficial ablataion for refractory and very extensive condylomas. Am J Obstet Gynecol 151:1047–1052

Schonfeld A, Schattner A, Crespi M et al. (1984) Intramuscular human interferon-B injections in treatment of condyloma acuminatum. Lancet I:1038–1041

Shevchuk MM, Richart RM (1982) DNA content of condyloma acuminta. Cancer 49:489–492

Sillman FH, Sedlis A, Boyce JG (1985) A review of lower intraepithelial neoplasia and use of topical 5 fluorouracil. Obstet Gynecol Surv 40:190–220

Staguet MJ, Viac J, Bustamante R et al. (1981) Human papilloma virus Type 1 purified from human genital wartzs. Dermatologia 162:213–219

Syrjanen KJ (1983) Immunocompetent cells in uterine cervical lesions of human papilloma virus origin. Gynecol Obstet Invest 16:327–340

Syrjanen KJ, Vayrynen M, Castren O et al. (1984) The relation between type of immunoreactive cells found in human papilloma virus (HPV) lesion of the uterine cervix and subsequent behaviour of these lesions. Arch Gynecol 234:189–196

Vallejos H, Del Mistro A, Kleinhaus S et al. (1987) Characterisation of human papilloma virus types in condyloma acuminata in children by in situ hybridization. Lab Invest 611–615

Walker PJ, Singer A, Dyson J et al. (1984) The natural history of cervical intraepithelial abnormalities in patients with vulval warts. Br J Vener Dis 59:327–329

Wilson J (1973) Extensive vulval condylomata acuminata necessitating Caesarean section. Aust N Z J Obstet Gynaecol 13:121–124

Squamous Papilloma

Ackerman AB, Kornberg R (1973) Pearly penile papules. Arch Dermatol 108:673–675

Grob JJ, Collet-Villette AM, Andrac L et al. (1987) Papillomatose hirsutoide de la vulve. Acta Derm Venereol (Stockh) 114:1235–1236

Growdon WA, Fu Y-S, Lebherz TB et al. (1985) Pruritic vulvar squamous papillomatosis: evidence for human papilloma virus etiology. Obstet Gynecol 66:564–568

Manoharan V, Sommerville JM (1985) Benign squamous papillomatosis: case report. Genitourin Med 63:393–395

Herpes Virus Infection

Adamas HG, Benson EA, Alexander ER et al. (1976) Genital herpetic infection in men and women: clinical course and effect of topical application of adenine arabinoside. J Infect Dis 133 [Suppl A]:151–159

Cabral GA, Marciane-Cabral F, Fry D et al. (1982) Expression of herpes simplex virus type antigens in premalignant and malignant human vulvar cells. Am J Obstet Gynecol 143:611-619

Corey L, Holmes KK (1983) Genital herpes simplex virus infections: current concept of diagnosis, therapy and prevention. Ann Intern Med 98:973–983

Guinan ME, McCalman J, Kern ER et al. (1981) The course of untreated recurrent genital herpes simplex infection in 27 women. N Engl J Med 304:759–763

Hertz K, Crawford PS, Chez RA et al. (1977) Herpes gestationalis: an update. Obstet Gynecol 49:733–735

Hill T, Blyth WA (1976) An alternative theory of herpes simplex recurrence and a possible role for prostaglandins. Lancet I:397–399

Kaufman RH, Bornstein J, Adam E et al. (1988) Human papilloma virus and herpes simplex virus in vulvar squamous cell carcinoma in situ. Am J Obstet Gynecol 158:862–871

Munoz N, Rabson A, Bedoya V et al. (1969) Infection of hamster spleen and thymus with herpes simplex virus in vitro and vivo. JNCI 42:165–174

Ng ABP, Reagan J, Lender E (1970) The cellular manifestations of primary and recurrent herpes genitalis. Acta Cytol (Baltimore) 14:124–129

Pazin GJ, Armstrong JA, Lam MT et al. (1978) Prevention of reactivated herpes simplex infection by human leucocyte interfern after operation on the trigenimal root. N Engl J Med 301:225–230

Reeves WC, Corey L, Adams HG (1981) Risk of recurrence after first episode of genital herpes. N Engl J Med 305:315–319

Wilbanks GD, Campbell JA, Kaufman LA (1970) Cellular changes of normal cervical epithelium infected in vitro with herpes hominis type 2 (herpes simplex). Acta Cytol (Baltimore) 538–543

Tuberculous Ulcer

Bhattacharya P (1978) Hypertrophic tuberculosis of the vulva. Obstet Gynecol 51 [Suppl]: 21–22

Corbet RM (1953) A case of tuberculosis of the vulva. J Obstet Gynaecol Br Emp 60:512–514

Lymphogranuloma Venereum

Douglas CP (1962) Lymphogranuloma venereum and granuloma inguinale of the vulva. J Obsteet Gynaecol Br Commonw 69:871–880

Holder WR, Duncan WC (1972) Lymphogranuloma venereum. Clin Obstet Gynecol 15: 1004–1009

Koteen H (1945) Lymphogranuloma venereum. Medicine (Baltimore) 24:1–69

Pund ER, Dick F Jr (1947) Lymphogranuloma venereum: pathologic basis of its various manifestations. Urol Cutaneous Rev 51:345–349

Schacter J (1978) Chlamydial infections. N Engl J Med 298:490–495

Swink RL (1949) Lymphogranuloma venereum associated with squamous cell carcinoma. South Med J 42:217–220

Lymphogranuloma Inguinale

Davis CM (1970) Granuloma inguinale. JAMA 211:632–636

Dodson RF, Fritz GS, Hubler WR et al. (1974) Donovanosis: a morphologic study. J Invest Dermatol 62:611–614

Garg BR (1978) Donovanosis of oral cavity. Br J Vener Dis 51:136–137

Hart G (1983) Chancroid, donovanosis and lymphogranuloma venereum. Dermatol Clin 1:75–83

Kirkpatrick DJ (1970) Donovanosis, a rare case of osteolytic bone lesions. Clin Radiol 21:101–106

Lal S, Garg BR (1980) Further evidence of the efficacy of co-trimoxazole in granuloma venereum. Br J Vener Dis 56:412–413

Milton MMA (1958) Donovanosis of the anus in the male: an epidermiological consideration. Br J Vener Dis 34:213–218

Pund ER, Botcher VA (1948) Granuloma venereum (granuloma inguinale) of uterus, tubes and ovaries. Surgery 3:34–40

Sehgal VN, Shyam-Prasad AL (1986) Donovanosis: current concepts. Int J Dermatol 25:8–16

Spagnolo DV, Coburn PR, Cream JJ et al. (1984) Extragenital granuloma inguinale (donovanosis) diagnosed in the United Kingdom: a clinical, histological and electron micrscopic study. J Clin Pathol 37:945–949

Stewart DB (1964) The gynecological lesions of lymphogranuloma venereum and granuloma inguinale. Med Clin North Am 48:773–786

Chancroid

Gaisin A, Heaton CL (1975) Chancroid alias soft chancre. Int J Dermatol 14:188–197

Mohanty KC (1988) Diagnosis and treatment of chancroid. Br J Sex Med 15:91–92

Ronald AR (1986) Chancroid: recent advances in treatment and control. Int J Dermatol 25:31–33

Sheldon WH, Heym,an A (1946) Studies on chancroid. I. Observations on the histology with an evaluation ob biopsy as a diagnostic procedure. Am J Pathol 22:415–426

Molluscum Contagiosum

Gudgel EF (1968) Can molluscum contagiosum be a venereal disease? US Armed Forces Med J 98:141–143

Lynch PJ, Minkin W (1968) Molluscum contagiosum of the adult: probable venereal transmission. Arch Dermatol 98:141–143

Reed RJ, Parkinson RP (1977) The histogenesis of molluscum contagiosum. Am J Surg Pathol 1:161–166

Wilkin JK (1977) Molluscum contagiosum venereum in a women's outpatient clinic: a venereally transmitted disease. Am J Obstet Gynecol 128:531–535

Amoebic Ulcer

Bhaduri KP (1957) Endamoeba histolytica in leukorrhoea and salpingitis. Am J Obstet Gynecol 74:434–435

Brandt H, Tamayo RP (1970) Pathology of human amoebiasis. Hum Pathol 1:351–385

Carter B, Jones CP, Thomas ML (1954) Invasion of the squamous carcinoma of the cervix uteri by endamoeba histolytica. Am J Obstet Gynecol 68:1607–1609

De Rivas D (1944) Amoebiasis of the uterus. Am J Trop Med 24:185–188

De Torres EF, Benitez-Bribiesca L (1973) Cytological detection of vaginal parasitosis. Acta Cytol (Baltimore) 17:252–257

Heinz KPW (1973) Amoebic infection of the female genital tract: a report of three cases. S Afr Med J 47:1795–1798

Hingorani V, Mahapatra LN (1964) Amoebiasis of the vagina and cervix. J Int Coll Surg 42:552–667

Majumdar B, Chaiken ML, Lee KU (1976) Amoebiasis of clitoris mimicking carcinoma. JAMA 236:1145–1146

Munguia H, Franco E, Valenzuela P (1966) Diagnosis of genital amoebiasis in women by standard papanicoloau technique. Am J Obstet Gynecol 94:181–188

Veliath AJ, Bansal R, Sankaran V et al. (1987) Genital amoebiasis. Int J Gynaecol Obstet 25:249–256

Schistosomiasis

Ad-Adnani MS, Saleh KM (1982) Extraurinary schistosomiasis in South Iran. Histopathology 6:747–6752

Attili VR, Hira SK, Dube MK (1983) Schistosomal genital granulomas: a report of 10 cases. Br J Vener Dis 59:269–272

Berry A (1966) A cytopathological and histopathological study of bilharziasis of the female genital tract. J Pathol Bacteriol 91:325–338

Berry A (1976) Multispecies schistosomal infections of the female genital tract detected in cytology smears. Acta Cytol (Baltimore) 20:361–365

Charlewood GP, Shippel S, Renton H (1949) Schistosomiasis in gynaecology. J Obstet Gynaecol Br Emp 56:367–385

Gelfand M, Ross MD, Blair DM et al. (1971) Distribution and extent of schistosomiasis in female pelvic organs with specvial reference to the genital tract as determined by autopsy. Am J Trop Med 20:846–849

McKee PH, Wright E, Hutt MS (1983) Vulval schistosomiasis. Clin Exp Dermatol 8:189–194

Wright ED, Chiphanwi, Hutt SR (1982) Schistosomiasis of the female genital tract: a histopathological study of 176 cases from Malawi. Trans R Soc Trop Med Hyg 76:822–829

Loxosceles Reclusa Spider Bite

Magrina JF, Masterson BJ (1981) Loxosceles reclusa spider bite: a consideration in the differential diagnosis of chronic nonmalignant ulcers of the vulva. Am J Obstet Gynecol 140:341–343

Granuloma Pyogenicum

Cooper PH, Mills AC (1982) Subcutaneous granuloma pyogenicum: lobular capillary haemangioma. Arch Dermatol 118:30–33

Kaufman RH, Gardner HL (1961) Benign mesodermal tumors. Obstet Gynecol 8:1953–1961

Ulbright TM, Santa-Cruz DJ (1980) Intravenous pyogenic granuloma: case report with ultrastructural findings. Cancer 45:1646–1652

Hidradenitis Suppuritivum

Bhatia NN, Bergman A, Boren EM (1984) Advanced hidradenitis suppuritiva of the vulva. J Reprod Med 29:436–440

Broadwater JR, Bryant RL, Petrino RA et al. (1982) Advanced hidradenitis suppuritiva: review of surgical treatment in 23 pat8ients. Am J Surg 144:668–670

Brown CF, Gallup DC, Brown VM (1988) Hidradenitis suppuritiva of the anogenital region: response to isotretionon. Am J Obstet Gynecol 158:12–15

Donsky HJ, Mendelson CG (1964) Squamous cell carcinoma as a complication of hidradenitis suppuritiva. Arch Dermatol 90:488–491

Jackman RJ (1959) Hidradenitis suppuritiva: diagnosis and surgical management of perianal manifestations. Proc R Soc Med 52 BSuppl:110–111

Masson JK (1969) Surgical treatment for hydradermitis suppurativa. Surg Clin N Am 49:1043–1062

Shaughnessy DM, Greminger RR, Margolis IE et al. (1972) Hidradenitis suppurativa: a plea for early operative treatment. JAMA 222:320–321

Stellon AJ, Wakeling M (1989) Hidradenitis suppuritiva associated with use of oral contraceptives. Br Med J 1:28–29

Thomas R, Barnhill D, Bibro M et al. (1985) Hidradenitis suppurativa: a case presentatiaon and review of the literature. Obstet Gynecol 66:592–595

Thornton JP, Abcarian H (1978) Surgical treatment of perianal and perineal hidradinitis suppurativa. Dis Colon Rectum 21:573–577

Vickeers MA Jr (1975) Operative management of chronic hidradenitis suppuritiva of the scrotum and perineum. J Urol 114:414–416

Pilonidal Sinus

Betson JR Jr, Chiffelle TL, George RP (1962) Pilonidal sinus involving the clitoris: a case report. Am J Obstet Gynecol 84:543–545

Palmer E (1957) Pilonidal cyst of the clitoris. Am J Surg 93:133–136

Smith TE (1951) Anterior or piecemeal pilonidal cyst. JAMA 136:973

Sclerosing Lipogranuloma

Kempson RL, Sherman AI (1968) Sclerosing lipogranuloma of the vulva. Am J Obstet Gynecol 101:854–856

Crohn's Disease

Ansell JD, Hogbin B (1973) Corhn's disease of the vulva. J Obstet Gynaecol Br Common w 80:376–378

Devroede G, Schlaeder G, Sanchez G et al. (1975) Crohn's disease of the vulva. Am J Clin Pathol 63:348–358

Donaldson LB (1976) Crohn's disease: its gynecologic aspects. Am J Obstet Gynecol 131:196–202

Gray BK, Lockhart-Mummery HE, Morson BC (1965) Crohn's disease of the anal region. Gut 6:515–524

Holland RM, Greiss FC Jr (1983) Perineal Crohn's disease. Obstet Gynecol 62:527–529

Holohan M, Coughlan M, O'Loughlin S et al. (1988) Crohn's disease of the vulva. Case report. Br J Obstet Gynaecol 95:943–945

Kao M-S, Paulson JD, Askin LB (1975) Crohn's disease of the vulva: Obstet Gynecol 46:329–333

Levine EM, Barton JJ, Grier EA (1982) Metastatic Crohn's disease of the vulva. Obstet Cynecol 60:395–397

McCallum DI, Kinmont PDC (1968) Dermatoalogical manifestataions of Crohn's disease. Br J Dermatol 80:1–8
Mountain JC (1970) Cutaneous ulceration in Crohn's disease. Gut 11:18–26
Parks AG, Morson BC, Pegum JS (1965) Crohn's disease with cutaneous involvement. Proc R Soc Med 58:241–242
Spiro HM (1983) Clinical gastroenterology, 3rd edn. McMillan, New York, pp 891–924
Williams JA (1971) Progress report: the place of surgery in Crohn's disease. Gut 12:739–745

Malakoplakia
Abdou NI, NaPombejara C, Sagawa A et al. (1979) Malakoplakia: evidence for monocyte lysosomal abnormality correctable by cholinergic agonist in vitro and in vivo. N Engl J Med 297:1413–1419
Almagro UA, Choi H, Caya JG et al. (1981) Cutaneous malakoplakia: report of a case and review of the literature. Am J Dermatopathol 3:295–301
Arul K, Emmerson RW (1977) Malakoplakia of the skin. Clin Exp Dermatol 2:131–135
Brown RC, Smith BH (1967) Malakoplakia of the testes. Am J Clin Pathol 47:135–147
Chalvardijan AC, Picard L, Shaw R et al. (1980) Malakoplakia of the female genital tract. Am J Obstet Gynecol 138:391–394
Chen KTK, Hendricks EJ (1985) Malakoplakia of the female genital tract. Obstet Gynecol 65 [Suppl]:84–87
Dockerty MB (1972) Primary malakoplakia of the colon. Mayo Clin Proc 47:114–116
Hoffman E, Garrido M (1964) Malakoplakia of the prostate. J Urol 92:311–313
Lewin KJ, Fair WR, Steigbigel RT et al. (1976) Clinical and laboratory studies into the pathogenesis of malakoplakia. J Clin Pathol 29:354–363
McClure J (1983) Malakoplakia. J Pathol 140:275–330
McClurg FV, D'Agostino AN, Martin JH et al. (1973) Ultrastructural demonstration of intracellular hacteria in three cases of malakoplakia of bladder. Am J Clin Pathol 60:780–788
Molnar JJ, Poliak A (1983) Recurrenct endometrial malakoplakia. Am J Clin Pathol 80:762–764
Moore WM III, Stokes TL, Cabanas VY (1973) Malakoplakia of the skin: report of a case. Am J Clin Pathol 60:218–221
Paquin ML, Davis JR, weiner S (1986) Malakoplakia of Bartholin's gland. Arch Pathol Lab Med 110:757–758
Price HM, Hanrahan JB, Florida RG (1973) Morphogenesis of calcium laden cytoplasmic bodies in malakoplakia of the skin: an electron microscopic study. Hum Pathol 4:381–394
Rao NR (1969) Malakoplakia of broad ligament and inguinal region. Arch Pathol 88:85–89
Sian CS, McCabe RE, Lattes CY (1981) Malakoplakia of skin and subcantenous tissue in a renal transplant recipient. Arch Dermatol 117:654–655
Thomas W Jr, Sadegieh B, Fresco R et al. (1977) Malakoplakia of the endometrium, a probable cause of post menopausal bleeding. Am J Clin Pathol 69:637–641
Wahl RW (1982) Malakoplakia of uterine cervix: report of two cases. Acta Cytol (Baltimore) 26:691–694
Willen R, Stendahl U, Willen H et al. (1983) Malakoplakia of the cervix and corpus uteri: a light microcopic, and X-ray microprobe analysis of a case. Int J Gynecol Pathol 2:201–208

17 Secondary Tumours

Secondary malignant tumours of the vulva are far less common than primary ones. In the series of Dehner (1973), secondaries constituted the third largest group of vulval malignant tumours. Cervical cancer was the most frequent primary. Burgess and Waymont (1987) noted metastatic deposits of a cervical carcinoma in an epidiotomy scar. Endometrial carcinoma, uterine malignant mixed mesodermal tumours (Dehner 1973), choriocarcinoma, carcinomas of the rectum and lung – all can metastasise to the vulva (Janovski and Douglas 1972). There are also reports of metastases from hypernephroma (Taussig 1938) and carcinoma of the breast (Mader and Friedrich 1982). Carcinoma of the vagina and urethra can involve the vulva by direct extension.

References

Burgess SP, Waymont B (1987) Implantation of a cervical carcinoma in an episiotomy site: case report. Br J Obstet Gynaecol 94:598–599

Dehner LP (1973) Metastatic and secondary tumours of the vulva. Obstet Gynecol 42:47–57

Janovski NA, Douglas CP (1972) Diseases of the vulva. Harper and Row, Hagerstown, p 104

Mader MH, Friedrich EG Jr (1982) Vulvar metastasis of breast carcinoma: a case report. J Reprod Med 27:169–171

Taussig FJ (1938) Metastatic tumors of vagina and vulva. Surg Clin North Am 18:1309–1314

18 Vulval Dystrophies

The multitude of terminology used for white patch or leukoplakia of the vulva is confusing. The International Society for the study of Vulval disease adopted the term vulval dystrophy as originally suggested by Jeffcoate (1966) to replace all other previously used terms such as kraurosis vulvae, atrophic dystrophy, leukoplakic vulvitis, leukoplakia, hyperplastic vulvitis, etc. The vulval dystrophies have been classified into:

(i) Hyperplastic dystrophy with or without atypia – In this there is acanthosis, elongation or blunting of the rete pegs and a varying degree of hyperkeratosis (Fig. 18.1). The granular layer may or may not be prominent. When atypia is present, it may be mild, moderate or severe. Chronic inflammatory cell infiltrates in the dermis, in varying numbers, are always seen.

(ii) Lichen sclerosus – Thinning of the squamous epithelium is the dominant feature. Hyperkeratosis is also present. A characteristic, acellular, homogeneous, eosinophilic layer of the dermis associated with variable oedema is seen just beneath the epidermis (Fig. 18.2). According to Hewitt (1986), this superficial hyalinisation, even if it is very thin and limited to the basement membrane or papillae, should be considered a significant point for the diagnosis of lichen sclerosus. There is a zone of lymphocyte and plasma cell infiltration below this acellular layer.

(iii) Mixed dystrophy with or without atypia – This shows areas of hyperplastic dystrophy as well as lichen sclerosus (Fig. 18.3). When atypia of the epithelial cells is present, it may be mild, moderate or severe.

18.1 Clinical Features

Hyperplastic dystrophy without atypia appears as a well-defined, localised, raised, white patch with an inflammatory background. Occasionally the lesions are ill-defined. Scratching may modify the appearances due to fissuring and excoriations.

Lichen sclerosus occurs occasionally in pre-menarchal girls (Lascano et al. 1964; Flynt and Gallup 1979), but the lesion resolves completely after the onset of menstruation. The lesion can involve any part of the vulva and may be multiple in up to 87% of patients (Hart et al. 1975). An hour-glass appearance, encircling the introitus and anus, when present, is seen only in lichen sclerosus (Douglas 1983). In occasional patients, sclerosis of the introitus causes dyspareunia.

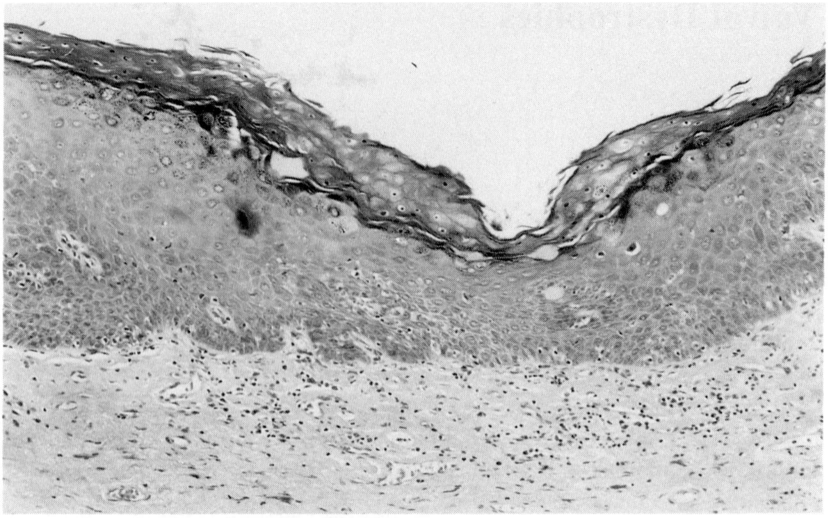

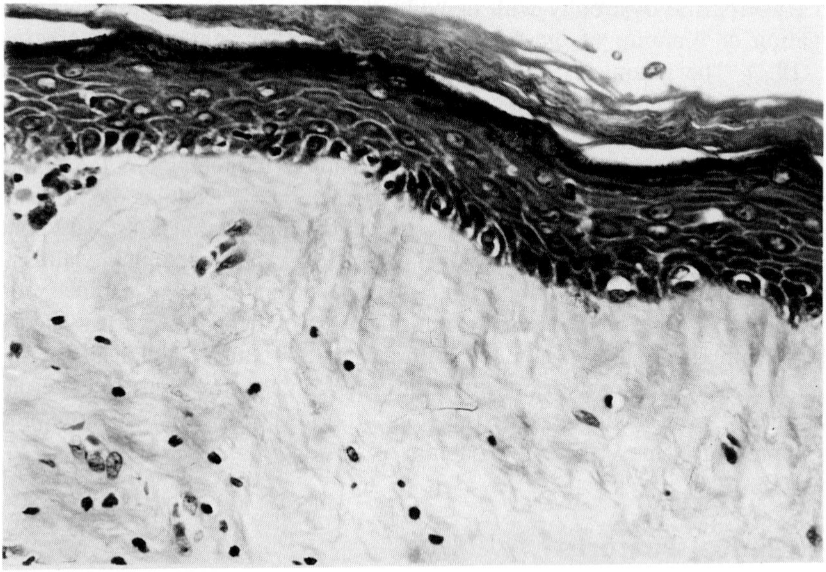

Fig. 18.1. Hyperplastic dystrophy: thickened epidermis and a zone of sub-epidermal chronic inflammatory cells

Fig. 18.2. Lichen sclerosus: hyalinised, acellular zone beneath the epidermis. The epidermis may be atrophied

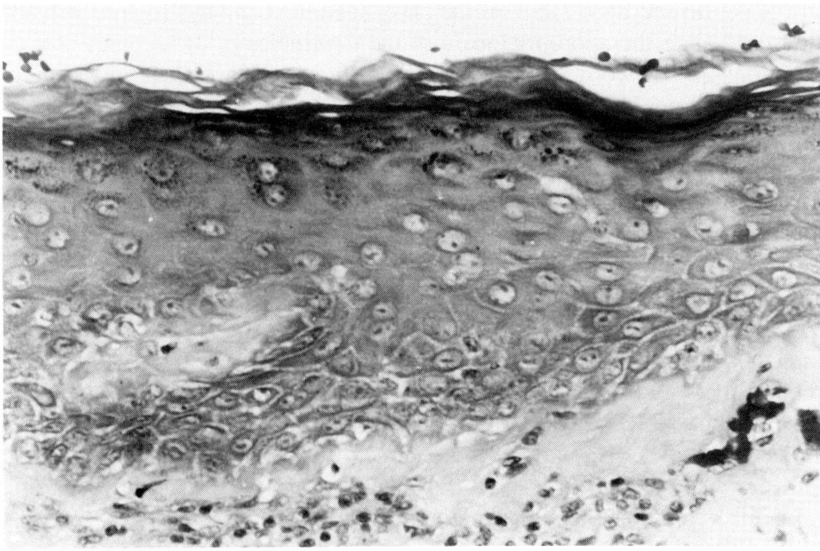

Fig. 18.3. Mixed dystrophy: a junctional area of hyperplastic epithelium and lichenoid change

Well-developed lichen sclerosus assumes a parchment or cigarette paper-like appearance. The early lesion may be irregular, white and flat-topped. Frequent association with comedo-like plugs or depressions differentiate this from hyperplastic dystrophy (Kaufman and Gardner 1978).

In mixed dystrophy features of both hyperplastic dystrophy and lichen sclerosus are present.

A modification of this classification by the ISSVS has recently been proposed (Lavery 1984).

In lichen sclerosus a sub-epithelial homogenous zone is not always present.

The homogeneous acellular zone, diagnostic of "lichen sclerosus", although found by Taussig (1929) and others in atrophic leukoplakia, has led to the abandonment of the term lichen sclerosus in favour of "atrophic dystrophy". It may be mentioned, however, that at least two studies using tritiated thymidine (Woodruff et al. 1965) and ^{32}P (Kaufman et al. 1967) have shown that the so-called atrophic lesions are not metabolically inert or hypoactive but are as active as normal vulval skin.

Recognition is given to the fact that atypical changes or even frank carcinoma may complicate the atrophic lesion.

Atrophic dystrophy (lichen sclerosus in the previous classification) can, therefore, be typed as without atypia (IIa) and with atypia (IIb). Similarly, hyperplastic dystrophy may be assigned 1a (without atypia) or 1b (with atypia), and mixed dystrophy IIA (without atypia) and IIIb (with atypia).

There is yet no full agreement on the classification of the dystrophies. Objection may be raised as to the appropriateness of the terminology "dystrophies" for these vulval lesions as the word "dystrophy" has different connotations in the medical literature for various pathological processes. Moreover, a wide variety of vulval dermatoses have been lumped in this group. In doing so, the importance of specific diagnosis and therapy has been somewhat compromised. It is probably more appropriate to recognise and separate these dermatoses under sub-categories if the term dystrophy is to be retained. At present it appears that the term has become firmly rooted in the literature just like the "dysplasia" of the uterine cervix. Also appropriately, all epithelial atypias should be included in the neoplastic group, albeit some of the reactive atypias may regress spontaneously.

The pathogenesis of vulval dystrophy is unknown. Friedrich (1976) proposed a metabolic theory to explain the genesis of this lesion. The role of trauma, infections, psychoneurosis and nutritional factors has not gained wide acceptance. A few recent studies (Goolamali et al. 1974; Bushkell et al. 1981; Harrington and Dunsmore 1981; Dickie et al. 1982) have demonstrated local deposits of immunoglobulin, complement and a high incidence of auto-antibodies against the thyroid cytoplasm and gastric parietal cells in the sera of patients with lichen sclerosus suggesting that an immunological phenomenon might be operative. Thomas et al. (1982) could not, however, confirm that these patients were at particular risk of developing autoimmune diseases. Lichen sclerosus has also been noticed among the siblings of two to three generations (Murphy et al. 1982; Friedrich and MacLaren 1984), pointing also to a genetic background. HLA-B40 antigen is significantly common in these patients (Harrington and Gelsthorpe 1981). Abnormal hormonal activity has also been suggested. The patients with vulval dystrophies were found to have low serum levels of dihydrotestosterone, free testosterone and androstenedione due to a 5α-reductase enzyme deficiency (Friedrich and Kalra 1984). After treatment the serum level of these hormones rose and exceeded the normal value (Friedrich and Kalra 1984). Recently, Lavery (Lavery 1984) postulated that a local homeostatic control mechanism mediated through the hormone somatostatin, a gastrointestinal peptide which causes achlorhydria and promotes epidermal cell growth, exists in the skin. Unopposed action of urogastrone causes hypertrophic dystrophy and that of somatostatin, an atrophic dystrophy (Lavery 1984). As early as 1936 Swift suggested that achlarhydria is an aetiological factor in leucoplakia vulvae. Subsequently, Jeffcoate (1962), in a series of 269 patients with vulval dystrophy, found histamine-fast achlorhydria in 23% of patients. To cause achlorhydria, a much higher level of urogastrone is required, and as such, hypertrophic dystrophy can occur without achlorhydria (Lavery 1984).

Yoshima et al. (1987) earlier demonstrated that there was a 50% reduction in hyaluronic acid in the dermal tissues of lichen sclerosus compared with that of normal skin. Elastic fibres are also affected and disappear from the upper dermis due to the action of an elastase-type protease which can be isolated from local fibroblasts (Godeau et al. 1982). Frances et al. (1983) have noticed alterations of the type I, III, IV collagen and linear laminin pattern at the dermo-epidermal junction, and disappearance of fibronectin. Whether these changes are due to the effects of various physical factors such as local irritations by sweat retention and infections, chemical agents like plastic, powders and deodorants or secondary to scratching from psychological irritations are at present conjectural. It is also uncertain whether the epidermal hyperplasia and atrophy are secondary to the dermal alterations. It may be that, in the early stage of the lesion in which the dermal changes are not microscopically apparent, the overlying epithelium reacts by hyperplasia. Later, with advanced dermal alterations, the epidermis atrophies.

Ultrastructural studies by Mann and Cowan (1973) have shown that there are holes and gaps in the basal lamina and passage of degenerate dermal material into the epidermis which contains an increased number of Langerhans' cells. The presence of collagen fibrils in the intercellular space (Kint and Geers 1975) with multilayering of basement membrane filaments tends to support the previous finding.

The recurrence of lichen sclerosus in the healthy myocutaneous graft on a vulva which was previously affected by lichen sclerosus and the disappearance of the lesion from the vulval skin when transferred to a healthy site (di Paola et al. 1982) point towards local factors such as warmth and moisture peculiar to the vulval environment, as suggested by Jeffcoate (1962), or to other factors yet unknown. Recently, HPV DNA has been demonstrated in atypical vulval dystrophy by Karram et al. (1988), who raised the possibility that the virus may not be casually associated. It appears at present that the aetiology of lichen sclerosus is multifactorial acting either synergistically or through several stages.

Pruritus vulvae is the most common symptom of the vulval dystrophies. In hyperplastic dystrophy, pruritus is severe, and in lichen sclerosus, pruritus is usually mild. Scratching causes excoriation and infection, which may in turn change the appearance of the lesion. Dyspareunia is experienced by some patients, particularly with lichen sclarosus which causes narrowing of the introitus.

In 1929 Taussig concluded that 50% of patients with leukoplakia of the vulva would ultimately develop invasive carcinoma. Subsequently, this view was supported by several authors (Bibby 1957; Green et al. 1958; Stening and Elliott 1959). Many other studies have, however, indicated that the risk of developing invasive carcinoma in the vulval dystrophies is small (Langley et al. 1951; Kaufman et al. 1974) and is in the order of 4%–5% over 3–25 years (Jeffcoate 1966). According to McAdams and Kistner (1958), 10% of leukoplakias progress to invasive carcinoma. In one follow-up study of 92 patients with lichen sclerosus, only 1 patient developed invasive carcinoma after 12 years (Hart et al. 1975). Progression to invasive carcinoma has also been noticed in the mixed dystrophies. Cario et al. (1984) reported squamous cell carcinoma developing from mixed dystrophy in an 18-year-old patient. According to Rodke et al. (1988), mixed dystrophy is not per se a separate disease but an associated process of lichen sclerosus. Hyperplastic changes following intense itching are somewhat at risk. It is more likely that the lesion showing atypical hyperplastic changes in the initial biopsy will have a higher risk of ultimately progressing to invasive carcinoma (Kaufman and Gardner 1978). Baird et al. (1978) observed multifocal, microinvasive lesions arising in the areas of lichen sclerosus in many of the vulvectomy specimens removed for invasive cancer.

18.2 Treatment

Multiple biopsies are important to establish the diagnosis of vulval dystrophy. The initial step, however, is to eliminate the source of irritations and exclude the possibility of infection, which if present should be treated first. Hydrocortisone ointment has been used with success in treating hypertrophic dystrophy and testosterone in lichen sclerosus. Intractable pruritus can be treated by local alcohol injection (Woodruff and Babaknia 1979) and CO_2 laser (Ovadia et al. 1984). Lesions with atypia should be excised with a wide margin showing no residual atypia (Kaufman and Gardner 1978).

References

Baird PJ, Russell P, Laverty CR (1978) A pathological study of the relationship between lichen sclerosus and squamous cell carcinoma of the vulva. Pathology 10:196

Bibby AVG (1957) Carcinoma of the vulva: a review of 71 cases. J Obstet Gynaecol Br Emp 64:263–266

Bushkell LL, Friedrich EG Jr, Jordan RE (1981) An apprisal of routine direct immunofluorescence in vulvar disorders. Acta Derm Venereol (Stockh) 61:157–161

Cario GM, House MJ, Paradinas FJ (1984) Squamous cell carcinoma of the vulva in association with mixed vulvar dystrophy in a 1 year old girl: case report. Br J Obstet Gynaecol 91:87–90

Dickie RJ, Horne CHW, Sutherland HW et al. (1982) Direct evidence of localised immunological damage in vulvar lichen sclerosis and atrophicus. J Clin Pathol 35:1395–1397

Di Paola GR, Rueda-Leverone NG, Belardi MG (1982) Lichen sclerosus of the vulva recurrent after myocutaneous graft: a case report. J Reprod Med 27:666–668

Douglas CP (1983) Vulvar dystrophy. In: Studd J (ed) Progress in obstetrics and gynecology, vol 3. Churchill Livingstone, London, pp 199–212

Flynt J, Gallup DG (1979) Childhood lichen sclerosus. Obstet Gynecol 53 [Suppl]:79–81

Frances C, Wechesler J, Meimon GT et al. (1983) Investigation of intercellular matrix macromolecules involved in lichen sclerosus. Acta Dermvenereol (Stockh) 63:483–490

Friedrich EG Jr (1976) Lichen sclerosus. J Reprod Med 17:147–154

Friedrich EG Jr, Kalra PS (1984) Serum levels of sex hormones in vulvar lichen sclerosus and effects of topical testosterone. N Engl J Med 310:488–491

Friedrich EG Jr, Maclaren NK (1984) Genetic aspects of vulvar lichen sclerosus. Am J Obstet Gynecol 150:161–166

Godeau G, Frances C, Hornebeck W et al. (1982) Isolation and partial characterisation of an elastase-type protease in human vulvar fibroblasts. Its probable involvement in vulvar elastic tissue destruction of patients with lichen sclerosus at atrophicus. J Invest Dermatol 78:270–275

Goolamali SK, Barnes EW, Irvine WJ (1974) Organ specific antibodies in patients with lichen sclerosus. Br Med J 4:78–79

Green TH Jr, Ulfelder H, Meigs JV (1958) Epidermoid carcinoma of the vulva: an analysis of 238 cases, pt 1: etiology and diagnosis. Am J Obstet Gynecol 75:834–847

Harrington CI, Dunsmore IR (1981) An investigation into the incidence of autoimmune disorders in patients with lichen sclerosus at atrophicus. Br J Dermatol 104:563–566

Harrington CI, Gelsthorpe K (1981) The association between lichen sclerosus at atrophicus and HLA-B40. Br J Dermatol 104:561–562

Hart WR, Norris HJ, Helwig EB (1975) Relation of lichen sclerosus et atrophicus of the vulva to the development of carcinoma. Obstet Gynecol 45:469–377

Hewitt J (1986) Histologic criteria for the diagnosis of lichen sclerosus of the vulva. J Reprod Med 31:781–787

Jeffcoate TNA (1962) The dermatology of the vulva. J Obstet Gynaecol Br Commonw 69:889–890

Jeffcoate TNA (1966) Chronic vulvar dystrophy. Am J Obstet Gynecol 95:61–74

Karram M, Tabor B, Smotkin D et al. (1988) Detection of human pailloma virus deoxyribonucleic acid from vulvar dystrophies and vulvar intraepithelial neoplastic lesions. Am J Obstet Gynecol 159:22–23

Kaufman RH, Gardner HL (1978) Vulvar dystrophies. Clin Obstet Gynecol 21:1081–1106

Kaufman RH, Gardner HL, Johnson PC (1967) P32 uptake in lichen sclerosus et atrophicus of the vulva. Am J Obstet Gynecol 98:312–319

Kaufman RH, Gardner HL, Brown DJ et al. (1974) Vulvar dystrophies: an evaluation. Am J Obstet Gynecol 120:363–367

Kint A, Geerts ML (1975) Lichen sclerosus et atrophicus: an electron microscopic study. J Cutan Pathol 2:30–34

Langley H, Hertig AT, Smith GVS (1951) Relation of leucoplakik vulvitis to squamous cell carcinoma of the vulva. Am J Obstet Gynecol 62:167–169

Lascano EF, Montes LF, Mazzini MA (1964) Lichen sclerosus et atrophicus in childhood: report of 6 cases. Obstet Gynecol 24:872–877

Lavery HA (1984) Vulval dystrophy: new approaches. Clin Obstet Gynecol 11:155–169

Mann PR, Cowan MA (1973) Ultrastructural changes in four cases of lichen sclerosus et atrophicus. Br J Dermatol 89:223–231

McAdams AJ Jr, Kistner RW (1958) The relationship of chronic vulvar disease, leukoplakia and carcinoma in-situ to carcinoma of the vulva. Cancer 11:740–757

Murphy FR, Lipa M, Haberman HF (1982) Familial vulvar dystrophy of lichen sclerosus. Arch Dermatol 118:329–331

Ovadia J, Levavi H, Edelstein T (1984) Treatment of pruritus vulvae by means of CO2 laser. Acta Obstet Gynecol Scand 63:265–267

Rodke G, Firedrich EG Jr, Wilkinson EJ (1988) Malignant potential of mixed dystrophy (lichen sclerosus associated with squamous cell hyperplasia). J Reprod Med 33:345–350

Stening M, Elliott P (1959) Primary carcinoma of the vulva with special reference to leukoplakia. J Obstet Gynaecol Br Emp 66:897–904

Swift BH (1936) Achlorhydria as an etiological factor in pruritus vulvae associated with kraurosis or leucoplakia. J Obset Gynaecol Br Emp 43:1053–1077

Taussig FJ (1929) Leukoplakic vulvitis and cancer of the vulva. Am J Obstet Gynecol 18:472–503

Thomas RHM, Holmes RC, Rowland Payne CME et al. (1982) The incidence of development of autoimmune diseases in women after the diagnosis of lichen sclerosus et atrophicus. Brt J Dermatol 107 [Suppl 22]:29

Woodruff JD, Babaknia A (1979) Local alcohol injection of the vulva. Discussion of 35 cases. Obstet Gynecol 54:512–514

Woodruff JD, Barkowf HI, Holzman GB et al. (1965) Metabolic activity in normal and abnormal vulvar epithelium: an assessment by the use of tzritiated nucleic acid precursos. Am Obstet Gynecol 91:809–819

Yoshima H, Shinkai H, Sanos S et al. (1978) Acidic glycosaminoglycans in the skin and urine of a patient with widespread lichen sclerosus et atrophicus. Arch Dermatol Res 263:59–66

Addendum

The International Society for the Study of Vulvar Disease has recommended the following new classification of non-neoplastic epithelial disorders and replaced old terminology 'dystrophy': Lichen sclerosus (replaces old 'lichen sclerosus et atrophicus'); Squamous cell hyperplasia (replaces old 'hyperplastic dystrophy'); Other dermatoses. (Ridley CM, Frankman O, Jones IS et al. (1989) New nomenclature for vulvar disease: International Society for the study of vulvar disease. Human Pathol 20:495–496).

Part II: The Vagina

19 Classification of the Tumours and Tumour-like Conditions of the Vagina

I. Cysts and Cyst-like Conditions

Cysts

Epidermal cyst
Endometriotic cysts
Developmental Cyst
  Paramesonephric duct cyst, Mesonephric duct cyst, Urogenital sinus cyst

Cyst-like conditions

Prolapsed fallopian tubes
Vaginitis emphysematosa
Hydrocolpos
Unilateral haematocolpos
Diverticulum of the urinary bladder

II. Polyps and Pseudopolyps

Pseudosarcomatous polyp
Cervical polyp presenting at the vaginal vault
Post-hysterectomy polyp
Carunculae myrtiformes (carunculae hymenales)
Adenomatous polyp

III. Tumours

Squamous cell origin

Squamous papilloma
Intraepithelial neoplasia
Microinvasive carcinoma
Invasive carcinoma
Verrucous carcinoma
Basal cell-like carcinoma

Glandular origin

DES-exposed adenosis
DES-exposed adenocarcinoma
Adenocarcinoma not related to DES

Naevi and melanoma

Mesenchymal and neural origin: benign
Leiomyoma
Neurofibroma
Rhabdomyoma
Glomus tumour

Mesenchymal and neural origin: malignant
Sarcoma botryoides
Leiomyosarcoma
Alveolar soft part sarcoma
Haemangiopericytoma
Aggressive angiomyxoma

Tumour-like conditions
Angiomyolipoma
Reactive fibrohistiocytic proliferation simulating histiocytoma

Lymphoma

Plasmacytoma

Granulocytic sarcoma

Neuroectodermal origin
Paraganglioma
Neuroepithelioma

Germ cell origin
Benign teratoma
Endodermal sinus tumour
Carcinoma of infant vagina (embryonal carcinoma)

Mesonephric and paramesonephric duct origin: benign
Mesonephric papilloma
Brenner tumour

Mesonephric and paramesonephric duct orogin: malignant
Malignant mixed mesodermal tumour
Endometrial stromal sarcoma
Gartner's duct carcinoma

Uncertain histogenesis
Malignant tumour resembling synovial sarcoma
Mixed tumour of vagina

Secondary tumours

IV. Inflammatory Conditions

Specific
Syphilis
Lymphogranuloma
Vaginal mass due to chlamydial proctitis

Non-specific
Crohn's disease
Diverticular disease of the colon eroding into the vagina

Inflammatory pseudotumour
Xanthogranuloma
Malakoplakia

20 Cysts and Cyst-like Conditions

20.1 Cysts

20.1.1 Epidermal Cysts

The inclusion cysts of the vagina are similar to the epidermal cysts of the vulva. They occur following trauma, vaginal or utero-vaginal surgery. The cysts are usually 1–4 cm in size, seen often near the introitus, vaults, lateral and posterior wall of the vagina. Cut sections reveal a single loculus containing caseaus and granular material. Occasionally, the cyst can be very large. Perl and Milles (1957) reported a squamous cell-lined large cyst of the vagina which occurred following hysterectomy and was large enough to cause urinary obstruction. Vulval epidermal cysts are very common among the Igbos of Nigeria who practice ritual circumcision of girls in infancy (Onuigbo 1976). Congenital epidermal cysts in newborn infants have also been occasionally noticed (Cohen et al. 1957). Meyer (1932) thought that these cysts were derived from mesonephric remnants and could be present early in fetal life. Many of these cysts in newborn infants are attached to the hymen (hymenal cysts) and have, therefore, been suggested to be of urogenital sinus origin (Merlob et al. 1978).

20.1.1.1 Microscopical Appearance

The cysts are lined by normal stratified squamous epithelium (Fig. 20.1). There are foreign body-type giant cell reactions when leakage occurs to the surrounding tissue.

20.1.2 Endometriotic Cysts

Endometriosis of the vagina is uncommon, and cystic endometriosis is rare. Like endometriotic cyst at any other sites, it is lined by columnar epithelium of the endometrial type and surrounded by stromal cells and pigment-laden macrophages (Fig. 20.2). Williams (1965) observed three forms of endometriosis occurring in the vagina:

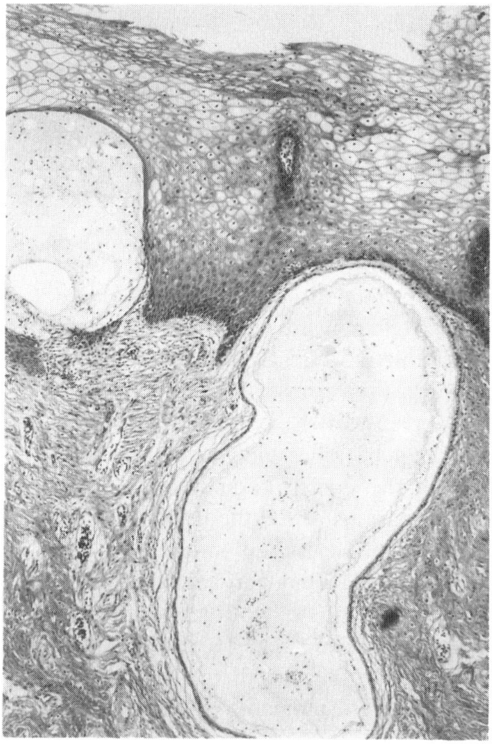

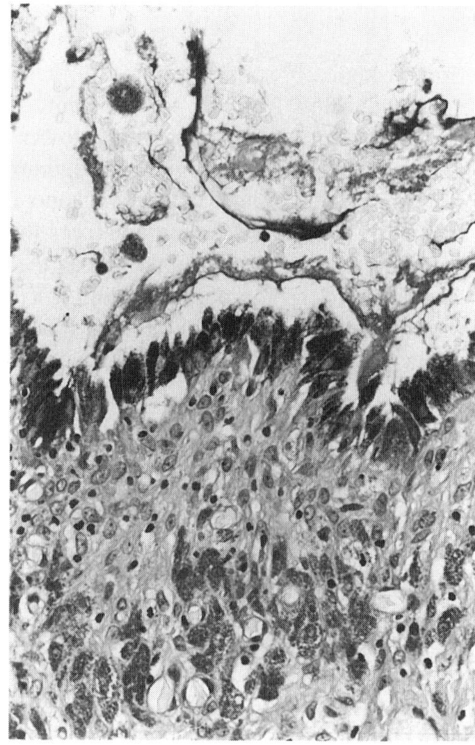

Fig. 20.1. Epidermal cyst: keratinous material within the cyst

Fig. 20.2. Endometriotic cyst: the cyst has an endometrial-type lining

(i) Endometriosis of the posterior formix occurs as an extension from the pouch of Douglas or uterosacral ligaments, and of the posterior wall of the vagina as an extension from the recto-vaginal septum. It consists of superficial bluish nodules which increase in size during the menstrual period and may bleed. The lesion, however, can be primary in this area without any focus in the pouch of Douglas or uterosacral ligaments (Studdiford 1957). Extensive lesions can cause dyspareunia and painful defaecation. Endometriosis of the posterior formix may extend laterally to infiltrate the sacral plexus and ureteral opening, causing more severe complications (Wolfe 1960).

(ii) Endometriosis implanted superficially can be diagnosed by careful inspection which reveals typical blood-filled blebs. The patient may present with intermenstrual bleeding.

(iii) Endometriosis may be implanted deeply in the damaged vagina. Symptoms may be more severe. Depositions of the endometrial tissue in the vaginal scar after hysterectomy are a notworthy example (Beebe and Edwards 1951; Brosset 1954).

Endometriosis of the vagina has occasionally been noticed at autopsy in postmenopausal women who are apparently asymptomatic during life (Sandberg 1968).

20.1.3 Developmental Cysts

Embryologically speaking, the fallopian tubes, uterus and upper two-thirds of the vagina develop from paramesonephric ducts. There are still some controversies regarding the development of the lower third of the vagina, which is considered generally to develop from the urogenital sinus. Müller's tubercle, which is the meeting point of the fused paramesonephric ducts and urogenital sinus, forms the hymen. It is believed by some authors that the inner lining of the hymen is derived from the vaginal epithelium whereas the outer lining is from the urogenital sinus. The origin of the vaginal epithelium is itself controversial. Bulmer (1957) suggested that the entire vaginal epithelium was derived from upward growth of the sinus epithelium, while others held that, under the inductive effects of the underlying stroma, the müllerian epithelium transformed into squamous epithelium (Robboy et al. 1982). In the embryo, mesonephric ducts appear earlier than paramesonephric ducts and open into the cloacal cavity, which later becomes the urogenital sinus. The remnants of these ducts may persist along the course beginning from the mesosalpinx close to the ovary along the lateral margins of the uterus, cervix and antero-lateral part of the vaginal wall up to the vestibule ending anteriorly in the labia. The vestibule is formed from the urogenital sinus and urogenital groove. Vaginal tumours can develop from vestigial remnants of the wolffian (Gartner's) ducts along their course. Paramesonephric cysts have been suggested, on the other hand, to result from incomplete fusion of the paramesonephric ducts (Evans and Paine 1981). Cysts can also develop from the aberrant remnants of these ducts, which may occasionally be present in the anterior wall of the vagina (Vilas 1934). Dislocated müllerian glands in the vaginal wall during embryonic development may also be the origin of paramesonephric cysts (Deppisch 1975). Although most common developmental cysts of the vagina have been believed in the past to be of mesonephric duct origin, histological evidence indicates that the majority are paramesonephric cysts (Evans and Hughes 1961; Junaid and Thomas 1981).

20.1.3.1 Paramesonephric Duct Cyst

The paramesonephric duct cyst occurs most commonly as a single cyst anywhere in the vaginal wall with a slight predilection for the anterior.

The patients are between 20 and 60 years old. The common symptoms are dyspareunia, pain and discharge. Some patients are asymptomatic.

20.1.3.1.1 Gross Appearance

The size of the cyst varies between 1 and 5 cm in diameter with an average of 3 cm. The cyst is unilocular and contains thin mucinous fluid. The wall is of moderate thickness and may be partly covered by smooth vaginal epithelium

20.1.3.1.2 Microscopical Appearance

Evans and Hughes (1961) sub-divided these cysts into three categories.

In the cervical type, the cysts are lined by tall columnar cells with basal nuclei and abundant cytoplasmic mucin (Fig. 20.3), imparting what is frequently labelled as the picket fence appearance. The epithelium may be cuboidal or flattened due to pressure effects of the contents and may partly undergo squamous metaplasia. In an occasional cyst, the epithelium may be thrown into short papillary folds. When the entire epithelium undergoes squamous metaplasia, it is impossible to distinguish it from an epithelial inclusion cyst.

In the fallopian tube type, the lining epithelium is columnar, partly ciliated and partly secretory, arranged irregularly on a poorly defined basement membrane. Ciliated cells are the predominant cell types.

The endometrial type of cyst is histologically similar to any genital or extra-genital endometriotic cyst. Characteristically, the cyst is located under the vaginal epithelium, and the lesion is primarily vaginal (Studdiford 1957) and not an extension from adjacent structures. In general, the epithelial lining of paramesonephric cysts, particularly the cervical and fallopian tube types, shows positive reactions with mucicarmine, periodic acid-Schiff reagents and alcian blue, in contrast to the lining of the mesonephric cysts, which give uniformly negative results (Janovski 1962).

20.1.3.2 Mesonephric Duct Cysts

These cysts are less common than the paramesonephric duct cysts and are located commonly on the anterior or antero-lateral wall of the vagina. They are asymptomatic and most often discovered incidentally during vaginal examination for other complaints.

An infrequent developmental anomaly consisting of unilateral renal hypoplasia or agenesis and a single vaginal ectopic ureter may be associated with mesonephric duct cyst (Gadbois and Duckett 1974; Currarino 1982). The ureteric buds which arise from the distal segment of the wolffian ducts have a separate opening into the cloaca due to incorporation of the ducts into the anterior part of the cloaca during the 6th to 8th week of embryonic development. Anomalies occurring before this separation of the ureteric bud and wolffian duct openings into the cloaca result in vaginal ectopic ureter, Gartner's duct cyst and renal agenesis (cephalad growth of ureteric bud induces formation of renal blastema) (Goldstein et al. 1973; Currarino 1982).

20.1.3.2.1 Gross Appearance

The cysts measure 1–2 cm in diameter and are unilocular with a moderately thick wall. The contents are a clear and thin watery fluid.

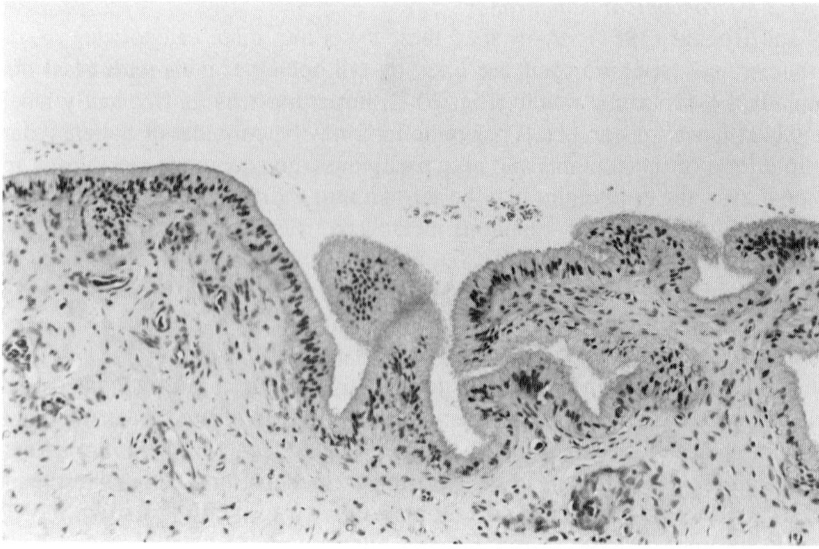

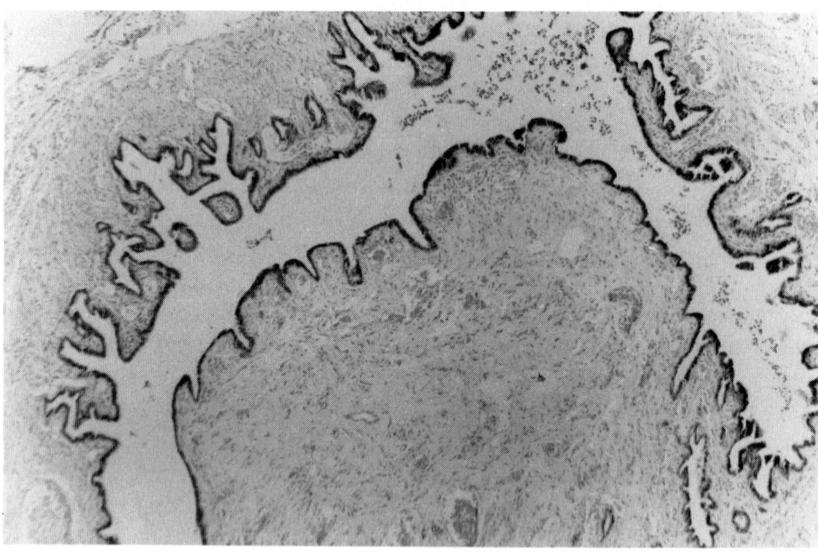

Fig. 20.3. Paramesonephric cyst: the cyst is lined by mucin-secreting columnar epithelium

Fig. 20.4. Mesonephric duct cyst: the cyst lining is thrown into short papillary folds

20.1.3.2.2 Microscopical Apperance
In contrast to the paramesonephric duct cysts, these cysts are lined by cuboidal, low cuboidal to low columnar epithelium with oval vesicular nuclei arranged on a basement membrane. The epithelium may occasionally be thrown into short papillary folds (Fig. 20.4) or flattened due to intra-cystic pressure. Cilia may be present but are unusual. The cells do not secrete mucin, and although PAS-positive granules may be present on the luminal border of the cells, mucicarmine and alcian blue reactions are uniformly negative. Areas of squamous metaplasia are not infrequent.

20.1.3.3 Urogenital Sinus Cysts (Mucous Cysts of the Vestibule)

The mucous cysts of the vestibular area are, unlike the paramesonephric duct cysts of the vagina, claimed to be of urogenital sinus origin (Friedrich and Wilkinson 1973). The common locations are the vestibular area beneath the clitoris, medial aspect of labia minora and Bartholin's gland areas. Development of these cysts seems to be under hormonal stimulation as they are not seen before puberty (Friedrich and Wilkinson 1973).

The patient may complain of dyspareunia, discomfort and pain.

20.1.3.3.1 Gross Appearance
The cysts average 2 cm in diameter and are unilocular, containing thick mucinous fluid.

20.1.3.3.2 Microscopical Appearance
The lining of these cysts is histologically similar to endocervical epithelium and the epithelium of the paraurethral glands. It also bears some similarity to the acinar epithelium of Bartholin's glands, which are derived from the urogenital sinus.

Ultrastructurally, the cells lining the cysts show prominent basal lamina, an apical junctional complex with interdigitations near the basal lamina, numerous secretory granules, cytoplasmic closely associated fibrillar bodies suggesting similarities to the cells of Bartholin's and paraurethral glands derived from the urogenital sinus (Oi and Munn 1982).

20.1.3.3.3 Treatment
A diverticulum of the urinary bladder is to be excluded by radiological examination before undertaking surgical removal of the cyst from the anterior vaginal wall. The smaller, superficially located cysts can be removed surgically without complications.

20.2 Cyst-like Conditions

20.2.1 Prolapsed Fallopian Tube

Prolapsed fallopian tube presents commonly as a firm polypoid mass at the apex of the vagina and may be mistaken for a malignant tumour (Silverberg and Frable 1974; Wheelock et al. 1985). It may occasionally be cystic. The lesion develops most commonly following vaginal total histerectomy and less commonly, abdominal histerectomy. About 70 casereports have so far appeared in the literature.

The common presenting symptoms are profuse bloody or vaginal discharge, abdominal pain, dyspareunia and occasionally salpingo-vaginal fistula at the vaginal vault (Tabrisky et al. 1972). Symptoms occur between 2 weeks (Hirsch and Wyatt 1961) and 4 years (Halpin 1971) but most commonly during the first 6 months after surgery (Ellsworth et al. 1973). A febrile course and profuse bleeding complicating the original surgery are thought to be predisposing factors (Silverberg and Frable 1974). The most common clinical diagnosis is granulation tissue. Adequate biopsy is, therefore, necessary to establish the diagnosis.

20.2.1.1 Microscopical Appearance

The tubal architecture may be distorted due to inflammation and granulation tissue. Reorganisation of the tubal epithelium may lead to the formation of pseudoglands (Sapan and Solbert 1973), and then the lesion has to be differentiated from endometriosis, adenosis or infected mesonephric cyst. With the clinical history of previous hysterectomy, it is often not difficult to establish the diagnosis. Insertion of a probe (Tabrisky et al. 1972) and instillation of contrast material (Beebe and Edwards 1951) are helpful additional measures.

20.2.1.2 Treatment

Treatment varies from simple cauterisation to abdominal salpingectomy (Symmonds et al. 1957). Trans-vaginal excisions with high ligation of the tube are usually practised (Sapan and Solbert 1973).

20.2.2 Emphysematous Vaginitis

Emphysematous vaginitis also known as colpohyperplasia cystica is a rare condition characterised by the presence of gas-filled cysts in the mucosa and submucosa, mostly of the upper part of vagina. In the earlier literature the condition was thought to be an entity of uncertain aetiology. The various aetiological factors suggested ranged from infections, hormonal influence, lymphatic stasis to embryological abnormalities (Bender and Jeffcoat 1950; Burt et al. 1954; Shenker and Blaustein 1963; Wilbanks and Carter 1963; Gardner and Fernet 1964). Nowadays, the condition is more a medical curiosity than disease entity (Fleury 1981). Although the exact mechanism of gas formation is not clear, the frequent demonstration of *Gardnerella vaginalis* and *Trichomonas vaginalis* in this condition has led us to believe that these organisms may have an important role.

20.2.2.1 Clinical Features

The condition has been noticed in patients ranging from 17 to 77 years old (Kramer and Tobon 1987). The overwhelming majority of them, however, are in the reproductive age group. The patients present with abnormal vaginal bleeding, white discharge, spotting and occasionally dysmenorrhoea and backache. Most of the patients are either pregnant or have a history of a recent pregnancy. It has been suggested that infections superimposed on the modified vaginal epithelium cause necrosis of the epithelial cells, which in turn form gas. Necrosis of the portio cervix can masquerade as carcinoma (McCallion and Parkin 1988). Cardiopulmonary disease (Gardner and Fernet 1964) and immunosuppression (Tjugum et al. 1986) have also been suggested as predisposing factors.

20.2.2.2 Gross Appearance

The size of the cyst varies from a pin head to about 2 cm. The cysts are discrete, shiny, tense, smooth and non-crepitant. The aggregates of tiny cysts are soft and friable and may appear granular to be mistaken at times as carcinoma (Buckingham and McLure 1954). Occasionally, the clusters of cysts resemble nabothian follicles (Gardner and Fernet 1964).

20.2.2.3 Microscopical Appearance

The vaginal epithelium is usually normal and intact but may be thickened and rarely ulcerated. The stroma beneath the epithelium shows scattered cysts of various sizes devoid of lining epithelium (Fig. 20.5). The cysts at times may be partly lined by squamous cells (Gardner and Fernet 1964). Multinucleate, foreign body-type giant cells in variable numbers can be seen around the cysts and occasionally line the cystic spaces. Leucocytes are almost always noticed in the connective tissue, particularly around the empty spaces.

20.2.2.4 Treatment

The disease may disappear without treatment (Zachariae 1956). Medical treatment with metranidazole eradicates *Trichmonas vaginalis* and *Gardnerella vaginitis* and causes disappearance of the blebs (Fleury 1981).

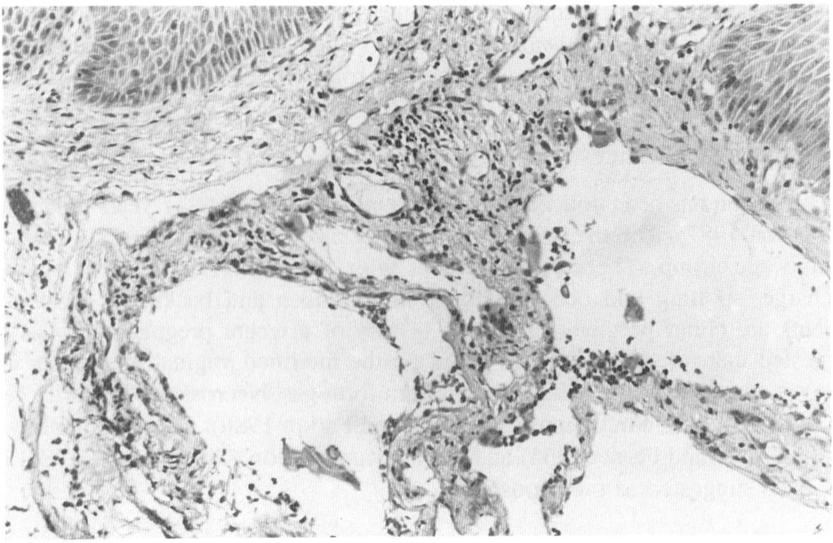

Fig. 20.5. Emphysematous vaginitis: irregular cystic spaceds devoid of lining epithelium beneath the epithelium

20.2.3 Hydrocolpos

Rarely, retention of sanguinal or non-sanguinal fluid due to atresia of the hymen and vagina, either congenital or following radiotherapy and surgery, may cause cystic distension of the vagina (Perl and Milles 1957; Radman et al. 1966; Hammen 1981). Diagnosis is made from the clinical history of abdominal pain, vaginal mass, fever, dysuria and inspection of the genitalia. Biopsy, which is rarely needed, reveals the benign character of the lesion.

20.2.4 Unilateral Haematocolpos

Unilateral haematocolpos develops from the accumulation of menstrual blood in one of the two vaginae which result from the malfusion of the caudal ends of the paramesonephric ducts. One of the vaginae has the normal opening, while the other vagina is a blind pouch. The latter becomes distended and forms a swelling (Evans and Paine 1965).

20.2.5 Diverticulum of the Urinary Bladder

Diverticulum of the urinary bladder is rare and may present as a cyst on the anterior vaginal wall. Congenital diverticulum is said to occur only in the male (Johnston 1976), while all such diverticulae in the female are acquired. Pre-operative radiological examination of the urinary bladder with opaque material is necessary to establish the diagnosis and avert formation of a vesico-vaginal fistula following excision of the vaginal cyst resulting from unawareness of the condition. Biopsy, which may be hazardous, is not recommended.

References

Epidermal Cyst

Cohen HJ, Klein MD, Laver MB (1957) Cysts of the vagina in newborn. Am J Dis Child 94:322–324

Merlob P, Bahari C, Liban E et al. (1978) Cysts of the female external genitalia in the newborn infant. Am J Obstet Gynecol 132:607–610

Meyer R (1932) Über Cysten der Vaginalwand von 3 Feten im Alter von 3 bis 5 Monaten. Arch Gynakol 151:576–586

Onuigbo EIB (1976) Vulval epidermal cysts in the Igbos of Nigeria. Arch Dermatol 112:1405–1406

Perl JI, Milles G (1957) Hydrocolpos after total hysterectomy. Am J Obstet Gynecol 73:1125–1128

Endometriotic Cyst

Beebe RA, Edwards EA (1951) Lesions of the vaginal vault following complete hysterectoma. Am J Obstet Gynecol 62:1034–1043

Brosset A (1954) Endrometriosis on the vaginal scar following vaginal hysterectomy for therapeutic abortion. Acta Obstet Gynecol Scand 33:445–456

Sandberg EC (1968) The incidence and distribution of occult vaginal adenosis. Am J Obstet Gynecol 101:322–334

Studdiford WE (1957) Vaginal lesions of adenomatous origin. Am J Obstet Gynecol 73:641–656

Williams GA (19654) Post surgical and post traumatic tumors. Clin Obstet Gynecol 8:1020–1034

Wolfe SA (1960) Endometriosis of the vagina: discussion and report of a polypoid form associated with rectovaginal endometriosis. Obstet Gynecol 15:612–615

Developmental Cysts

Blumer D (1957) The development of human vagina. J Anat 91:490–509

Deppisch LM (1975) Cysts on the vagina: classification and clinical correlations. Obstet Gynecol 45:632–637

Evans DMD, Hughes H (1961) Cysts of the vaginal wall. J Obstet Gynaecol Br Commonw 68:247–253

Evans DMD, Paine CG (1965) Benign cysts tumors of developmental origin. Clin Obstet Gynecol 8:997–1019

Junaid TA, Thomas SM (1981) Cysts of the vulva and vagina, a comparative study. Int J Gynaecol Obstet 19:239–243

Robboy SJ, Taguchi O, Cunha GR (1982) Normal development of the human female reproductive tract and alterations resulting from experimental exposure to diethylstilbestrol. Hum Pathol 13:190–198

Vilas E (1934) Cysten in der Scheide von Feten. Arch Gynakol 158:1–13

Paramesonephric Cyst

Evans DMD, Hughes H (1961) Cysts of the vaginal wall. J Obstet Gynaecol Br Commonw 68:247–253

Janovski NA, Weir JH (1962) Comparative histologic and histochemical studies of mesonephric derivatives and tumors. Obstet Gynecol 19:57–63

Studdiford WE (1957) Vaginal lesions of adenomatous origin. Am J Obstet Gynecol 73:641–656

Mesonephric Cyst

Currarino G (1982) Single vaginal ectopic ureter and Gartner's duct cyst with ipsilateral renal hypoplasia and dysplasia (or agenesis). J Urol 128:988–993

Gadbois WF, Duckett JW Jr (1974) Gardner's duct cyst and unilateral renal agenesis. Urology 4:720–721

Goldstein AI, Eckerman ES, Woodruff R et al. (1973) Vaginal and cervical communication with mesonephric duct remnants. Relationship to unilateral renal agenesis. Am J Obstet Gynecol 116:101–105

Urogenital Sinus Systs

Friedrich EG Jr, Wilkinson EJ (1973) Mucous cysts of the vulvar vestibule. Obstet Gynecol 42:407–414

Oi RH, Munn R (1982) Mucous cysts of the vulvar vestibule. Hum Pathol 13:584–586

Prolapsed Fallopian Tube

Beebe RA, Edwards EA (1951) Lesions of the vaginal vault following complete hysterectomy. Am J Obstet Gynecol 62:1034–1043

Ellsworth HS, Harris JW, McQuarrie HG et al. (1973) Prolapse of the fallopian tube following vaginal hysterectomy. JAMA 224:891–892

HalpinTF (1971) Prolapse of the fallopian tube following abdominal hysterectoma, a report of one case. Am J Obstet Gynecol 110:880–881

Hirsch H, Wyatt L (1961) Prolapse of a fallopian tube after total abdominal hysterectomy, a report of one case. Am J Obstet Gynecol 82:938–939

Sapan IP, Solbert NS (1973) Prolapse uterine tube after abdominal hysterectomy. Obstet Gynecol 42:26–32

Silverberg SG, Frable WJ (1974) Prolapse of fallopian tube into vaginal vault after hysterectoma. Arch Pathol 97:100–173

Symmonds RE, Counsellor VS, Pratt JH (1957) Prolapse of a fallopian tube as a complication of hysterectomy. Am J Obstet Gynecol 74:214–217

Tabrisky J, Mallin LP, Smith JA (1972) Pneumoperitoneum after coitus; a complication due to uterine tube prolapse after vaginal hysterectomy. Obstet Gynecol 40:218–220

Wheelock JB, Schneider V, Goplerud DR (1985) Prolapsed fallopian tube masquerading as adenocarcinoma of the vagina in a postmenopausal woman. Gynecol Oncol 21:369–375

Vaginitis Emphysematous

Bender S, Jeffcoat TNA (1950) Vaginitis emphysematosa. J Obstet Gynaecol Br Emp 57:432–436

Buckingham JC, McLure JH (1954) Vaginitis emphysematosa. Obstet Gynecol 4:331–334

Burt EP, Rorak P, Couri PJ (1954) Vaginitis emphysematosa, a report of a case. Obstet Gynecol 4:335–338

Fleury FJ (1981) Adult vaginitis. Clin Obstet Gynecol 24:407–438

Gardner HL, Fernet P (1964) Etiology of vaginitis emphysematous: report of 10 cases and review of literature. Am J Obstet Gynecol 88:650–694

Kramer K, Tobon H (1987) Vaginitis emphysematosa. Arch Pathol Lab Med 111:746–749

McCallion JS, Parkin DE (1988) Emphysematous vaginitis masquerading as carcinoma of the cervix: case report. Br J Obstet Gynaecol 95:309–311

Shenker L, Blaustein A (1963) Emphysematous vaginitis: a theory of its pathogenesis and report of a case. Obstet Gynecol 22:295–300

Tjugum J, Jonassen F, Olsson J-H (1986) Vaginitis emphysematosa in a renal transplant patient. Acta Obstet Gynecol Scand 65:377–378

Wilbanks GD, Carter B (1963) Vaginitis emphysematous: report of 4 patients. Obstet Gynecol 22:301–309

Zachariae F (1956) Vaginitis emphysematosa. Acta Obstet Gynecol Scand 35:393–403

Hydrocolpos

Hammen S (1981) Hydrocolpometra. Acta Obstet Gynecol Scand 60:89–90

Perl JI, Milles G (1957) Hydrocolpos after total hysterectomy. Am J Obstet Gynecol 73:1125–1128

Radman HM, Askin JA, Kolodner LJ (1966) Hydrocolpometrocolpos and hematocolpometrocolpos. Obstet Gynecol 27:2–6

Unilateral Haematocolpos

Evans DMD, Paine CG (1965) Benign cysts and tumors of developmental origin. Clin Obstet Gynecol 8:997–1019

Diverticulum of the Urinary Bladder

Johnston JH (1976) Congenital abnormalities of the bladder and uretha. In: Blandy J (ed) Urology. Blackwell, Oxford, pp 619–671

21 Polyps and Pseudopolyps

21.1 Polyps

21.1.1 Fibroepithelial Polyp

Although tumours and inflammatory lesions may protrude into the vaginal canal as polypoid masses, true polyps composed of a fibrovascular core covered by vaginal epithelium are rare. The fibroepithelial polyp is a benign polypoid mass 1–2 cm in average diameter occurring usually in adult women. The polyp is histologically similar to a fibroepithelial polyp of the vulval and anal region. It grows from the fornix or wall of the vagina. The squamous epithelium covering the polyp is normal but may be thickened (Fig. 21.1) and infected by HPV (Maenpaa et al. 1988). Polyps with an atypical connective tissue component have been labelled pseudosarcomatous polyp.

The treatment is excision.

21.1.2 Pseudosarcomatous Polyp

Pseudosarcomatous polyps are uncommon vaginal lesions which have been reported under various names, such as pseudosarcoma botryoides (Elliott et al. 1967; O'Quinn et al. 1982), sarcoma botryoides-like lesions (Norris and Taylor 1966), vaginal polyps with pseudosarcomatous features (Miettinen et al. 1983), polyps of the vagina (Chirayil and Tobon 1981) and fibroepithelial polyps of the vagina (Burt et al. 1976). Some authors prefer the term pseudosarcomatous polyp as better, firstly because it makes pathologists and clinicians aware of the benign nature of the condition and cautions against the possible diagnosis of sarcoma (botryoides), and secondly the vaginal squamous cells are not components of the lesion. The term fibroepithelial polyp which connotes epithelial participation, is not a proper designation of this polyp. Ostor et al. (1988) have recently suggested fibroepithelial polyp with atypical stromal cells.

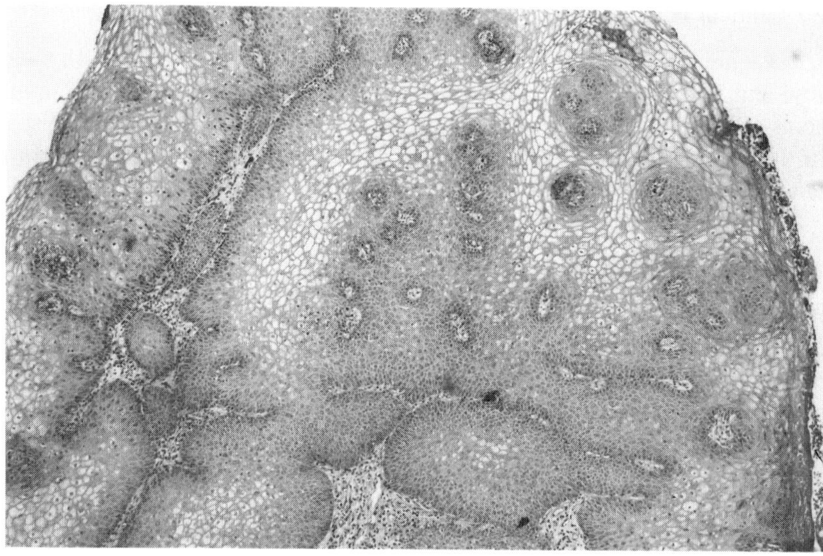

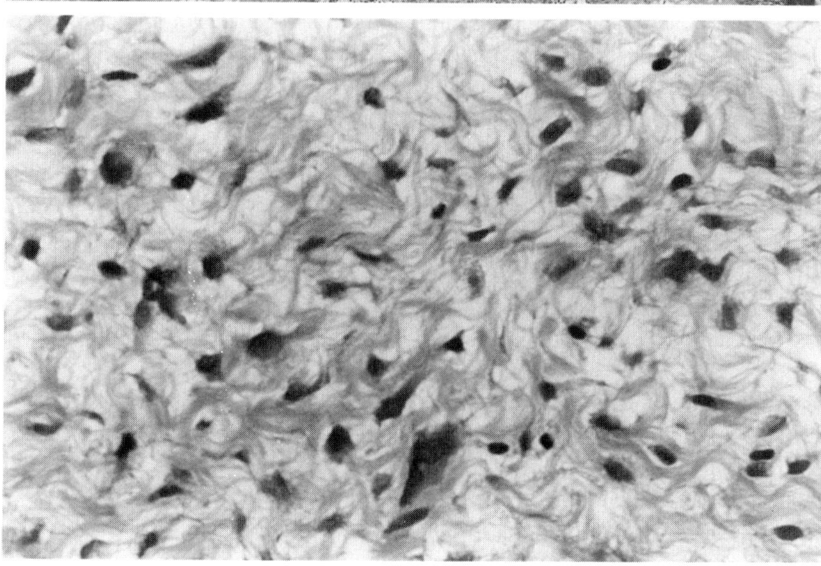

Fig. 21.1. Fibroepithelial polyp: the polyp is lined by thickened squamous epithelium

Fig. 21.2. Pseudosarcomatous polyp: atypical cells with cytoplasmic processes scattered in oedematous stroma

21.1.2.1 Clinical Features

The patients are of wide age range, 18–86 years, with a median age of 48.5 years (Chiraryl and Tobon 1981). One-third of the patients are asymptomatic. The main symptoms are vaginal bleeding, vaginal growth and in occasional patients dyspareunia or dysuria. Approximately one-quarter of the patients are pregnant when the lesions are discovered.

21.1.2.2 Pathological Features

The polyps are mostly single and may be located anywhere along the vaginal canal, although a predielection for the lateral wall was noted in one series (Norris and Taylor 1966). Grossly, the polyps are round, oval or globular in shape, with a soft to rubbery consistency and 0.5–3.5 cm in size. The surface is usually smooth and moist, the colour ranging from grey-pink to tan.

21.1.2.3 Microscopical Appearance

The polyps are covered by normal vaginal squamous epithelium and composed of loose oedematous and dense fibroconnective tissue containing abundant blood vessels of various sizes. Scattered in and intimately mixed with the fibrocollagenous tissue are many plump atypical cells and bizarre giant cells possessing abundant eosinophilic cytoplasm and hyperchromatic abnormal nuclei (Fig. 21.2). The cytoplasm of these cells lack cross-striations but display multiple irregular processes. The abnormal nuclei may take binucleate, multinucleate and giant forms. Mitotic figures may be seen but are usually fewer in number. The hypocellular connective tissue displays variable myxoid changes and is often infiltrated by a variable number of lymphocytes. The sub-epithelial zone is usually fibrotic but may occasionally contain focal areas of increased cellularity. The cambium layer of sarcoma botryoid is not seen.

Immunoperoxidase studies (Ostor et al. 1988) have shown positive reactions with histiocytic markers (α_1-antitrypsin and α_1-antichymotrypsin) in the giant cells and atypical mononuclear cells.

Ultrastructural studies confirm the fibroblastic nature of the bizarre cells (Miettinen et al. 1983). The component spindle cells with cytoplasmic processes which extend into the adjacent collagen contain numerous membrane-bound vesicles, abundant microsomes, occasional stacks of rough endoplasmic reticulum, Golgi apparatus and poorly developed mitochondria. The nuclear membrane is irregular due to invaginations (Mitchell et al. 1987). A basal lamina is absent. Cachaza et al. (1986) demonstrated eosinophilic inclusions with similarities to cytoplasmic microfibrils.

21.1.2.4 Aetiology and Biological Behaviour

The aetiology is at present unknown. Association with pregnancy (Elliott and Elliott 1973) and post-menopausal hormone treatment suggest a hormonal stimulus. In spite of the startling histological appearances, the lesion is not aggressive but benign.

21.1.2.5 Treatment

Complete excision is curative.

21.1.3 Post-hysterectomy Polyp

21.1.3.1 Gross Appearance

Following hysterectomy, polyps may develop as conical or horn-shaped projections from the surgical scar (Williams 1965). They are exuberant, firm, hypovascular scar tissues covered by vaginal epithelium and usually asymptomatic. Some patients may experience dyspareunia.

21.1.3.2 Microscopical Appearance

The polyps consist of fibrocollagenous tissue covered by squamous epithelium which is continuous with the vaginal lining. Giant cell reactions around the buried suture material may be noticed (Williams 1965).

21.1.3.3 Treatment

Surgical excision under local anaesthesia if symptomatic suffices.

21.1.4 Carunculae Myrtiformes (Curuncula Hymenalis)

These are remnants of hymen and usually asymptomatic. Inflammation and coital trauma can produce symptoms of dyspareunia and dysuria.

21.1.4.1 Gross Appearance

Carunculi are small, polypoid lesions of an average 0.5–1 cm in size, located at the level of the hymenal ring.

21.1.4.2 Microscopical Appearance

The lesion is similar to a benign polyp containing a fibroconnective tissue core and lined externally by normal squamous epithelium.

21.1.4.3 Treatment

Treatment involves excision or cauterisation under local anaesthesia (Williams 1965), followed by sexual rest.

21.1.5 Villous Adenoma of the Vagina

Villous adenomas with histological features indistinguishable from colonic villous adenomas have been reported from the urinary bladder (Assor 1978; Miller et al. 1983), urethra (Howells et al. 1985) and uterine cervix (Michal et al. 1986). They occur in both elderly men and women. Symptoms vary according to the location of the tumour. Women may present with haematuria, watery vaginal discharge, frequency of micturition and dysuria. One patient with a vaginal lesion was 72 years old and presented with vaginal irritation. Polyps were discovered in the introitus as well as in the anus.

21.1.5.1 Pathological Features

The polyps vary in size between 1 and 3 cm and display an irregular, lobulated surface.

21.1.5.2 Microscopical Appearance

They are composed of papillary fronds similar to the villous adenomas of the colon and rectum. The papillae are supported on a stalk, and their fibrovascular cores are covered usually by a single layer of columnar epithelium with scattered, mucus-secreting cells interposed between them. The neoplastic cells may display stratification and contain mildly hyperchromatic and pleomorphic nuclei. Invasion of the stalk has not been noticed.

21.1.5.3 Histogenesis

Villous adenomas of the urinary bladder have been suggested to arise from metaplastic transitional cells (Susmano et al. 1971) and urachal remnants (Thomas et al. 1971), and the urethral tumour, from the metaplastic epithelium of the paraurethral glands (Howells et al. 1985). The incomplete closure of the rectovaginal septum during embryological development might allow occurrence of a polyp in the septum and vagina from endodermal mucosa.

21.1.5.4 Treatment

Complete excision of the polyp with a marghin of normal vaginal epithelium around its base is adequate. The corresponding rectal mucosa should be examined for adenomatous changes and excised. The vaginal tumour reported was treated by wide en block dissection, partial resection of the vagina and excision of the rectal mucosa (Giano et al. 1987).

References

Fibroepithelial Polyp

Maenpaa J, Soderstrom T, Salmi T et al. (1988) Large atypical polyp of the vagina during pregnancy with concomitant human papilloma virus infection. Eur J Obstet Gynecol Reprod Biol 27:65–69

Pseudosarcomatous Polyp

Burt RL, Prichard RW, Kim BS (1976) Fibroepithelial polyp of the vagina. Obstet Gynecol 47 [Suppl]:52–54

Cachaza JA, Cabellero JJL, Fernandez JA et al. (1986) Endocervical polyp with pseudosarcomatous pattern and cytoplasmic inclusions: an electron microscopic study. Am J Clin Pathol 85:633–635

Chirayil SJ, Tobon H (1981) Polyps of the vagina: a clinicopathological study of 18 cases. Cancer 47:2904–2907

Elliott GB, Elliott JDA (1973) Superficial stromal reactions of lower genital tract. Arch Pathol 95:100–101

Elliott GB, Reynolds HA, Fidler HK (1967) Pseudosarcoma botryoides of the cervix and vagina in pregnancy. J Obstet Gynaecol Br Commonw 74:728–733

Miettinen M, Wahlstrom T, Vesterinen E et al. (1983) Vaginal polyps with pseudosarcomatous features: a clinicopathological study of seven cases. Cancer 51:1148–1151

Mitchell M, Talerman A, Sholl JS et al. (1987) Pseudosarcoma botryoides in pregnancy: report of a case with ultrastructural observations. Obstet Gynecol 70:522–526

Norris HJ, Taylor HB (1966) Polyps of the vagina: a benign lesion resembling sarcoma botryoides. Cancer 19:227–232

O'Quinn AG, Edwards CL, Gallger HS (1982) Pseudosarcoma botryoides of the vagina in pregnancy. Gynecol Oncol 13:237–241

Ostor AG, Fortune DW, Riley CB (1988) Fibroepithelial polyps with atypical stromal cells (Pseudosarcoma botryoides) of vulva and vagina. Int J Gynecol Pathol 7:351–360

Post Hysterectomy Polyps

Williams GA (1965) Postsurgical and post-traumatic tumors. Clin Obstet Gynecol 8:1020–1034

Carunculae Myrtiformis

Williams GA (1965) Postsurgical and post-traumatic tumors. Clin Obstet Gynecol 8:1020–1034

Villous Adenoma

Assor D (1978) A villous tumor of the bladder. J Urol 119:287–288

Giano PS, Antonioli DA, Critclow J et al. (1987) Villous adenoma presenting as a vaginal polyp in a rectovaginal tract. Hum Pathol 18:863–866

Howells MR, Baylis MS, Howell S (1985) Benign urethral villous adenoma: case report. Br J Obstet Gynaecol 92:1070–1071

Michael H, Sutton G, Hull M et al. (1986) Villous adenoma of the uterine cervix associated with invasive adenocarcinoma: a histologic, ultrastructural and immunohistochemical study. Int J Gynecol Pathol 5:163–169

Miller DC, Gang DL, Gavris V et al. (1983) Villous adenoma of the urinary bladder: a morphologic or biologic entity? Am J Clin Pathol 79:728–731

Susmano D, Rubenstein AB, Dakin AR et al. (1971) Cystitis glandularis and adenocarcinoma of the bladder. J Urol 105:671–674

Thomas DG, Ward AM, Williams JL (1971) A study of 52 cases of adenocarcinoma of the urinary bladder. Br J Urol 43:4–15

22 Tumours

22.1 Squamous Cell Origin

22.1.1 Squamous Papilloma

Squamous papillary lesions of the vagina comprise a spectrum of squamous lesions with simple warts at one end and giant condyloma at the other. They are all manifestations of the same squamous proliferative process associated with HPV infection. With the recognition of papillary condylomata of wart virus origin in the cervix and other organs, the interrelationship among these lesions became more obvious. Meyer (1921) originally classified papillary lesions of the cervix into two separate groups – the true neoplastic papilloma and the condyloma-like papillary lesion due to infections. This subdivision has been, in general, adhered to up until now; it recognises that true neoplastic papilloma exists (Woodruff and Peterson 1958; Qizilbash 1974). WHO (1975) has defined squamous papilloma as a benign neoplasm composed of papillary processes with a core of fibrous tissue covered by stratified squamous epithelium. The distinction between condyloma acuminatum and true squamous papilloma has been made on the basis that the condylomatous lesions are multiple and occur in a younger age group whereas the true papilloma is single and occurs in older patients. Condyloma acuminatum displays cytoplasmic vacuolations in the squamous cells of the upper epidermis, whereas these vacuolar changes are minimal or absent in true papilloma, and instead precancerous changes may be present. This distinction appears mostly artificial, as it is known that condyloma can be single and may show malignant changes and histological evolution with increasing age (Schmauz and Owar 1980).

22.1.2 Vaginal Intra-epithelial Neoplasia

While invasive carcinoma of the vagina constitutes 1%–2% of all primary gynaecological malignancies, vaginal intra-epithelial neoplasia (VAIN) is much less frequent and according to Henson and Tarone (1977) occurs only in about 3 to 4 per million women. It has also been estimated to make up only 0.4% of all genital tract lesions in women (Cramer and Cutler 1974). An increased number of case reports since the early 1960s (Samuel et al. 1961; Moran and Robinson 1962; Ferguson and Maclure 1963; Copenhaver et al. 1964; Gray and Christopherson 1969; Hummer et al. 1970; Oliver 1979; Hernandez-Linares et al. 1980; Woodruff 1981; Benedet and Sanders 1984) indicates an increased awareness of the condition (Lee and Symmonds 1978) and a rise in incidence.

The aetiology of this condition is not exactly known. It is generally held that intra-epithelial neoplasia of the cervix (CIN) predisposes to carcinoma-in-situ of the vagina. It has been estimated that 1%–6% of patients with CIN develop VAIN following hysterectomy for CIN (Parker et al. 1960; Petrilli et al. 1980; Woodman et al. 1984). According to some authors, in about 70%–80% of patients, there is a previous history of hysterectomy for benign and malignant diseases of the cervix and radiation therapy for cervical carcinoma (Sockel et al. 1961; McIndoe and Green 1969: Gallup and Morley 1975; Geelhoed et al. 1976; Benedet and Sanders 1984; Lenehan et al. 1986). A latent period as long as 22 years after surgery (Rutledge 1967) and 17–24 years after radiation therapy (Koss et al. 1961; Lenehan et al. 1986) has been noted. Many of the post-hysterectomy lesions are residuals of direct extension of cervical lesions (Schiffer et al. 1972), and the unsuspected vaginal epithelial abnormality could have been overlooked and buried during surgery (Ireland and Monaghan 1988). The high incidence of synchronous neoplasia at another part of the lower genital tract and the occurrence of intra-epithelial neoplasia and invasive carcinoma in the artificial vagina (Ramming et al. 1970; Duckler 1972; Rotmensch et al. 1983; Lathrop et al. 1985; Imrie et al. 1986; Gallup et al. 1987) and graft tissues may be due to the same local carcinogenic environment (Lathrop et al. 1985), "field carcinogenesis" (Marcus 1960) or expression of oncogenic potential of the graft (Ramming et al. 1970). The graft tissue in the vagina assumes the same characteristics (Whitacre and Wang 1944) and acquires the same vulnerability as the local tissue. Immunosuppression as in renal transplant patients (Simpkins and Hull 1974) is also recognised as a high-risk factor for the development of a cervical intra-epithelial lesion (Kay et al. 1970). The incidence of VAIN is also significantly high amongst them (Simpkins and Hull 1974). In recent years, HPVs have been increasingly incriminated in cervical pre-invasive and invasive carcinomas. In about one-third of the patients with VAIN, histopathological evidence of condylomatous features is found (Lenehan et al. 1986), indicating that HPVs may also play an important role in the causation of vaginal pre-invasive and invasive lesions. Some authors object to the diagnosis of all lesions comprising acanthosis, papillomatosis and perinuclear halols with mild to moderate nuclear atypia as an HPV infection (Nuovo et al. 1988), because in only a small number of such cases can HPV DNA be detected. It is also held that in the absence of an antecedent or synchronous cervical lesion VAIN is uncommon, and the majority of VAIN occur de novo (Ruez-Moreno et al. 1987).

22.1.2.1 Clinical Features

The age of the patients ranges from 17 to 77 years (Lenehan et al. 1986) with an average of 54 years (Benedet and Sanders 1984). Patients with VAIN are older than patients with CIN (Gallup and Morley 1975; Woodruff 1981). The majority of patients are asymptomatic, and the lesions are usually discovered after abnormal smears and colposcopic biopsies. Symptomatic patients complain of dyspareunia, post-coital spotting, burning sensation of the vagina, leucorrhoea and, rarely, sanguinous discharge (Gallup and Morley 1975; Lee and Symmonds 1978).

22.1.2.2 Gross Appearance

The lesions are pink "blush" or granular in appearance (Gray and Christopherson 1969). On colposcopic examination after application of 3% acetic acid, the lesions appear whitish with punctation and mosaic patterns of the sub-epithelial blood vessels. In the overhwelming majority of patients the lesions are located in the upper third of the vagina (Benedet and Sanders 1984; Lenehan et al. 1986). About 40% of the lesions are multicentric.

22.1.2.3 Microscopical Appearance

The histological appearance is similar to CIN. The entire thickness of the vaginal epithelium is occupied by neoplastic squamous cells displaying pleomorphism, nuclear atypia and mitoses (Figs. 22.1, 22.2). In VAIN I the deeper and outer third, in VAIN II the outer and deeper two-thirds and in VAIN III the entire thickness of the epithelium is replaced by dedifferentiated neoplastic cells.

These lesions are still relatively uncommon, and their biological behaviour is mostly unknown. The likelihood is that they behave similarly to their cervical counterparts. Spontaneous regression has been reported (Petrilli et al. 1980).

22.1.2.4 Treatment

Surgical treatment in the form of wide local, partial or total vaginectomy has been used with success (Benedet and Sanders 1984). Where sexual function is to be maintained, local excision and skin grafts have been advocated (Rutledge 1967). Pre-operative local oestrogen therapy, application of iodine and colposcopy are helpful in the delineation of the lesion (Gallup and Morley 1975; Veridiano et al. 1978; Oliver 1979). As clear excision margins are an important safeguard against recurrence, the margins of the surgical specimens should be examined carefully to exclude any residual lesions.

5-Fluorouracil cream has been used with various success rates (Woodruff et al. 1975; Ballon et al. 1979; Piver et al. 1979; Daly and Ellis 1980; Caglar et al. 1981; Pride and Chumpervich 1982; Kirwan and Naftalin 1985; Lathrop et al. 1985). The duration of treatment has ranged from 10 to 20 weeks (Kirwan and Naftalin 1985).

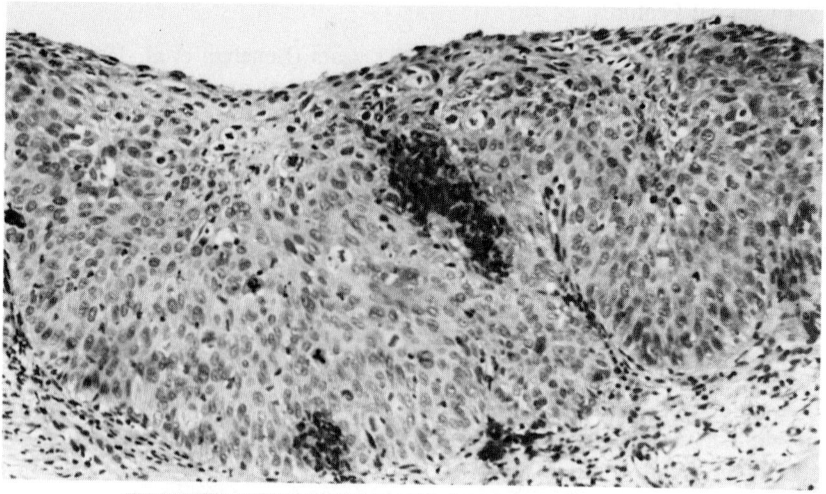

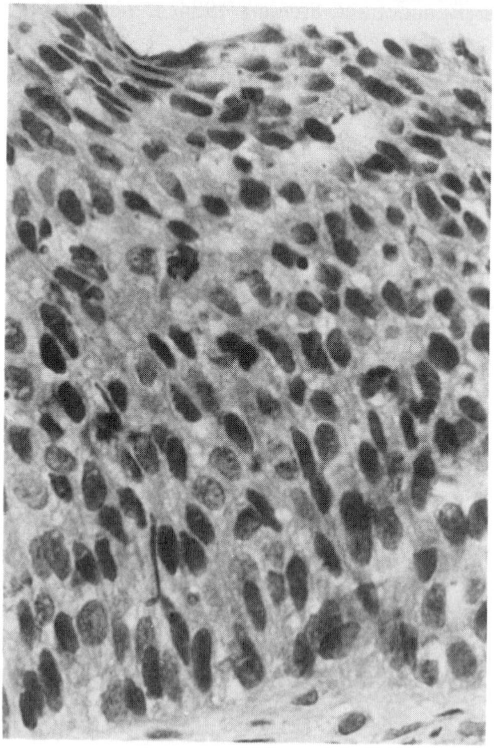

Fig. 22.1. Vaginal intra-epithelial neoplasia: full thickness of the epithelium is replaced by dedifferentiated cells

Fig. 22.2. Vaginal intra-epithelial neoplasia: high power view of a detail of Fig. 22.1

Radiation in the form of local application of radium has been found to be effective in selected group of patients (Hummer et al. 1970; Hernandez-Linares et al. 1980; Punnonen et al. 1981; Woodman et al. 1988), but it is not without complications. In sexually active women, vaginal retraction may occur. Also, patients who have been treated previously by radiotherapy are not suitable (Hernandez-Linares et al. 1980). Carbon dioxide laser therapy in recent years has become increasingly popular for treating intra-epithelial neoplasia because of its effectiveness and minimal complications (Townsend et al. 1982; Jobson and Homesley 1983; Stanhope et al. 1983; Curtin et al. 1985; Lenehan et al. 1986). Stafl et al. (1977) stressed the advantage of laser treatment over electrodiathermocautery and cryosurgery, which are known to be associated with post-operative complications of scarring, stenosis and fistula formation.

Following any form of treatment, a long follow-up of the patient is essential.

22.1.3 Microinvasive Carcinoma

Although there is still some disagreement regarding the diagnostic criteria, microinvasive carcinoma of the uterine cervix is a recognised entity. Considering the different and unpredictable behaviour of the similar condition in the vulva, the term stage 1a carcinoma rather than microinvasive has been recommended (Kneale 1984) for vulval lesions. In earlier as well as recent reports on vaginal carcinomas, the existence of an early invasive phase, although recognised (Douglas 1954; Lewis and Brady 1967; Jimerson and Merrill 1976; Barclay 1979), has only been cursorily mentioned. Recently, attention has been drawn to this lesion, and there is renewed interest regarding its aetiology, biological behaviour and treatment. Some authors consider it to be a distinct stage in the evolution of vaginal carcinoma (Dini and Park 1984; Peters et al. 1985) similar to the microinvasive phase in the life history of cervical carcinoma. As microinvasive carcinoma of vagina is much less frequent than the cervical microinvasive lesion, and reports on vaginal lesions are only few, its biological behaviour is still mostly undetermined. Criteria for their diagnosis are therefore based on the diagnostic criteria of cervical microinvasive carcinoma. It is still, however, uncertain whether the diagnostic criteria should be the same or whether a different set of criteria would better suit. The six cases of microinvasive carcinoma reported by Peters et al. (1985) were diagnosed on the criteria of less than 3 mm stromal invasion from the overlying epithelial surface. The patients were 10 years younger than those with invasive carcinoma, and three of them had had previous treatment for invasive carcinoma of the cervix. In all patients, the lesions were thought to have progressed from the intra-epithelial phase. Treatment was by partial or total vaginectomy. None of the patients experienced recurrence in 51–125 months of follow-up. One of the two patients reported by Dini and Park (1984) had had a vaginal hysterectomy 15 years earlier for carcinoma-in-situ of the cervix. She developed carcinoma-in-situ of the vagina, which was treated by colpectomy and skin graft. During a subsequent follow-up, microinvasive carcinoma was detected

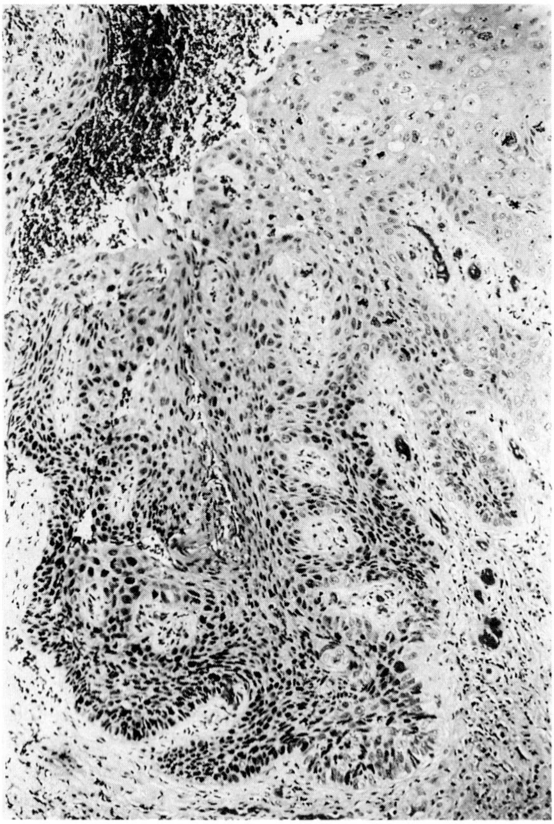

Fig. 22.3. Microinvasive carcinoma: an irregular column of atypical cells showing early invasion less than 3 mm from the most superficial layer of epithelium

at the vault of the neovagina. The patient was free of recurrence 3 years after the resectionn of the neovagina.

The number of cases reported so far is small. It is not known with certainty whether microinvasive carcinoma of vagina arises from pre-existing intra-epithelial carcinoma or de novo. The majority of these patients had had previous treatment for cervical carcinoma, which raises a strong suspicion of incomplete excision of the cervical lesion and inadvertent overlooking of the vaginal lesion at the time of treatment. It nevertheless stresses an obligatory follow-up of all patients with cervical and vulval carcinoma for subsequent vaginal intra-epithelial and invasive lesions.

At present it appears that until we understand the natural history more clearly from studies of many more patients, the diagnostic criteria for vaginal microinvasive carcinoma will be similar to those used for the cervical lesion (Fig. 22.3).

22.1.4 Invasive Squamous Cell Carcinoma

Primary invasive carcinoma of the vagina constitutes about 1%–2% of all gynaecological malignancies (Dunn and Napier 1966; Rutledge 1967; Frick et al. 1968) and ranks as the second rarest malignancy of the female genital tract after primary carcinoma of the fallopian tube. In an analysis of cervical, corporeal and vulval cancers over a 20-year period at M.D. Anderson Hospital in Texas, Rutledge (1967) observed a ratio of 1:60 for vaginal to cervical cancer, 1:12 to corporeal cancer and 1:3 to cancer of the vulva. The low incidence of vaginal squamous cell carcinoma has been attributed to the inclusion of many vaginal cancers as cervical cancers when the malignancy involves the lower cercix and upper vagina (W.G. Smith 1981). A definite aetiology and predisposing factors are not known. There are reports suggesting (Bivens 1953; Marcus 1960a; Perez et al. 1973; Prempree et al. 1977) as well as denying (Kaiser 1952; Underwood and Smith 1971) racial background as a predisposing factor. Chronic irritations from wearing pessaries for prolapse (Blunt 1965; Rutledge 1967; Herbst et al. 1970; Daw 1971), irritating chemicals and leucorrheal discharges have been incriminated, but no conclusive evidence about their role has been substantiated (Singh 1951). The role of previous hysterectomy for benign and malignant lesions of the cervix to the subsequent development of vaginal cancer has been discussed in numerous reports (Dunster and Bennett 1953; Berthelsen 1957; May 1958; Carter et al. 1961; Gray and Christopherson 1969; Adduci 1972; Schiffer et al. 1972; Hummer et al. 1970; Barclay 1979; Payne and Moolgasker 1981; Stuart et al. 1981; Choo and Anderson 1982; Bell et al. 1984; Leneham et al. 1986). Herman et al. (1986) have concluded recently that the probability of hysterectomy as a risk factor when age and cervical diseases are controlled for is, in fact, low. The association of VAIN with antecedent CIN or VIN is well recognised (Schiffer et al. 1972; Gallup and Morley 1975; Ramussen and Diernaes 1983). In the majority of patients incomplete excision of CIN (Carter et al. 1961; Copenhaven et al. 1964; Jimerson and Merrill 1976; Barclay 1979; Woodruff 1981) is believed to be the reason for the persistence and recurrence of the lesion in the vagina. The vaginal recurrence rate of carcinoma-in-situ after hysterectomy has been estimated to vary between 1% (McIndoe and Green 1969) and about 7% (Funnell and Merrill 1969). Some intra-epithelial neoplasias have a multicentric origin involving the cervix, vagina and vulva due to the effects of common carcinogenic agents as proposed in the "field" theory (Marcus 1960b). The squamous epithelia of the cervix, vulva, vagina and perianal skin are parts of a general field of epithelium which reacts as a single tissue to a carcinogenic stimulus or stimuli (Jimerson and Merrill 1970). The malignant changes in these organs may be both synchronous and metachronous (Kanbour et al. 1974). The metachronous development of invasive carcinoma in the cervix and vagina after a variable interval may be due to the field change which may be focal, evolving through the continuum of mild intra-epithelial change to invasive carcinoma (Geelhoed et al. 1976). Carcinoma-in-situ of the vagina may behave in a similar manner to that of the cervix and vulva by being invasive after a variable period (Rutledge 1967).

The occasional development of carcinoma in the neovagina (Steffanoff 1953; Ramming et al. 1970; Rotmensch et al. 1983; Hopkins and Morley 1987) indicates a persistent local carcinogenic stimulus or stimuli operative on the graft tissue. These patients are usually younger than the patients with typical vaginal carcinoma. The atypical epithelial changes and carcinoma-in-situ of the vagina following radiotherapy for cancer of the cervix may progress to invasive cancers (Koss et al. 1961; Rutledge 1967; Hummer et al. 1970; Piver et al. 1979). In recent years wart virus infections occurring in the female lower genital tract are being diagnosed with increasing frequency. Different strains of this virus have been identified in the spectrum of lesions ranging from flat condyloma to invasive carcinoma. Vaginal carcinoma can develop in a similar manner to that in cervical and vulval condylomas (Beck 1984). HPV has also been identified in verrucous carcinoma of the vagina (Okagaki et al. 1984), which is considered to be a part of the spectrum of the neoplastic squamous lesion.

22.1.4.1 Clinical Features

The age of the patients ranges from 35 (Singh 1951) to 87 years (Marcus 1960a), peak incidence occurring between 50 and 70 years (Herbst et al. 1970). The youngest patient reported was 14 years old (Siddall 1949). The most common symptom is abnormal vaginal bleeding. Many patients complain of brown discharge, post-coital bleeding and urinary trouble such as dysuria, frequency and retention. An occasional patient may be asymptomatic, and the diagnosis is made as an incidental finding during pelvic examination. Paraneoplastic hypercalcaemia was reported in one patient (O'Neil and Mikuta 1970).

Clinically, the vaginal tumours must be clearly identified, and to establish the diagnosis of a primary carcinoma of the vagina, the following criteria have to be satisfied (Kottmeir 1963; Rutledge 1967; Gray and Christopherson 1969; Perez et al. 1974): (i) the primary site of growth must be in the vagina, (ii) the uterine cervix must be intact (negative cervical biopsies are preferable), and (iii) there must be no clinical evidence of a primary carcinoma elsewhere. The tumours can arise anywhere in the vagina, but the upper one-third and posterior wall apear to be the most common sites (Singh 1951; Bivens 1953; Palmer and Biback 1954; Merrill and Bender 1958; Palumbo et al. 1969; Perticucci 1972; Benedet et al. 1983; Johnston et al. 1983). The upper third has been found to be the most common site for post-hysterectomy and the lower third in multifocal genital lesions (Usherwood 1975). The distal and middle thirds are affected in 23% and 4%, respectively (Gallup et al. 1987).

Clinical staging of invasive cancers of FIGO (Kottmeier 1976):

Stage 0: Carcinoma-in-situ, intra-epithelial carcinoma
Stage I: Carcinoma is confined to the vaginal wall
Stage II: Carcinoma has infiltrated the sub-vaginal tissue but has not extended to the pelvic wall
IIa: Sub-vaginal infiltration not extending into the parametrium

IIb: Parametrial infiltration not extending to the pelvic wall
Stage III: Carcinoma has extended to the pelvic wall
Stage IV: Carcinoma has extended outside the true pelvis or infiltrated the bladder or rectum. A bullous oedema as such does not permit allotment of a patient to stage IV
IVa: Spread of the growth to adjacent organs
IVb: Spread to distant organ

22.1.4.2 Gross Appearance

Three types of carcinoma are seen:

(i) Exophytic, everting or papillary form, the most common type, is a large fungating friable mass which may undergo necrotic changes and turn into crater-like ulcers with everted edges. Initially, when the tumour is small, it may appear as a wart.

(ii) Infiltrative or indurated type is an indurated mass which extends diffusely into the subvaginal tissue with irrgular margins. Ulceration is a late event.

(iii) Solitary nodulo-ulcerative form presents as a solitary indurated nodule which becomes ulcerated with well-defined margins.

Occasionally, the tumours may be annular and constricting, converting the vagina in to a rigid tube (Bivens 1953). In a small number of patients, the tumour may appear as an elevated, well-demarcated, firm patch without ulceration (Whelton and Kottmeir 1962).

22.1.4.3 Microscopical Appearance

Squamous cell carcinoma accounts for about 93%–97% of vaginal malignancies (Rutledge 1967; Herbst et al. 1970; Hummer et al. 1970; Brown et al. 1971; Prempree et al. 1977). The tumours are usually moderately differentiated and nonkeratinising, but well-differentiated keratinising (Fig. 22.4) and non-keratinising types are not infrequent. Both the keratinising and non-keratinising carcinomas are arranged in irregular sheets, strands and single columns of polygonal cells with hyperchromatic oval and round nuclei containing prominent nucleoli. The keratinising carcinomas display cytoplasmic keratins with a tendency to form epithelial pearls.

In the exophytic tumours the neoplastic cells are arranged in papillary configurations, being supported on central fibrovascular cores. The epithelium adjacent to the squamous cell carcinoma may show carcinoma-in-situ over a wide area. Scattered mitotic figures can be seen within the thickened and somewhat verrucoid epithelium. A small percentage of tumours are undifferentiated and may show markedly bizarre cells with many atypical mitotic figures. A more aggressive small cell carcinoma which has been identified in different organs in recent years has also been recognised in the vagina (Peters et al. 1985). Some of these tumours may belong to the category of neuroendocrine tumours. The reported transitional cell-type carcinomas (Brack et al. 1958; Merrill and Bender 1958; Palumbo et al. 1969) probably

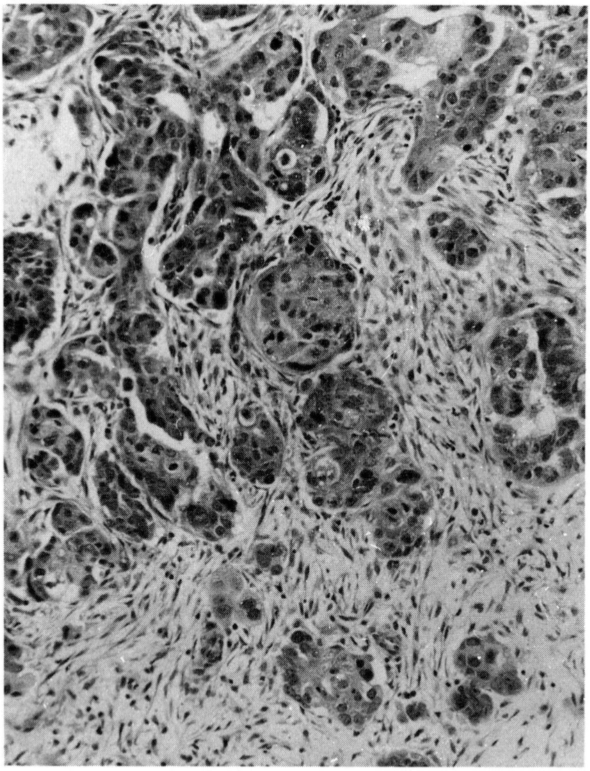

Fig. 22.4. Squamous cell carcinoma: well-differentiated keratinising carcinoma

belong to the poorly differentiated group (Whelton and Kottmeir 1962). It is also possible that some of them are truly transitional carcinomas and arise from the cloacal epithelium which is shared embryologically by the vulva, vagina and anus. Like papillary transitional carcinoma of the urinary bladder, these tumours also contain central cores of vascular connective tissue. The cloacogenic transitional cell carcinoma may contain squamous as well as mucus-secreting cells (Rhatigan and Mojadidi 1973). In some tumours, the superficial layer of squamous cells is normal, but the deeper layer shows loss of polarity, pleomorphism and mitoses with irregular tongues of invasion in the underlying stromal tissue. This has been labelled by Murad et al. (1975) as sub-mucosal-type carcinomna. Amyloid-producing squamous cell carcinoma of the vagina has recently been reported (Hsueh and Kuo 1986).

22.1.4.4 Spread of the Tumours

The tumour spreads by local infiltration of sub-epithelial, paravaginal and parametrial tissue. It may extend upwards to involve the cervix and infrequently downwards to the vulva. Recto-vaginal or vasico-vaginal fistulae can occur in the advanced stage.

The vagina is richly supplied by lymphatics, but the lymphatic spread of vaginal carcinoma has not been documented in detail. The lymphatic drainage from the upper third of the vagina is similar to that of the cervix and from the lower third, to that of the vulva. The middle third drains both ways.

The incidence of nodal metastases appears to be low (Douglas 1954) and occurs in about 6%–7% of patients (Whelton and Kottmeir 1962). The risk particularly increases when the size of the lesion is greater than 3 cm (W.G. Smith 1981). Haematogenous spread is rare and occurs commonly to the lung and bone. Metastases to the lungs can also occur due to retrograde involvement of the thoracic duct or diaphragmatic lymphatic system due to peritoneal seeding from upper third vaginal carcinoma (Koenigs et al. 1983). The lesion of the lower third shows a propensity to metastasise to the inguinal nodes (Houghton and Iversen 1982). Most local recurrences occur generally during the first year following treatment (Rubin et al. 1985), and the recurrence rate is higher in the high grade tumours and in tumours which involve a wide area of the vagina (Chu and Beechinor 1984).

22.1.4.5 Treatment

Early recognition of the lesion, routine biopsy of all innocent-looking vaginal lesions (Decker 1950) and routine smear and colposcopy in patients with a previous history of CIN or invasive lesions will undoubtedly ensure a higher success rate.

Individualisation of the treatment for vaginal invasive carcinoma has been emphasised by many workers (Herbst et al. 1970; W.G. Smith 1981; Johnston et al. 1983). Radiotherapy appears to have been the mainstay of treatment and has been used extensively either as the sole modality or in conjunction with surgery since 1950 (Fricke and Bowing 1950; F.R. Smith 1955; Whelton and Kottmeir 1962; Chau 1963; Rutledge 1967; Frick et al. 1968; Palumbo et al. 1969; Brown et al. 1971; Whelton and Kottmeier 1962; Perez et al. 1974; Prempree et al. 1977; Reddy et al. 1982; Benedet et al. 1983; Kuchera et al. 1985). This modality of treatment has shown good results in stages I and II of the disease (Brown et al. 1971). Combined interstitial and intra-cavitary radium with external supervoltage beam, especially to the parametrium and pelvic wall, have also shown very encouraging results (Prempree et al. 1977). Integrated external and interstitial irradiation has been found to be effective in the treatment of early as well as advanced carcinoma (Puthawala et al. 1983). In advanced tumours involving the bladder or rectum, a combination of pre-operative radiation and surgery may be considered (Prempree et al. 1977). Others have managed by a combination therapy of whole pelvic irradiation and brachytherapy (Manetta et al. 1988). Radical surgery in some patients has also yielded good results (Rubin et al. 1985). Katib et al. (1985) reported an advanced

Table 2. 5-year survival rates in percentage according to the stage of vaginal invasive squamous cell carcinoma in some series

	No. of patients	Stage I	Stage II	Stage III	Stage IV	Overall survival
Perez and Camel (1982)	105	81	42	30	9	50
Prempree (1982)	80	78	57	39	–	48
Benedet et al. (1983)	75	71	50	15	–	45
Nori et al. (1983)	36	71	66	33	–	42
Puthawala et al. (1983)	27	100	75	22	0	56
Chu and Beechinor (1984)	53	88	44	35	–	–
Gallup et al. (1987)	28	100	50	–	25	42.8
Reddy et al. (1987)	32	100	72	0	–	–
Manetta et al. (1988)	29	71	47	33	33	48

carcinoma treated by combination chemotherapy with bleomycin, methotrexate and cis-platinum prior to radiotherapy in the form of teletherapy and brachytherapy. This led to the complete disappearance of the primary tumour and inguinal nodes.

22.1.4.6 Survival Rate

In 1954, Palumbo reviewed the world literature, which revealed a dismal 5-year survival rate of only 12.3%. The results improved significantly in the 1960s. Whelton and Kottmeir (1962), Murphy and Bozzini (1963) and Rutledge (1967) achieved 5-year cure rates of 50%–60% for stage I, 30% for stage II and 20% for stage III disease.

Survival rate in some series is given in Table 2.

22.1.5 Verrucous Carcinoma

Verrucous carcinoma is a well-defined variant of squamous cell carcinoma and is known to occur at different anatomical sites. Considering the female genital tract, the vagina is a rare site, occupying third place after the vulva and cervix. In a report of 105 patients with verrucous carcinoma, Kraus and Perez-Mesa (1966) found only

1 in the vagina. Subsequently, a few more instances were published (Ramzy et al. 1976; Powell et al. 1978; Wood et al. 1978; Faaborg et al. 1979; Stehman et al. 1980; Jones et al. 1981). One of the reported cases occurred in an artificial vagina (Abrenio et al. 1977). True incidence, however, is difficult to estimate, as many of these lesions have been diagnosed under different names such as giant condyloma of Buschke-Löwenstein, giant papillary carcinoma, papillary squamous carcinoma, well-differentiated squamous cell carcinoma and pseudoepitheliomatous hyperplasia. The aetiology is unknown. Chronic irritation, poor oral hygiene and ill-fitting dentures have been incriminated for the oral form of varrucous carcinoma. In recent years, HPV-DNA (Ubben et al. 1979) and several strains of HPV have been demonstrated in condylomata acuminata, pre-invasive and invasive squamous neoplastic lesions as well as verrucous carcinoma of the lower female genital tract (Boshart et al. 1984; Crum et al. 1986). HPV-1 and 6 have been detected in vaginal verrucous carcinoma (Okagaki et al. 1984).

The patients are post-menopausal and over 50 years old. The main symptoms are vaginal discharge and vaginal bleeding.

22.1.5.1 Gross Appearance

The tumours are warty, fungating, cauliflower-like masses varying in size from 2 to 10 cm and may be ulcerated. The cut surface displays a grey-white bulbous appearance with sharp demarcation of the deeper margins.

22.1.5.2 Microscopical Appearance

The tumours are made of well-differentiated squamous cells thrown into papillary folds which are covered by layers of hyperkeratotic and parakeratotic cells. The squamous cells are uniform in size and shape and possess abundant eosinophilic cytoplasm and vesicular nuclei. Mitoses are rare. The deeper margins are well delineated and formed of bulbous rete ridges consisting of well-differentiated squamous cells (Fig. 22.5). Due to their wider bases, the bulbous ridges impart a pushing appearance at the tumour connective tissue interfaces. A zone of chronic inflammatory cells are almost always seen along the deeper margin.

The tumours are to be differentiated from invasive squamous cell carcinoma, condylomata acuminata and pseudoepitheliomatous hyperplasia. Condylomata acuminata contain fibrovascular cores extending from the stroma to the surface, while verrucous carcinoma lacks the central connective tissue support of the papillae (Kraus and Perez-Mesa 1966). The deeper margins of pseudoepitheliomatous hyperplasia are elongated, narrow and pointing. The clinical presentation should also be taken into consideration for the final diagnosis. The tumours, if left untreated, will grow slowly and ultimately be invasive (Kraus and Perez-Mesa 1966). They have a high tendency to recur and display a marked freedom to metastasise to the lymph nodes.

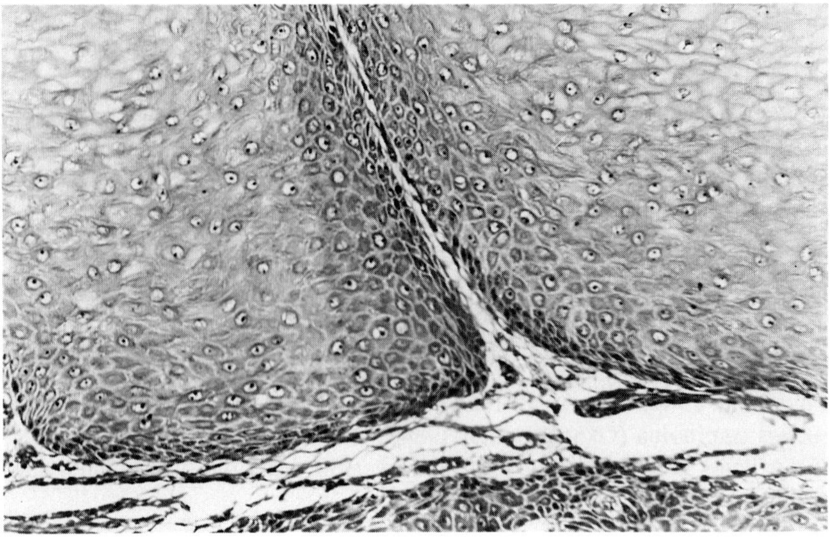

Fig. 22.5. Verrucous carcinoma: bulbous rete ridges consisting of well-differentiated squamous cells

22.1.5.3 Treatment

Wide local excision is advocated by most authors (Foye et al. 1969; Jennings and Barclay 1972; Lucas et al. 1974; Ramzy et al. 1976) as the treatment of choice. Radiotherapy has not been found particularly useful. Moreover, a high incidence of transformation to a more aggressive lesion has been reported with radiotherapeutic treatment (Demian et al. 1973). Similarly, bleomycin has been ineffective (De Graaff and van der Harten 1975).

22.1.6 Basal Cell-like Carcinoma in the Upper Third of the Vagina

Whelton and Kottmeier (1962) mentioned about "a most unusual basalioma" in their reported series of vaginal carcinoma. This was not elaborated on and presumably was a similar tumour to that reported by Naves et al. (1980). The tumour was 0.8 cm in largest diameter, projecting into the upper third of the posterior vaginal wall, and had microscopic features similar to that of a basal cell epithelioma of the skin. The tumour was thought to arise in the superficial or glandular epithelium.

References

Squamous Papilloma
Meyer R (1921) Papilloma of uterine cervix. Arch Gynakol 115:167–183

Qizilbash AH (1974) Papillary squamous tumors of uterine cervix. Am J Clin Pathol 61:508–520

Schmauz R, Owor R (1980) Condymatous tumours of vulva, vagina and penis. J Clin Pathol 33:1039–1046

WHO (1975) Poulsen HE, Taylor CW, Sovin LH (eds) Histologic typing of female genital tumors. WHO, Geneva

Woodruff JD, Peterson WF (1958) Condyloma acuminata of cervix. Am J Obstet Gynecol 75:1354–1362

Intraepithelial Carcinoma

Ballon SC, Roberts JA, Lagasse LD (1979) Topical 5 fluorouracil in the treatment of intraepithelial neoplasia of vagina. Obstet Gynecol 54:163–166

Benedet JL, Sanders BH (1984) Carcinoma-in-situ of the vagina. Am J Obstet Gynecol 148:695–700

Caglar H, Hertzog RW, Hreshchyshyn MM (1981) Topical 5 fluorouracil treatment of vaginal intraepithelial neoplasia. Obstet Gynecol 58:580–583

Copenhaver EH, Salzman FA, Wright KA (1964) Carcinoma-in-situ of the vagina. Am J Obstet Gynecol 89:962–969

Cramer DW, Cutler SJ (1974) Incidence and histopathology of malignancies of the female genital organs in the United States. Am J Obstet Gynecol 118:443–460

Curtin JP, Twiggs LB, Julian TM (1985) Treatment of vaginal intraepithelial neoplasia with CO2 laser. J Reprod Med 30:942–944

Daly JW, Ellis GF (1980) Treatment of vaginal dysplasia and carcinoma in situ with topical 5-fluorouracil. Obstet Gynecol 55:350–352

Duckler L (1972) Squamous cell carcinoma developing in an artifical vagina. Obstet Gynecol 40:35–38

Ferguson JH, Maclure JK (1963) Intraepithelial carcinoma, dysplasia and exfoliation of cancer cells in vaginal mucosa. Am J Obstet Gynecol 87:326–336

Gallup DG, Morley GW (1975) Carcinoma in situ of the vagina: a study and review. Obstet Gynecol 46:334–340

Gallup DG, Castle CA, Stock RJ (1987) Recurrent carcinoma in situ of the vagina following split thickness skin graft vaginoplasty. Gynecol Oncol 26:98–102

Geelhoed GW, Henson DE, Taylor PT et al. 1976) Carcinoma in situ of the vagina following treatment for carcinoma of the cervix: a distinctive clinical entity. Am J Obstet Gynecol 124:510–516

Gray LA, Christopherson WM (1969) In situ and early invasive carcinoma of the vagina. Obstet Gynecol 34:226–230

Henson D, Tarone R (1977) An epidemiological study of cancer cervix, vagina and vulva based on the Third National Cancer Survey in the United States. Am J Obstet Gynecol 129:525–532

Hernandez-Linares W, Puthawala A, Nolan JF et al. (1980) Carcinoma in situ of vagina – past and present management. Obstet Gynecol 56:356–360

Hummer WK, Hussey E, Decker DG et al. (1970) Carcinoma in situ of the vagina. Am J Obstet Gynecol 108:1109–1116

Imrie JEA, Kennedy JH, Holmes JD et al. (1986) Intraepithelial neoplasia arising in an artifical vagina. Case report. Br J Obstet Gynaecol 93:886–888

Ireland D, Monaghan JM (1988) The management of the patient with abnormal vaginal cytology following hysterectomy. Br J Obstet Gynaecol 95:973–975

Jobson VW, Homesley HD (1983) Treatment of vaginal intraepithelial neoplasia with carbondioxide laser. Obstet Gynecol 62:90–93

Kay S, Frable WJ, Hume DH (1970) Cervical dysplasia and cancer developing in women on immunosuppression therapy for renal homotransplantation. Cancer 26:1048–1052

Kirwan P, Naftalin NJ (1985) Topical 5fl. in treatment of vaginal intraepithelial neoplasia. Br J Obstet Gynaecol 92:287–291

Koss LG, Melamed MR, Daniel WW (1961) In situ epidermoid carcinoma of the cervix and vagina following radiotherapy for cervical cancer. Cancer 14:353–360

Lathrop JC, Ree HJ, McDuff HC Jr (1985) Intraepithelial neoplasia of the neovagina. Obstet Gynecol 65 [Suppl]:91–94

Lee RA, Symmonds RE (1978) Recurrent carcinoma in situ of vagina in patients previously treated for in situ carcinoma cervix. Obstet Gynecol 48:61–64

Lenehan PM, Meffe F, Lickerish GM (1986) vaginal intraepithelial neoplasia. Biologic aspects of management. Obstet Gynecol 68:333–337

Marcus SL (1960) Multiple squamous cell carcinoma involving the cervix, vagina and vulva. The theory of multicentric origin. Am J Obstet Gynecol 80:802–812

McIndoe WA, Green GH (1969) Vaginal carcinoma in situ following hysterectomy. Acta Cytol (Baltimore) 13:158–161

Moran JP, Robinson HJ (1962) Primary carcinoma in situ of the vagina: report of 2 cases. Obstet Gynecol 20:405–409

Nuovo GJ, Blanco JS, Silverstein SJ et al. (1988) Histologic correlates of papillomavirus infection of the vagina. Obstet Gynecol 72:770–774

Oliver JA Jr (1979) Severe dysplasia and carcinoma in situ of the vagina. Am J Obstet Gynecol 134:133–137

Parker RT, Cuyler WK, Kaufmann LA et al. (1960) Intraepithelial (stage 0) cancer of the cervix. Am J Obstet Gynecol 80:693–710

Petrilli ES, Townsend DE, Morrow CP et al. (1980) Biologic aspects and treatment with topical 5-fluorouracil and carbon di-oxide laser. Am J Obstet Gynecol 138:321–328

Piver MS, Barlow JJ, Tsukuda Y et al. (1979) Post irradiation squamous cell carcinoma in situ of the vagina, treatment by topical 20% 5-fluorouracil cream. Am J Obstet Gynecol 135:377–380

Pride GL, Chuprevich TW (1982) Topical 5-fluorouracil treatment of transformation zone intraepithelial neoplasia of cervix and vagina. Obstet Gynecol 60:467–472

Punnonen R, Gronroos M, Meurman L et al. (1981) Diagnosis and treatment of primary vaginal carcinoma in situ and dysplasia. Acta Obstet Gynecol Scand 60:513–514

Ramming KP, Pilch YH, Powell RD Jr et al. (1970) Primary carcinoma in an artificial vagina. Am J Obstet Gynecol 120:108–112

Rotmensch J, Rosenthal N, Dillon M et al. (1983) Carcinoma arising in neovagina. Case report and review of the literature. Obstet Gynecol 61:534–536

Ruiz-Moreno JA, Garcia-Gomz R, Vargas-Salano A et al. (1987) Vaginal intraepithelial neoplasia: report of 14 cases. Int J Gynaecol Obstet 25:359–362

Rutledge F (1967) Cancer of the vagina. Am J Obstet Gynecol 97:635–655

Samuel B, Bradburn DM, Johnson CG (1961) Primary carcinoma in situ of the vagina. Am J Obstet Gynecol 82:393–396

Schiffer MA, Mackles AM, Greene HJ (1972) Carcinoma in situ of the vagina after hysterectomy. Surg Gynecol Obstet 134:652–654

Schneider A, de Villiers EM, Schneider V (1987) Multifocal squamous neoplasia of the female genital tract: significance of human papilloma virus infection of the vagina after hysterectomy. Obstet Gynecol 70:294–298

Simpkins PB, Hull MGR (1974) Intraepithelial carcinoma of the vagina following immunosuppression treated with 5 fluorouracil. Proc R Soc Med 67:589–590

Sockel PW III, Collier FC, Jones WN et al. (1961) Relation of carcinoma in situ of the vagina to the early diagnosis of vaginal cancer. Am J Obstet Gynecol 82:397–400

Stafl A, Wilkinson EJ, Mattingly RF (1977) Laser treatment of cervical and vaginal neoplasia. Am J Obstet Gynecol 128:128–136

Stanhope CR, Phibbs GD, Stuart GCE et al. (1983) Carbon dioxide laser surgery. Obstet Gynecol 61:624–636

Townsend DE, Levine RU, Crum CP et al. (1982) Treatment of vaginal carcinoma in situ with the carbon dioxide laser. Am J Obstet Gynecol 143:565–568

Veridiano NP, Gomez-Leon G, Tancer ML (1978) The colposcope and vulvovaginal neoplasia. Gynecol Oncol 6:487–493
Whitacre FE, Wang Y-Y (1944) Biologic changes in squamous epithelium transferred to the pelvic connective tissue. Surg Gynecol Obstet 79:192–194
Woodman CBJ, Jordan JA, Wade-Evans T (1984) The management of vaginal intraepithelial neoplasia after hysterectomy. Br J Obstet Gynaecol 91:707–711
Woodman CB, Mould JJ, Jordan JA (1988) Radiotherapy in the management of vaginal intraepithelial neoplasia after hysterectomy. Br J Obstet Gynaecol 95:976–979
Woodruff JD (1981) Carcinonma in situ of the vagina. Clin Obstet Gynecol 24:485–501
Woodruff JD, Parmley TH, Julian CG (1975) Topical 5-fluorouracil in the treatment of vaginal carcinoma in situ. Gynecol Oncol 3:124–132

Microinvasive Carcinoma

Barclay DL (1979) Carcinoma of the vagina after hysterectomy for severe dysplasia or carcinoma in situ of the cervix. Gynecol Oncol 8:1–11
Dini MM, Park JM (1984) Microinvasive squamous cell carcinoma of the vagina. J Nat Med Assoc 78:709–711
Douglas GW (1954) Observations on the pathology of primary carcinoma of the vagina and its relation to therapy. Surg Gynecol Obstet 98:456–466
Jimerson GK, Merrill JA (1976) Cancer and dysplasia of the post hysterectomy vaginal cuff. Gynecol Oncol 4:328–334
Kneale BL (1984) Recommendations of the 7th International Congress. International Society for the Study of Vulvar Disease. Gynecol Oncol 18:134
Lewis GD Jr, Brady L (1967) Carcinoma of the vagina. Clin Obstet Gynecol 10:655–663
Peters WA III, Kumar NB, Morley GW (1985) Microinvasive carcinoma of the vagina: a distinct clinical entity. Am J Obstet Gynecol 153:505–507

Invasive Carcinoma

Adduci J (1972) Carcinoma of the vagina. Treatment by combined excision and cryosurgery. Geriatrics 27:121–123
Barclay DL (1979) Carcinoma of the vagina after hysterectomy for severe dysplasia or carcinoma in situ of the cervix. Gynecol Oncol 8:1–11
Beck I (1984) Vaginal carcinoma arising invaginal condylomata. Case report. Br J Obstet Gynaecol 91:503–505
Bell J, Sevin BU, Averette H et al. (1984) Vaginal cancer after hysterectomy for benign disease: value of cytologic screening. Obstet Gynecol 64:699–702
Benedet JL, Murphy JK, Fairey RN et al. (1983) Primary invasive carcinoma of the vagina. Obstet Gynecol 62:715–719
Berthelsen HG (1957) Vaginal carcinoma associated with prolapse. Acta Obstet Gynecol Scand 36:257–261
Bivens MD (1953) Primary carcinoma of the vagina. A report of forty six cases. Am J Obstet Gynecol 65:390–399
Blunt VAW (1965) Primary carcinoma of the vagina. Aust NZ J Obstet Gynaecol 5:29–33
Brack CB, Merritt BI, Dickson RJ (1958) Primary carcinoma of the vagina. Obstet Gynecol 11:3–11
Brown GR, Fletcher GH, Rutledge FN (1971) Irradiation of in-situ and invasive squamous cell carcinomas of the vagina. Cancer 28:1278–1283
Carter ER, Salvaggio AT, Jarokowski TL (1961) Squamous cell carcinoma of the vagina following vaginal hysterectomy for intraepithelial carcinoma of the cervix. Am J Obstet Gynecol 82:401–404
Chau PM (1983) Radiotherapeutic management of malignant tumours of vagina. Am J Roentgenol Radium Ther Nucl Med 89:502–503
Choo YC, Anderson D (1982) Neoplasms of the vagina following cervical carcinoma. Gynecol Oncol 14:125–132

Chu AM, Beechinor R (1984) Survival and recurrence patterns in radiation treatment of carcinoma of the vagina. Gynecol Oncol 19:298–307

Copenhaven E, Salzman EA, Wright KA (1964) Carcinoma in situ of the vagina. Am J Obstet Gynecol 89:962–969

Davis PC, Franklin EW III (1975) Cancer of the vagina. South Med J 68:1239–1242

Daw E (1971) Primary carcinoma of the vagina. Obstet Gynaecol Br Commonw 78:853–856

Decker DG (1950) Radiation therapy of primary carcinoma and other malignant lesions of the vagina. Am J Roentgenol 64:86–94

Douglas GW (1954) Observations on the pathology of primary carcinoma of the vagina and its relation to therapy. Surg Gynecol Obstet 98:456–466

Dunn LJ, Napier JG (1966) Primary carcinoma of the vagina. Am J Obstet Gynecol 96:1112–1116

Dunster M, Bennett D (1953) Primary carcinoma of the vaginal vault following total hysterectomy for non malignant conditions. J Obstet Gynaecol Br Em 66:126–128

Frick HC, Jacox HW, Taylor HC (1968) Primary carcinoma of the vagina. Am J Obstet Gynecol 101:695–703

Fricke RE, Bowing HH (1950) Radium therapy of primary carcinoma and other malignant lesions of the vagina. Am J Roentgenol 64:86–94

Funnell JD, Merrill JA (1969) Recurrence after treatment of carcinoma in situ of the cervix. Surg Gynecol Obstet 117:15–19

Gallup DG, Morley GW (1975) Carcinoma in situ of the vagina. Obstet Gynecol 46:334–340

Gallup DG, Talledo OE, Shah K et al. (1987) Invasive squamous cell carcinoma of the vagina. Obstet Gynecol 69:782–785

Geelhoed GW, Hanson DE, Taylor PT et al. (1976) Carcinoma in situ of the vagina following treatment for carcinoma cervix: a distinctive entity. Am J Obstet Gynecol 124:510–516

Gray LA, Christopherson WM (1969) In situ and early invasive carcinoma of the vagina after hysterectomy. Obstet Gynecol 34:226–230

Herbst AL, Green TH Jr, Ulfelder H (1970) Primary carcinoma of the vagina: an analysis of 68 cases. Am J Gynecol 106:210–218

Herman JM, Homesley HD, Dignan MB (1986) Is hysterectomy a risk factor for genital cancer? JAMA 256:601–603

Hopkins MP, Morley GW (1987) Squamous cell carcinoma of the neovagina. Obstet Gynecol 69:525–527

Houghton CRS, Iversen T (1982) Squamous cell carcinoma of the vagina: a clinical study of the location of the tumor. Gynecol Oncol 13:365–372

Hsueh S, Kuo T-T (1986) Amyloid in squamous cell carcinoma of the vagina. Immunohistochemical study with monoclonal anti-keratin antibodies. Int J Gynecol Pathol 5:357–361

Hummer WR, Mussey E, Decker DG et al. (1970) Carcinoma in situ of the vagina. Am J Obstet Gynecol 108:1109–1116

Jimerson GK, Merrill JA (1970) Multicentric squamous malignancy involving both cervix and vulva. Cancer 26:150–155

Jimerson GK, Merrill JA (1976) Cancer and dysplasia of the post hysterectomy vaginal cuff. Gynecol Oncol 4:328–334

Johnston GA, Klotz J, Boutselis JG (1983) Primary invasive carcinoma of the vagina. Surg Gynecol Onstet 156:34–40

Kaiser IH (1952) Primary carcinoma of the vagina. Cancer 5:1146–1160

Kanbour AI, Klionsky B, Murphy AI (1974) Carcinoma of the vagina following cervical cancer. Cancer 34:1838–1841

Katib S, Kuten A, Steiner M et al. (1985) The effectiveness of multidrug treatment by bleomycin, methotrexate, cis-platinum in advanced vaginal carcinoma. Gynecol Oncol 21:101–102

Koenigs KP, Campbell DR, Magrina J et al. (1983) Pulmonary lymphangitis carcinomatosis from vaginal carcinoma presenting as congestive heart failure. Obstet Gynecol 61:760–763

Koss LG, Melamed MR, Daniel WW (1961) In situ epidermoid carcinoma of the cervix and vagina following radiotherapy for cervical cancer. Cancer 14:353–360
Kottmeier HL (1963) The classification and clinical staging of carcinoma of the uterus and vagina. Int J Gynecol Obstet 1:83–93
Kottmeier HL (1976) International federation in obstetrics and gynecology. Annual report on the results of treatment. In: Carcinoma of the uterus, vagina and ovary. Radiumhemmet, Stockholm, Vol. 16
Kuchera H, Langer M, Smekal G et al. (1985) Radiotherapy of primary carcinoma of the vagina: management and results of different therapy schemes. Gynecol Oncol 21:87–93
Leneham PM, Meffe F, Lickerish GM (1986) Vaginal intraepithelial neoplasia, biologic aspects of management. Obstet Gynecol 68:333–337
Manetta A, Pinto JL, Larson JE et al. (1988) Primary invasive carcinoma of the vagina. Obstet Gynecol 72:77–81
Marcus SL (1960a) Primary carcinoma of the vagina. Obstet Gynecol 15:673–689
Marcus SL (1960b) Multiple squamous cell carcinoma involving the cervix, vagina and vulva, the theory of multicentric origin. Am J Obstet Gynecol 80:802–812
May HC (1958) Carcinoma in situ of the vagina subsequent to hysterectomy for carcinoma in situ of the cervix. Am J Obstet Gynecol 76:807–811
McIndoe WA, Green GH (1969) Vaginal carcinoma in situ following hysterectomy. Acta Cytol (Baltimore) 13:158–162
Merrill JA, Bender WT (1958) Primary carcinoma of the vagina. Obstet Gynecol 11:3–11
Murad TM, Durant JR, Maddox WA et al. (1975) The pathologic behavior of primary vaginal carcinoma and its relationship to cervical cancer. Cancer 35:787–794
Murphy WT, Bozzini MA (1963) End results in the irradiation of primary carcinoma of the vagina. Radiology 80:566–567
Nori D, Hilaris BS, Stanimir G et al. (1983) Radiation therapy of primary vaginal carcinoma. Int J Radiat Oncol Biol Phys 9:1471–1475
Okagaki T, Clark BA, Zachow KR et al. (1984) Presence of human papilloma virus in verrucous carcinoma (Ackerman) of the vagina. Arch Pathol Lab Med 108:567–570
O'Neil RT, Mikuta JJ (1970) Reversible hypercalcaemia in squamous cell carcinoma of the vagina. Obstet Gynecol 36:458–461
Palmer JP, Biback SM (1954) Primary cancer of the vagina. Am J Obstet Gynecol 67:377–397
Palumbo L (1954) Primary carcinoma of the vagina. South Med J 47:356–362
Palumbo L Jr, Shingleton HM, Fishbourne JI Jr et al. (1969) Primary carcinoma of the vagina. South Med J 62:1048–1053
Payne PR, Moolgasker AS (1981) Vaginal vault cancer following hysterectomy. J R Coll Surg Edinb 26:99–100
Perez CA, Camel HM (1982) Long term follow up in radiotherapy of carcinoma of the vagina. Cancer 49:1308–1315
Perez CA, Arneson AM, Galakatos A et al. (1973) Malignant tumours of the vagina. Cancer 31:36–44
Perez CA, Arneson AM, Dehner LP et al. (1974) Radiation therapy in carcinoma of the vagina. Obstet Gynecol 44:862–872
Perticucci S (1972) Diagnostic, prognostic and therapeutic considerations in invasive carcinoma of the vagina. Obstet Gynecol 40:843–850
Peters WA III, Kumar NB, Moreley GW (1985) Carcinoma of the vagina. Factors influencing treatment outcome. Cancer 55:892–897
Piver MS, Barlow JJ, Tsukada Y et al. (1979) Postirradiation squamous cell carcinoma in situ of the vagina. Treatment by topical 20% 5-fluorouracil cream. Am J Obstet Gynecol 135:377–380
Prempree T, Viravathana T, Slawson RC et al. (1977) Radiation management of primary carcinoma of the vagina. Cancer 40:109–118

Pride GL, Buchler DA (1977) Carcinoma of vagina 10 or more years following pelvic irradiation therapy. Am J Obstet Gynecol 127:513–517

Puthawala A, Syed AMN, Nalick R et al. (1983) Integrated external and internal radiation therapy for primary carcinoma of the vagina. Obstet Gynecol 62:367–372

Ramming KP, Pilch YH, Powell RD Jr et al. (1970) Primary carcinoma in an artificial vagina. Am J Surg 120:108–112

Rasmussen J, Diernaes E (1983) Neoplasia in the vagina following hysterectomy for dysplasis or carcinoma in situ of the uterine cervix. Acta Obstet Gynecol Scand 62:437–441

Reddy KS, Robert L, Rao R et al. (1982) Radiation therapy in primary carcinoma of the vagina. Acta Radiol Oncol 21:191–201

Reddy S, Graham JE, Yorden EL et al. (1987) Radiation therapy in primary carcinoma of the vagina. Gynecol Oncol 26:19–24

Rhatigan RM, Mojadidi Q (1973) Adenosquamous carcinoma of the vulva and vagina. Am J Clin Pathol 60:208–217

Rotmensch J, Rosenhein N, Dillon M et al. (1983) Carcinoma arising in the neovagina. Case report and review of the literature. Obstet Gynecol 61:534–536

Rubin S, Young J, Mikuta JJ (1985) Squamous carcinoma of the vagina. Treatment complications and long term follow up. Gynecol Oncol 20:346–353

Rutledge F (1967) Cancer of the vagina. Am J Obstet Gynecol 97:635–655

Schiffer MA, Mackles AM, Green HS (1972) Carcinoma in situ of the vagina after hysterectomy. Surg Gynecol Onstet 134:652–654

Siddall RS (1949) Vaginal carcinoma in a girl 14 years of age treated by radiation. Am J Obstet Gynecol 57:396–397

Singh BP (1951) Primary carcinoma of the vagina. Cancer 4:1073–1082

Smith FR (1955) Primary carcinoma of the vagina. Am J Obstet Gynecol 69:525–537

Smith WG (1981) Invasive carcinoma of the vagina. Clin Obstet Gynecol 24:503–514

Steffanoff DN (1953) Late development of squamous cell carcinoma in a skin graft lining a vagina. Plast Reconstr Surg 51:454–456

Stuart GCE, Allen HH, Anderson RJ (1981) Squamous cell carcinoma of the vagina following hysterectomy. Am J Obstet Gynecol 139:311–315

Underwood PB, Smith RT (1971) Carcinoma of the vagina. JAMA 217:46–52

Usherwood MM (1975) Management of vaginal carcinoma after hysterectomy. Am J Obstet Gynecol 122:352–354

Whelton J, Kottmeier HL (1962) Primary carcinoma of the vagina. Acta Obstet Gynecol Scand 41:22–40

Woodruff JD (1969) Treatment of recurrent carcinoma in situ in the lower genital canal. Clin Obstet Gynecol 8:757–770

Woodruff JD (1981) Carcinoma in situ of the vagina. Clin Obstet Gynecol 24:485–501

Verrucous Carcinoma

Abrenio JK, Chung HI, Pomante R (1977) Verrucous carcinoma arising from an artificial vagina. Obstet Gynecol 50 [Suppl]:18–21

Boshart M, Gismann L, Ikenberg H et al. (1984) A new type of papilloma virus DNA, its presence in genital cancer biopsies and in cell lines derived from cervical cancer. EMBO J 3:1151–1157

Crum CP, Nagai N, Levine RU et al. (1986) In situ hybridisation analysis of HPV 16 DNA sequences in early cervical neoplasia. Am J Pathol 123:174–182

De Graaff, van der Harten JJ (1975) Ineffectiveness of bleomycin in verrucous carcinoma of the vulva. Eur J Obstet Gynecol Reprod Biol 5/6:327–330

Demian SDE, Bushkin FL, Echevarria RA (1973) Perineural invasion and anaplastic transformation of verrucous carcinoma. Cancer 32:395–401

Faaborg LL, Smith ML, Newland JR (1979) Uterine cervical and vaginal verucous squamous cell carcinoma. Gynecol Oncol 8:104–109 Foye G, Marsh MR, Minkowitz S (1969) Verrucous carcinoma of the vulva. Obstet Gynecol 34:484–488

Jennings RH, Barclay DL (1972) Verrucous carcinoma of the cervix. Cancer 30:430–434
Jones MJ, Levin HS, Ballard LA (1981) Verrucous squamous cell carcinoma of the vagina: case report. Cleve Clin Q 48:305–313
Kraus FT, Perez-Mesa C (1966) Verrucous carcinoma: clinical and pathologic study of 105 cases involving oral cavity, larynx, genitalia. Cancer 19:26–38
Lucas WE, Benirischke K, Lebherz TS (1974) Verrucous carcinoma of the female genital tract. Am J Obstet Gynecol 119:435–440
Okagaki T, Clark BA, Zachow KR et al. (1984) Presence of human papilloma virus in verrucous carcinoma (Ackerman) of the vagina. Arch Pathol Lab Med 108:567–570
Powell JL, Franklin EW III, Nickerson FJ et al. (1978) Verrucous carcinoma of the female genital tract. Gynecol Oncol 6:565–573
Ramzy I, Smout MS, Collins JA (1976) Verrucous carcinoma of the vagina. Am J Clin Pathol 65:644–653
Stehman FB, Castaldo TW, Charles EH et al. (1980) Verrucous carcinoma of the vulva. Int J Gynaecol Obstet 17:523–525
Ubben K, Krzyzek R, Ostrow R et al. (1979) Human papilloma virus DNA detected in verrucous carcinoma. J Invest Dermatol 72:195
Wood WG, Gustin FG, Sohn S et al. (1978) Verrucous carcinoma of the vagina. South Med J 71:368–371

Basal Cell Carcinoma Like Lesion
Naves AE, Monti JA, Chiconi E (1980) Basal cell like carcinoma in the upper third of the vagina. Am J Obstet Gynecol 137:136–137
Whelton J, Kottmeier HL (1962) Primary carcinoma of the vagina: a study of a Radiumhemmet series of 145 cases. Acta Obstet Gynecol Scand 41:22–40

22.2 Gland Cell Origin

22.2.1 Vaginal Adenosis

In 1877 von Preuschen first noticed the presence of endocervical type glands in the sub-mucosa of the vagina in 4 of 36 adult women at autopsy. In 1910 Bonney and Glendining first reported in a 42-year-old woman a vaginal lesion in which the vaginal epithelium was replaced by endocervical type glands and which they called adenomatosis vaginae. Subsequent publications focussed mainly on the clinico-pathological and aetiological aspects of the condition (Plaut and Dreyfuss 1940; Studdiford 1957; Stabler 1961: Sandberg et al. 1965), and it was not until 1971 when Herbst et al. published the report of their observations of a significant association of adenocarcinoma in young girls with maternal administration of stilbestrol that a renewed interest was generated worldwide on the subject. Subsequent publications not only confirmed such an association (Greenwald et al. 1971; Silverberg and DeGiorgi 1972; Tsukada et al. 1972) but also revealed that there was a high frequency of occurrence of vaginal adenosis and lower genital tract abnormalities in girls exposed to synthetic oestrogen in utero (Herbst et al. 1972; Sherman et al. 1974; Stafl et al. 1974; Antonioli and Burke 1975; Sandberg 1976; Robboy et al. 1979; Jefferies et al. 1984).

Vaginal adenosis has been defined as the presence of benign müllerian glandular tissue (Kurman and Scully 1974; Antonioli and Burke 1975; Hart et al. 1976a), mucus-secreting columnar cells or secretory products in the vagina (Zermer et al. 1980): The glands may be mucus-secreting, similar to those of the endocervix, or may be non-mucinous, being lined by endometrial or tubal type epithelium. These glands are always found in a superficial location either lining the vaginal surface or lying in the lamina propria.

22.2.1.1 Clinical Features

Vaginal adenosis also occurs in women who have not been exposed to stilbestrol in utero but the incidence of such lesions is at present uncertain. Sandberg (1968) was able to demonstrate adenosis in 41% of 35 post-pubertal women at autopsy, whereas Kurman and Scully (1974) could find adenosis in only 8 vaginas from 100 fetuses and women up to 25 years of age, also at autopsy. The incidence among the stillborn and neonates exposed in utero was 10% in comparison with 4% among unexposed offspring (Johnson et al. 1979). According to Robboy et al. (1986) an average of 2.3 cases of adenosis per year used to be diagnosed microscopically among women born before the DES era in the Massachussets General Hospital.

The incidence of adenosis among women exposed in utero has varied in different series from 14.1% (Fowler and Edelman 1978) to over 90% (Sherman et al. 1974; Stafl et al. 1974). This variation has been attributed to the different criteria for diagnosis and anatomical delineation of vaginal and cervical boundaries used by different workers (Fowler and Edelman 1978).

The age of patients born before the DES era ranged in one series from 24 to 88 years with a median age of 44 (Robboy et al. 1986). The youngest patient reported among the non-exposed groups was 14 years old (Hansen and Egholm 1975). In the exposed group, the range was from 11 to 28 years with a median age of 21 years, 95% falling between 13 and 26 years (Burke and Antonioli 1976).

The majority of patients (73%) are asymptomatic (Fowler and Edelman 1978). Some patients present with vaginal discharge, vaginal bleeding, dyspareunia and local discomfort.

22.2.1.2 Gross Appearance

Vaginal adenosis may present as a red, granular, erythroplakic area, which may be multiple with "strawberry" appearances (Stafl et al. 1974). Some lesions may be cystic and papillary. Sandberg et al. (1965) proposed a clinical classification which also embraced the histological spectrum of the lesions, namely occult (presence of non-cystic glands in the sub-mucosa), small cystic (accumulation of mucin with cystic distension of one or more of the glands), effluent (generalised sprinkling of red raw patches replacing the vaginal mucosa), adenomatous (papillary or ulcerative with tumorous overgrowth of the glands, as in endocervical polyp) and adenocarcinomatous (exophytic and ulcerative). In some patients, the lesions may not be altogether visible. The vaginal mucosa may be intact, and only careful digital palpation detects the sub-mucous nodules of adenosis (Strauss et al. 1973).

The lesions are seen commonly in the vaginal fornices near the cervix (Ostergard 1981). All parts of the vagina may be involved. The anterior vagina is more frequently affected than the posterior, and the upper vagina is involved more than the lower half (Ng et al. 1977). The lesions are seen in the lower third of the vagina only when the upper and middle thirds also harbour the lesion, and they are almost always confluent (O'Brien et al. 1979).

Non-staining areas or abnormal staining with Schiller's iodine test have been reported in from 60% to over 90% of patients (Sherman et al. 1974). The value of this test as a screening procedure has been, however, questioned in several quarters (Gunning and Ostergard 1976). The colposcopic findings which were abnormal in about 90% of cases (Burke et al. 1974; Stafl et al. 1974; Fowler and Edelman 1978) were described as white, masoic, both white and mosaic in appearance and punctations (Burke and Antonioli 1976; Welch et al. 1978). Stafl et al. (1974) noticed grape-like structures of the columnar epithelium and nabothian cysts in the transformation zone at colposcopic examination.

Cytological screening of patients with a history of intra-uterine exposure to stilbestrol has yielded variable positive results in different series from about 45% (Hart et al. 1976b) to 71% (Ng et al. 1975). When the scrapes are taken from each quadrant of the vagina, columnar and/or metaplastic cells of adenosis can be seen in as high as 88% of the case without visible lesions (Vooijs et al. 1973; Ng et al. 1975). Bibbo et al. (1975) confirmed the efficacy of the cytological technique to detect DES-related epithelial changes.

22.2.1.3 Microscopic Appearance

Adenosis may be superficially on the surface, in which the vaginal epithelum is focally or diffusely replaced by flat or pseudostratified columnar epithelium. Two types of columnar cells are seen, mucin secreting similar to the endocervical and non-mucinous, ciliated or non-ciliated, light and dark cells of the endometrium and fallopian tubes, occasionally thrown into short papillary folds. In some instances, the columnar cells are seen overlying a thick layer of squamous cells, indicating the process of squamous metaplasia (Fig. 22.6), which with the evolution of the lesion may replace the entire layer of columnar epithelium and may bring about regression. In the early stage of squamous metaplasia, the immature squamous cells are poor in glycogen and can be identified by the sharp vertical or oblique line of demarcation separating the areas of immature and mature squamous cells (Sherman et al. 1974; Hart et al. 1976a). The sub-mucous adenosis consists of glands which may be simple, complex or cystic types (Sandberg et al. 1985). The simple glands are tubular and complex glands with papillary infolding have the appearance of clustered and crowded small glands on cross section. The cystic glands are the results of dilatation to various sizes (Antonioli and Burke 1975) due to secretions. The glands, which are located in the lamina propria, are seen mostly within 2 mm from the surface mucosa. These glands are frequently lined by the tubo-endometrial type of epithelium with or without cilia (Fig. 22.7). Cyst formations are rare in the tubo-endometrial glands because of serous-type secretory products within the

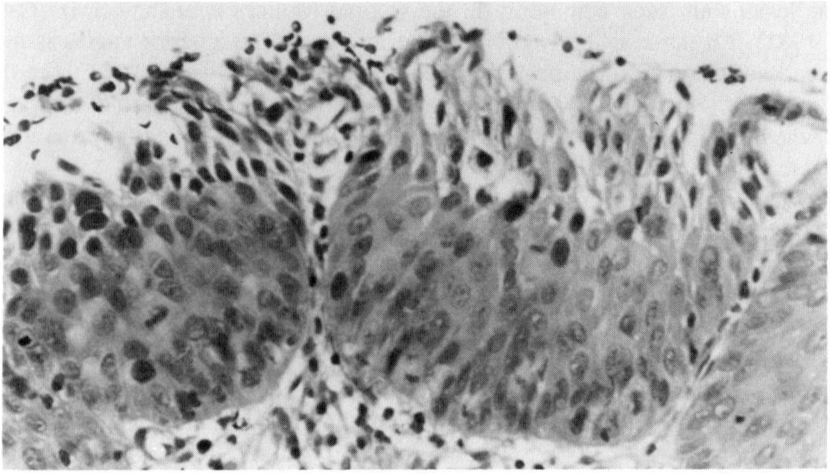

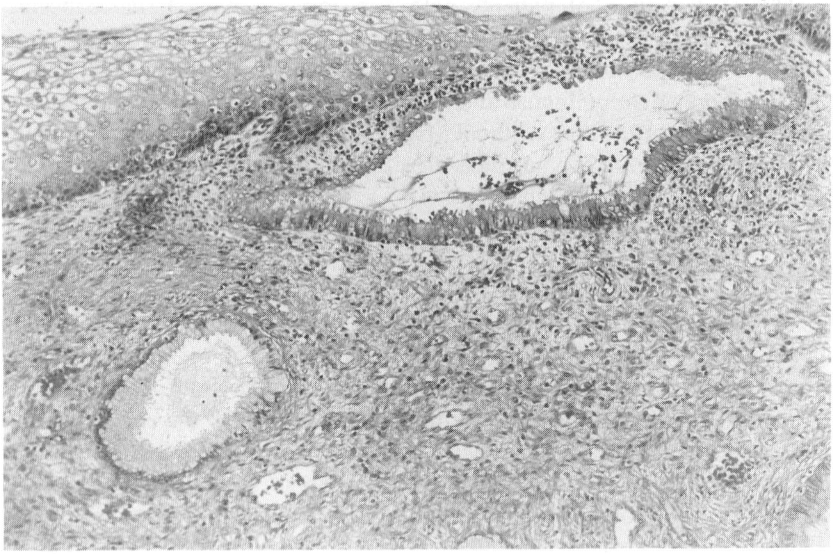

Fig. 22.6. Vaginal adenosis: squamous epithelium growing under columnar epithelium

Fig. 22.7. Vaginal adenosis: sub-mucosal glands lined by mucinous and endometrial-type epithelium

lumen, in contrast to the mucinous glands which are more prone to be distended by the inspissated mucin obstructing the neck of the glands (Robboy et al. 1986). The tubo-endometrial type of epithelium is found in 20% of specimens harbouring adenosis from the upper vagina, 31% from the mid-vagina and 100% from the lower vagina (Robboy et al. 1979). Occasionally, microglandular hyperplasia is seen in adenosis that grossly appears to be a cauliflower-like nodule, polyp or granular area (Robboy and Welch 1977). Microscopically, it consists of closely packed glands displaying honeycomb or reticular patterns and may be mistaken for an adenocarcinoma. The glands are uniform and small (Fig. 22.8) and lined by cuoidal or low columnar cells containing intra-cytoplasmic mucin in contrast to the cells of adenocarcinoma which contain intra-cytoplasmic glycogen but not mucin (Robboy and Welch 1977). Variable chronic inflammatory cell infiltrates are common in the lamina propria around the glands. Squamous metaplasia, which can be found in the columnar epithelium of the vagina in over 90% of patients (Ng et al. 1977), occurs also in these glands. When the glands are replaced completely by metaplastic cells, the evidence of antecedent glandular tissue may only be demonstrable by the entrapped residual mucin or occasional mucinous cells within the metaplastic cells. The metaplastic squamous epithelium of the glands may be continuous with the metaplastic epithelium of the vaginal mucosa, which appears as elongated rete pegs. The presence of "eddies" with a concentric arrangement of the metaplastic squamous cells in the pegs marks the sites of gland openings (Hart et al. 1976a). Here also, the poorly glycogenated metaplastic cells eventually mature to stratified squamous cells.

22.2.1.4 Follow-up

With colposcopic follow-up over a period of 3 years, Noller et al. (1983) noticed a decrease in the epithelial changes (adenosis) in about 30% of patients, an increase in 7% and no change in 53%. Histologically, the progression of metaplastic changes was confirmed in 85% of the biopsies taken at intervals up to 5 years, and it was concluded that the magnitude of changes correlated with the length of time (Burke et al. 1981). By 25 years of age, squamous metaplasia, which became more extensive, could be seen in all women, suggesting that adenosis regresses as the women grow old (Ng et al. 1977).

Atypical squamous epithelial changes amounting to dysplasia and carcinoma-in-situ have been observed in the metaplastic areas (Fig. 22.9). Although the incidence has varied from 6% (Bibbo et al. 1975; Burke et al. 1978) to 18% (Mattingly and Stafl 1976) in different series, it is generally recognised that these changes are infrequent, occurring in about 2% of patients and in the overwhelming majority of them, are mild (Robboy et al. 1978; Veridiano et al. 1976). Cytological examination of 575 DES-exposed patients revealed a mild dysplasia in 4% and moderate dysplasia to carcinoma-in-situ in only 1% (Robboy et al. 1976). It has, however, been suggested that there was some bias in the estimation of frequency of dysplasia (Robboy et al. 1978), as a significant number of referrals had a higher incidence of dysplasia than unselected patients (Robboy et al. 1978). Nevertheless, Mattingly

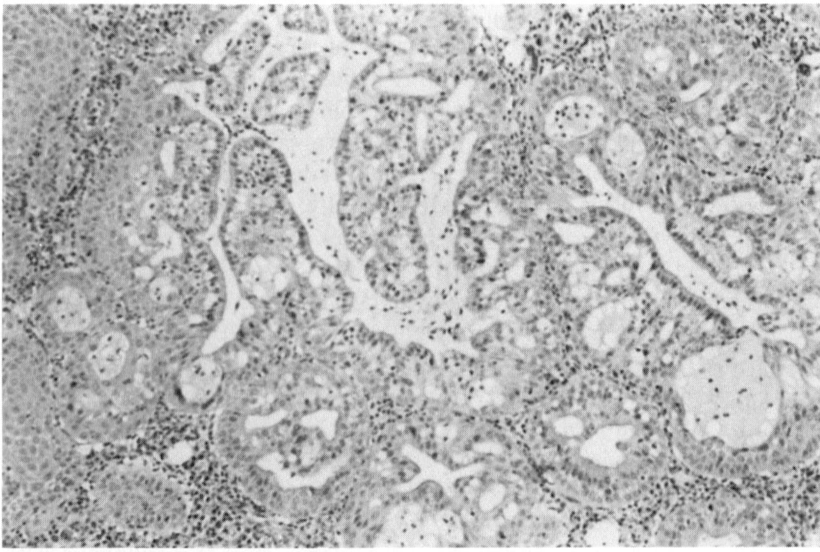

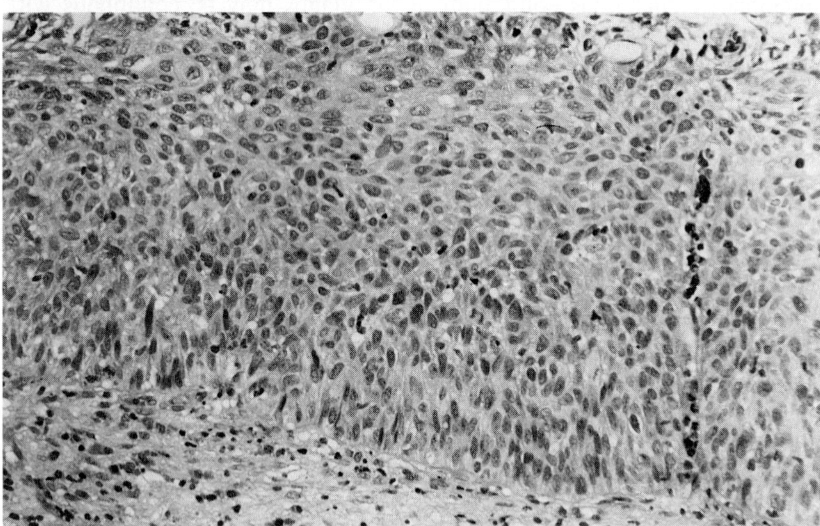

Fig. 22.8. Vaginal adenosis: microglandular hyperplasia showing group of small glands lined by low columnar epithelium

Fig. 22.9. Vaginal adenosis: carcinoma-in-situ in a metaplastic area: Residual glands can be seen at the upper part of the lesion

and Staffl (1976) observed nearly a five times higher prevalence rate of both vaginal and cervical carcinoma-in-situ in the exposed than in unexposed women. The DNA study of squamous cell abnormalities (Fu and Robboy 1978) showed that dysplasias with euploid or polypoid DNA content rarely persisted, whereas persistence was common in aneuploid dysplastic lesions, indicating neoplastic potential. Squamous cell carcinoma can no doubt occur in association with adenosis (Mattingly and Stafl 1976; Veridiano et al. 1976) but risk does not seem to be high (Robboy et al. 1977a).

Atypical changes in the glandular epithelium have been noticed less frequently (Barber and Sommers 1974; Antonioli et al. 1979). Although atypical glands have been identified near the periphery of an adenocarcinoma, a transition from the former to the latter has rarely been demonstrated (Blaikley et al. 1971; Robboy et al. 1977b; Ghosh and Cera 1983). Doubt has been expressed on this ground as well as on the basis of histochemical and nuclear DNA analysis as to whether adenocarcinoma develops at all from adenosis. Whereas the endocervical-type epithelium is the most common type of epithelium in vaginal adenosis, is mucin secreting and PAS-positive, the clear cell carcinoma, which is rare, is uniformly PAS- and mucin negative (Ng et al. 1977). The analysis of nuclear DNA demonstrated a diploid pattern of vaginal adenosis, whereas adenocarcinomas were aneuploid (Lewis et al. 1973). The tubo-endometrial type cells of vaginal adenosis are ultrastructurally similar to the endometrial glandular cells in their proliferative phase (Antonioli et al. 1979). At nuclear DNA analysis they are occasionally aneuploid, demonstrating greater proliferative potentials than the endocervical cells (Fu et al. 1979). Whether these tubo-endometrial glands are precursors of adenocarcinomas is not known. The frequent presence of tubo-endometrial-type glands adjacent to adenocarcinoma and the occurrence of adenocarcinoma in the non-mucinous endometrial glands in older women have led to the speculation that these glands may provide a scaffold for the development of malignancy (Robboy et al. 1982).

22.2.1.5 Other Changes in the Vagina

Other than vaginal adenosis, several structural abnormalities in both the upper and lower genital tracts have been noticed in DES-exposed women. They include protruding partial or complete transverse ridges, circumferential bands obliterating the upper vagina (Herbst et al. 1972; Sherman et al. 1974), also called a vaginal hood (Pomerance 1973) and constriction bands (Barber and Sommers 1974). Microscopical examination of the ridges show a connective tissue core and surface lined by either mucinous or tubo-endometrial type of epithelium (Robboy et al. 1975). Sandberg (1976) listed these abnormalities under different names with the addition of several more such as corolla-like mucosal elevation, fibrous band, apical narrowing and forniceal obliteration, unusual cervical size, unusual diameter and form of external os and pericervical fibrous collars. The corolla-like nucosal elevations are sharply demarcated, discrete, 1–2 cm broad multipetated elevations of the vaginal mucosa; the thin wire-like fibrous band encircles the vagina partially or completely; the apical narrowing of the upper part of the vagina appears as a conical constriction occasionally associated with the small cervix, and the forniceal obliteration is characterised by the absence or obliteration of a vaginal fornix (Sandberg 1976).

Non-neoplastic changes also occur in the cervices of DES-exposed women and have been described as erythroplakia (Stafl et al. 1974), cervical Cock's comb-like lesion (Pomerance 1973; Stafl et al. 1974), cervical ridges (Herbst et al. 1972; Sherman et al. 1974), strawberry cervix with granular portio, cervical pseudopolyp (Herbst et al. 1972; Shane and Perlmutter 1973; Sherman et al. 1974) and snub nose-like cervices (Sherman et al. 1974).

22.2.1.6 Pathogenesis

The pathogenesis of vaginal adenosis has been a controversial issue. Siders et al. (1965) thought it to be an acquired metaplastic change (prosoplasia) in the vaginal epithelium. It has also been suggested that vaginal adenosis arises in the wolffian residue, which is preserved by stilbestrol (Editorial 1972), and stimulated later to develop adenosis by unknown carcinogens. Embryologically, the müllerian epithelium of the vagina is replaced by cephalad growth of squamous epithelium of the urogenital sinus, and in vaginal adenosis stilbestrol or some other factors prevent this cephalad growth or cause the persistence of müllerian epithelium. Experimental injections of oestradiol into the neonate mice inhibit the transformation of pseudocolumnar epithelium of the vaginal anlage to squamous epithelium. Similar changes have been suggested to occur in the human fetus under the effects of oestrogens (Forsberg 1972) causing persistence of the müllerian epithelium of the vagina. Robboy (1983) has hypothesised that it is the stroma of the vaginal wall which normally provides a scaffold for the urogenital sinus to grow upwards to replace the müllerian epithelium and which under the effects of DES becomes hostile to this process resulting in the persistence of residual patches of glandular epithelium at the interface of the mesenchyme and squamous lining of the vaginal wall. Cunha (1976) suggested a similar mechanism and emphasised the role of stromal tissue in relation to the epithelium. In a recent ultrastructural study by Roberts et al. (1988), two types of stromal-epithelial interaction in vaginal adenosis were documented. In one, the epithelial cells send cytoplasmic processes to the fibroblasts and at times are completely fused with them. In the second type, mast cells act as intermediaries between the epithelial and stromal cells. Squamous metaplasia of the vaginal adenosis probably occurs through these processes.

22.2.1.7 Treatment

There is no well-established modality of management of vaginal adenosis. Barber and Sommers (1974) suggested that if adenocarcinoma is excluded by biopsy, the area of adenosis should be removed by surgery, cautery or cryosurgery. Sherman et al. (1974) advocated complete excision of the lesion. When a large area is removed, a skin graft may be necessary (Herbst et al. 1972). Some lesions may regress spontaneously (Studdiford 1965; Siders et al. 1965; Burke et al. 1981) but as previously mentioned, several reports suggest that dysplasia and carcinoma-in-situ could complicate the lesion (Barber and Sommers 1974; Fetherston 1975; Antonioli et al. 1979), and therefore, vaginal adenosis should be followed up closely (Robboy et al. 1978). In general, treatment is not warranted unless the patient is symptomatic due to excessive vaginal discharge and local infections (Ostergard 1981), or the lesion is complicated by intra-epithelial neoplasia. Cautery and cryosurgery are less frequently associated with post-operative complications than local excisions. Laser treatment has been stated to be similarly useful in the management of the lesion with much less tissue damage than cautery or cryosurgery (Stafl et al. 1977).

22.2.2 Clear Cell Adenocarcinoma

The registry of clear cell adenocarcinoma established in 1971 in the USA to investigate different aspects of clear cell adenocarcinoma of the genital tract in young women estimated that 0.014%–0.14% of the women exposed in utero to DES were at high risk to develop this lesion up to the age of 24 years old. The peak incidence was 19 years, and the women born between 1951–1953 had the highest incidence rates because 1%–10% of pregnant women were exposed to DES during this period in the USA (Herbst et al. 1977). It was also observed that women exposed to DES early in the intra-uterine life were at a higher risk of tumour development than those exposed later in gestational life (Herbst et al. 1979a; Jefferies et al. 1984). Clear cell adenocarcinoma has not been observed in any girl under the age of 7 years (Welch et al. 1978). About two-thirds of these tumours occur in the vagina and one-third, in the cervix. The tumour involves particularly the upper third of the anterior wall (Scully et al. 1974; Welch et al. 1978), although any part of the vagina can be affected.

The histogenesis of this malignancy is unknown. DES has been thought to be teratogenic and to some degree carcinogenic. The carcinogenic role of this agent is also not clearly understood. It has been suggested recently that DES is not a complete carcinogen and that some other factors are involved (Melnick et al. 1987). In the studies on nuclear DNA (Lewis et al. 1973; Fu et al. 1979), atypical adenosis (Fu et al. 1979) and adenocarcinomas (Lewis et al. 1973) have been found to be aneuploid, suggesting a possible link between these two conditions. Such a link, however, is yet to be clarified.

22.2.2.1 Gross Appearance

The tumours vary in size from the minute 2 mm × 2 mm (Chambers et al. 1978) to more than 10 cm and are mostly polypoid or nodular. They are usually soft, haemorrhagic and friable with variegated appearance. They may also be flat and ulcerated with an indurated base. Most tumours are superficially located, penetrating less than 3 mm into the vaginal or cervical wall (Robboy et al. 1975).

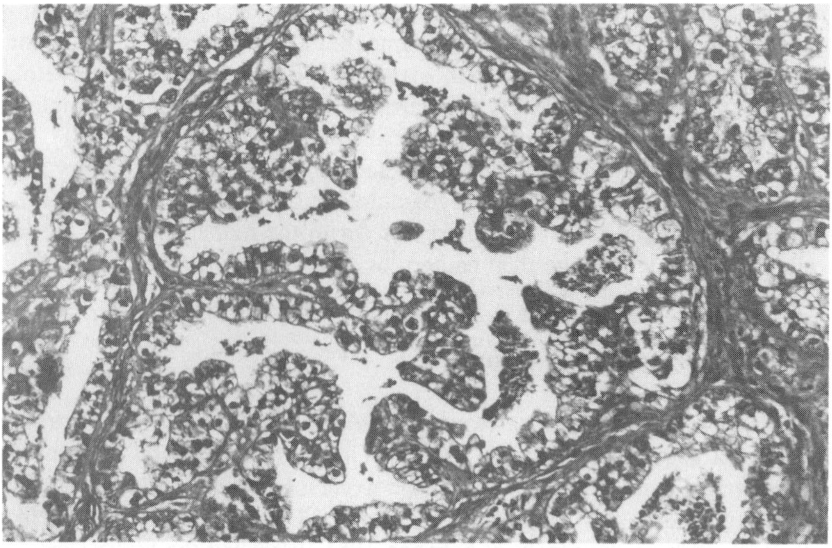

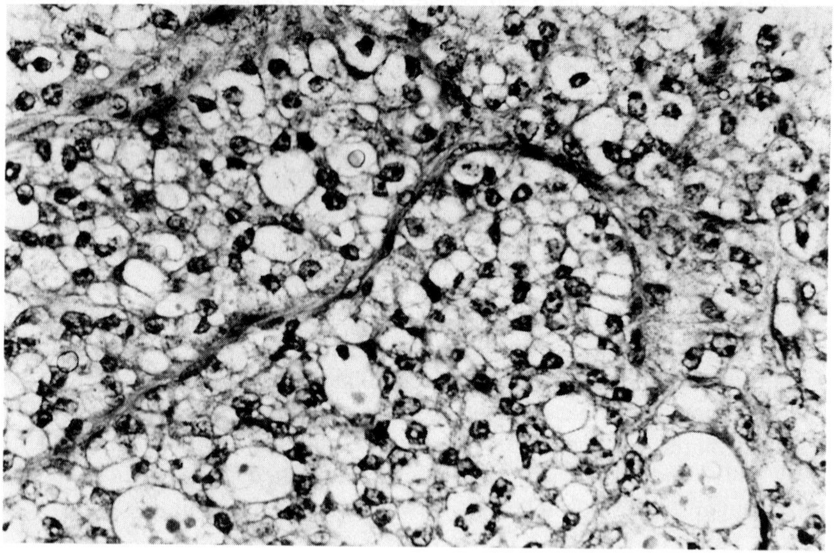

Fig. 22.10. Clear cell carcinoma papillary pattern: the papillae are lined by clear cells

Fig. 22.11. Clear cell carcinoma solid pattern: clear cells may be arranged in a solid sheet

22.2.2.2 Microscopical Appearance

Of the several microscopical patterns – solid, tubular, cystic and papillary (Herbst et al. 1974) – the papillary (Fig. 22.10) and solid patterns (Fig. 22.11) are seen predominantly in biopsy fragments, whereas the tubular and cystic patterns are more common in excised specimens (Herbst et al. 1972). The common cell types are clear cells, with abundant clear cytoplasm, and hobnail cells, with bulbous nuclei protruding into the cystic spaces and lumens of the tubules. The nuclei are hyperchromatic and contain prominent nucleoli. Mitotic figures vary from 0 to 16 per 10 high power fields (Herbst et al. 1974). While the cytoplasm of clear cells contains abundant glycogen, mucin can be present in the luminal borders of the epithelium lining the cysts and tubules. The solid pattern consists of sheets of clear cells with scattered cystic spaces which may contain occasional papillary structures. These features resemble microscopically those of renal cell carcinoma. In some tumours the clear cells and hobnail cells may be absent, and the tumours may resemble poorly differentiated adenocarcinoma of the corpus uteri (Scully et al. 1974).

Ultrastructurally, these tumours demonstrate short, thick microvilli, cell attachments by desmosomes and interdigitating cytoplasmic processes, abundant cytoplasmic glycogen and stacked parallel rows of granular endoplasmic reticulum (Silverberg and DeGiorgi 1972). These features are suggestive of a müllerian origin of these tumours.

22.2.2.3 Treatment

About 60% of patients ase clinically in stage I, yet regional nodal metastases were noted in 17%, indicating the virulent nature of the tumour. Even a minute tumour has been found to metastasise to the pelvic lymphnodes (Chambers et al. 1978).

Local excisions have been tried in a few cases, but the recurrence rates are high (Herbst et al. 1979b). Although several methods of treatment have been employed, vaginectomy and hysterectomy with pelvic node dissections leaving the adnexae and adjuvant radiation has been the most frequently followed modality (Scully et al. 1974; Jones et al. 1987).

The tumour spreads locally to the pelvis and distally to the lungs and follows a general pattern of spread by endometrial adenocarcinoma rather than squamous cell carcinoma of the vagina and cervix (Robboy et al. 1974). Recurrences were frequent in those tumours which were large (more than 1 cm in size) and incompletely excised and which had penetrated more than 3 mm into the vaginal wall (Robboy et al. 1974). With an overall recurrence rate of 23% at 5 years, most recurrences appeared in the pelvis, lungs and supraclavicular nodes (Herbst and Anderson 1979; Holt and Herbst 1982). Of the various types of therapy employed in stage 1 disease, radical hysterectomy with partial or complete vaginectomy and pelvic node dissection has been associated with the lowest rates of recurrence (Herbst and Anderson 1979). Radiation therapy has also been found effective in stage 1 lesions (Herbst et al. 1974) and pelvic recurrences (Herbst and Anderson 1979).

Chemotherapy has not been very effective in the advanced disease, although an objective response has been noted in a few cases (Herbst and Anderson 1979).

The actuarial survival rate for stage I disease is 87%, stage II 76%, stage III 30% and stage IV less than 30 months (Herbst and Anderson 1979).

22.2.3 Primary Vaginal Adenocarcinoma Not Related to DES

Primary adenocarcinoma of the vagina is far less common than secondary adenocarcinoma. Although almost every report of invasive carcinoma of the vagina mentioned adenocarcinoma, the exact incidence of these lesions is difficult to estimate. Most of the reports either lacked an adequate histological description and precise location of the lesions or included the lesions which were located at the vaginal apex in continuity with the cervix. According to some authors, the estimated incidence ranges between 1% and 5% of all vaginal malignancies (Daw 1971; Davis and Franklin 1975; Ledward 1972). The histogenesis of adenocarcinomas not related to stilbestrol is most often uncertain. Most of the tumours are thought to arise from any of the following sources: (i) wolffian rests (Way 1948), (ii) periurethral glands (Frick et al. 1968), (iii) misplaced mesenchymal mesonephric remnants (Marcus 1960), (iv) endometriosis (Palumbo et al. 1969), (v) aberrant cervical glands (Plaut and Dreyfuss 1940) or (vi) cloacogenic epithelium (Rhatigan and Mojadidi 1973). Vaginal adenosis can occur congenitally without the background of intra-uterine exposure to DES (Sandberg et al. 1965; Kurman and Scully 1974), and it occasionally transforms to malignancy (Plaut and Dreyfuss 1940; Barbosa 1956; Blaikley et al. 1971; Wade-Evans 1976; Ballon et al. 1979; Ray and Ireland 18985). For the patient described by Mawad and Latour (1974), the lesion have originated from an occult adenosis. Three primary carcinomas mentioned by Livingstone (1950) could have arisen from a similar source. Primary adenocarcinoma has also been reported to arise in the neovagina (Ritchie 1929; Andryjowicz et al. 1985). One of the two patients reported by Andryjowicz et al. (1985) previously had borderline endometrioid carcinoma of the ovary, endometrial carcinoma, squamous carcinoma-in-situ of the vaginal vault and early invasive carcinoma of the residual vagina. The patient was treated at different stages by surgery, radiation, chemotherapy and lastly by vaginal reconstruction. The other patient was 26 years old and had had reconstruction of the vagina with an ileal loop at the age of 13 years (Ritchie 1929). Multiple aetiological factors were probably operative in the genesis of adenocarcinoma in the neovagina.

Since Sampson's original description in 1925, the association of endometriosis, particularly in the ovary, with the development of adenocarcinoma has been well recognised. About 40 patients with adenocarcinoma occurring in extra-ovarian endometriosis have been reported, and in about one-third a lesion developed in the rectovaginal septum and posterior vaginal wall (Dockerty et al. 1954; Ferreira and Clayton 1958; Lash and Rubenstone 1959; Bamford 1967; Young and Gamble 1969; Brooks and Wheeler 1977; Hayman 1977; Goldberg et al. 1978; Addison et al. 1979; Mostoufizadeh and Scully 1980; Kapp et al. 1982).

22.2.3.1 Clinical Features

The majority of the patients are between 40 and 50 years old, with the age ranging from 35 to 60 years. The main complaints are irregular vaginal bleeding, pain and vaginal mass. About a third of the patients are multiparous.

22.2.3.2 Gross Appearance

The tumour is usually single and presents as a friable fungating mass (Strachan 1932), an indurated area, plaque, hard, raised nodule or polypoid, rubbery, cystic mass with a reddish-tan appearance. The size varies from 1.5 to 5 cm. The tumour may be ulcerated.

22.2.3.3 Microscopical Appearance

The appearance is similar to that of the classic adenocarcinomas arising in the endometrium. The crowded neoplastic glands of various sizes lined by stratified columnar epithelium may show papillary tufting and squamous differentiation (adenosquamous). Clear cell carcinoma composed predominantly of clear cells with vacuolated cytoplasm and hyperchromatic nuclei has also been noticed (Brooks and Wheeler 1977; Goldberg et al. 1978). Any histological type of tumour which can be found in the endometrium may also occur in an endometriosis. Typical endometrioid carcinoma is by far the most common histological type. Adenocarcinoma with a malignant squamous component similar to adenosquamous carcinoma of the endometrium can also be seen (Rhatigan and Mojadidi 1973). Foci of endometriosis with or without atypia in the glands can usually be demonstrated intermixed with adenocarcinomas or adjacent to or in continuity with the lesion. Granai et al. (1984) reported an endometriotic focus evolving through adenomatous hyperplasia to adenocarcinoma in a patient on continuous, unopposed, oestrogen therapy. The foci of endometriosis may be overgrown by the neoplastic glands, and the stigma of previous endometriosis may then disappear altogether. Under these circumstances, clinical suspicion of pelvic endometriosis or knowledge of a previous vaginal lesion could provide the only clue. Adenocarcinoma is known to develop in extra-gonadal endometriosis after a 14-year, symptom-free period following total hysterectomy and bilateral salpingo-oopherectomy for endometriosis (Samsuddin et al. 1979). According to Sampson (1925), three criteria needed to be fulfilled before establishing that a particular lesion developed in endometriosis: (i) evidence of endometriosis at the site of malignancy, (ii) no other primary site for a similar malignancy being found and (iii) demonstration of transition of endometriosis to adenocarcinoma. According to some authors, the last criterion is not absolutely necessary (Scott 1959; Brooks and Wheeler 1977).

Although the endometrioid type is the most common adenocarcinoma of the vagina, a rare variety of mixed adenocarcinoma has also been noticed. Fukushima et al. (1986) reported a mixed intestinal and argentaffin carcinoma of the vagina, consisting of an adenocarcinoma with occasional goblet cells on the surface and small cell carcinoma beneath the adenocarcinomatous area. Ultrastructurally, the small cells demonstrated neurosecretory granules.

22.2.3.4 Treatment

In all vaginal adenocarcinomas a thorough investigation to exclude a primary lesion should be made in the genital and entire gastrointestinal tract including the gall bladder, kidney, breast and thyroid (Lewis and Brady 1967). The treatment so far tried has been mainly surgical, i.e. total abdominal hysterectomy, bilateral salpingo-oopherectomy or vaginal resection supplemented by radiotherapy and in some patients also by lymph node dissection (Brooks and Wheeler 1977). The number of patients is small, and long-term follow-up data are not usually available to draw a valid conclusion on the prognosis. Kapp et al. (1982) reported one patient still well 7 years after treatment by intra-vaginal and external beam radiotherapy.

References

Vaginal Adenosis

Antonioli DA, Burke L (1975) Vaginal adenosis: an analysis of 325 biopsy specimens from 100 patients. Am J Clin Pathol 64:625–638

Antonioli DA, Rosen S, Burke L et al. (1979) Glandular dysplasia in diethylstilbestrol associated vaginal adenosis: a case report and review of the literature. Am J Obstet Gynecol 71:715–721

Barber HRK, Sommers SC (1974) Vaginal adenosis, dysplasia and clear cell adenocarcinoma after diethylstilbestrol treatment in pregnancy. Obsteet Gynecol 43:645–652

Bibbo M, Ali I, Al-Naqueeb M et al. (1975) Cytologic findings in female and male offspring of DES treated mothers. Acta Cytol (Baltimore) 19:568–572

Bibbo M, Gill WB, Azizi F et al. (1978) Follow up of male and female offsprings of DES exposed mothers. Obstet Gynecol 132:537–455

Blaikley JB, Dewhurst CJ, Ferreira HP et al. (1971) Vaginal adenosis: clinical and pathological features with special reference to malignant change. J Obstet Gynaecol Br Commonw 78:1115–1122

Bonney V, Glendining B (1910) Adenosis vaginae: a hitherto undescribed condition. Proc R Soc Med 4:18–25

Burke L, Antonioli D (1976) Vaginal adenosis: factors influencing detection in a colposcopic evaluation. Obstet Gynecol 48:413–421

Burke L, Antonioli D, Knapp RC et al. (1974) Vaginal adenosis: correlation of colposcopic and pathologic findings. Obstet Gynecol 44:257–264

Burke L, Antonioli D, Rosen S (1978) Vaginal and cervical squamous cell dysplasia in women exposed to diethylstilbestrol in utero. Am J Obstet Gynecol 132:537–544

Burke L, Antonioli D, Friedman EA (1981) Evolution of diethylstilbestrol associated genital tract lesions. Obstet Gynecol 57:79–84

Cunha GR (1976) Epithelial-stromal interactions in development of the urogenital tract. Int Rev Cytol 47:137–194

Editorial comments (1972) Obstet Gynecol Surv 27:462

Fetherston WC (1975) Squamous neoplasia of vagina related to DES syndrome. Am J Obstet Gynecol 122:176–181

Forsberg J-G (1972) Estrogen, vaginal cancer and vaginal development. Am J Obstet Gynecol 113:83–87

Fowler WC Jr, Edelman D (1978) In utero exposure to DES: evaluation and follow up of 199 women. Obstet Gynecol 51:459–463

Fu Y-S, Robboy SJ (1978) Nuclear DNA study of vaginal and cervical squamous cell abnormalities in DES exposed progeny. Obstet Gynecol 52:129–137

Fu Y-S, Reagan JW, Richart RM et al. (1979) Nuclear DNA and histologic studies of genital lesions in diethylstilbestrol exposed progeny. II Intraepithelial glandular abnormalities. Am J Clin Pathol 72:515–520

Ghosh TK, Cera PJ (1983) Transition of benign adenosis to clear cell carcinoma. Obstet Gynecol 61:126–130

Greenwald P, Barlow JJ, Nasca PC et al. (1971) Vaginal cancer after maternal treatment with synthetic estrogen. N Engl J Med 285:390–392

Gunning JE, Ostergard DR (1976) Value of screenign procedures for detection of vaginal adenosis. Obstet Gynecol 47:268–271

Hansen R, Egholm M (1975) Diffuse vaginal adenosis. Acta Obstet Gynecol Scand 54:287–292

Hart WR, Townsend DE, Aldrich JO et al. (1976a) Histopathological spectrum of vaginal adenosis and related changes in stilbestrol exposed females. Cancer 37:763–775

Hart WR, Zahrov I, Kaplan BJ et al. (1976b) Cytologic findings in stilbestrol exposed females with emphasis on detection of vaginal adenosis. Acta Cytol (Baltimore) 20:7–14

Herbst AL, Kurman RJ, Scully RE (1972) Vaginal and cervical abnormalities after exposure to stilbestrol in utero. Obstet Gynecol 40:287–298

Herbst AL, Ulfelder H, Poskanzer DC (1971) Adenocarcinoma of the vagina: association of maternal stilbestrol therapy with tumor appearance in young women. N Engl J Med 284:878–881

Jefferies JA, Robboy S, O'Brien PC et al. (1984) Structural anomalies of the cervix and vagina in women enrolled in diethylstilbestrol adenosis (DESAD) project. Am J Obstet Gynecol 148:59–66

Johnson LD, Driscoll SG, Hertig AT (1979) Vaginal adenosis in stilborns and neonates exposed to diethylstilbestrol and sterioidal estrogens and progestins. Obstet Gynecol 53:671–679

Kurman RJ, Scully RE (1974) The incidence and histogenesis of vaginal adenosis: an autopsy study. Hum Pathol 5:265–276

Lewis JL Jr, Nordqvist SRB, Richart RM (1973) Studies of nuclear DNA in vaginal adenosis and clear cell adenocarcinoma. Am J Obstet Gynecol 115:737–750

Mattingly RF, Stafl A (1976) Cancer risk in diethylstilbestrol exposed offsprings. Am J Obstet Gynecol 126:543–548

Ng ABP, Regan JW, Hawliczek K et al. (1975) Cellular ditection of vaginal adenosis. Obstet Gynecol 46:323–328

Ng ABP, Regan JW, Nadji M et al. (1977) Natural history of vaginal adenosis in women exposed to diethylstilbestrol in utero. J Reprod Med 18:1–13

Noller KL, Townsend DE, Kaufman RH et al. (1983) Maturation of vaginal and cervical epithelium in women exposed in utero to diethylstilbestrol (DESAD Project). Am J Obstet Gynecol 146:279–285

O'Brien PC, Noller KL, Robboy SJ et al. (1979) Vaginal epithelial changes in young women enrolled in the National co-operative diethylstilbestrol adenosis (DESAD) project. Obstet Gynecol 3:300–308

Ostergard DR (1918) DES related vaginal lesions. Clin Obstet Gynecol 24:379–394

Plaut A, Dreyfuss ML (1940) Adenosis of the vagina and its relation to primary adenocarcinoma of the vagina. Surg Gynecol Obstet 71:756–765

Pomerance W (1973) Post-stilbestrol secondary syndrome. Obstet Gynecol 42:12–18

Robboy SJ (1983) A hypothetic mechnaism of diethylstilbestrol (DES) induced anomalies in prenatally exposed women. Hum Pathol 14:831–833

Robboy SJ, Welch WR (1977) Microglandular hyperplasia in vaginal adenosis associated with oral contraceptives and prenatal diethylstilbestrol exposure. Obstet Gynecol 49:430–434

Robboy SJ, Scully RE, Herbst AL (1975) Pathology of vaginal and cervical abnormalities associated with prenatal exposure to diethylstilbestrol (DES). J Reprod Med 15:13–18

Robboy SJ, Friedlander IM, Welch WR et al. (1976) Cytology of 575 young women with prenatal exposure to diethylstilbestrol. Obstet Gynecol 48:511-515

Robboy SJ, Prat J, Welch WR et al. (1977a) Squamous cell neoplasia controversy in the female exposed to diethylstilbestrol. Hum Pathol 8:483–485

Robboy SJ, Scully RE, Welch WR et al. (1977b) Intrauterine diethylstilbestrol exposure and its conequences: pathologic characteristics of vaginal adenosis, clear cell adenocarcinoma and relatred lesions. Arch Pathol Lab Med 101:1–5

Robboy SJ, Keh PC, Nickerson RJ et al. (1978) Squamous dysplasia and carcinoma in situ of the cervix and vagina after prenatal exposure to diethylstilbestrol. Obstet Gynecol 51:528–535

Robboy SJ, Kaufman RH, Prat J et al. (1979) Pathologic findings in young women enrolled in the National co-operative diethylstilbestrol adenosis (DESAD) project. Obstet Gynecol 53:309–317

Robboy SJ, Young RH, Herbst AL (1982) Female gential tract changes related to prenatal diethylstilbestrol exposure. In: Blaustein A (ed) Pathology of the female genital tract, 2nd edn. Springer, Berlin Heidelberg New York, pp 99–118

Robboy SJ, Hill EC, Sandberg EC et al. (1986) Vaginal adenosis in women born prior to the diethylstilbestrol era. Hum Pathol 17:488–492

Roberts DK, Walter NJ, Parmley TH et al. (1988) Interaction of epithelial and stromal cells in vaginal adenosis. Hum Pathol 19:855–861

Sandberg EC (1968) The incidence and distribution of occult vaginal adenosis. Am J Obstet Gynecol 101:322–334

Sandberg EC (1976) Benign cervical and vaginal changes associated with exposure to stilbestrol in utero. Am J Obstet Gynecol 125:777–789

Sandberg EC, Danielson RW, Cawet RW et al. (1965) Adenosis vaginae. Am J Obstet Gynecol 93:209–222

Shane JM, Perlmutter JF (1973) Pseudopolyp of the uterine cervix. Am J Obstet Gynecol 115:273–274

Sherman AI, Goldrath M, Berlin A et al. (1974) Cervical vaginal adenosis after in-utero exposure to synthetic estrogens. Obstet Gynecol 44:531–545

Siders DB, Parrott MH, Abell MR (1965) Gland cell prosoplasia (adenosis) of vagina. Am J Obstet Gynecol 91:190–203

Silverberg SG, DeGiorgi LS (1972) Clear cell carcinoma of the vagina: a clinical pathologic and electron microscopic study. Cancer 29:1680–1690

Stabler F (1961) Adenosis vaginae. J Obstet Gynaecol Br Commenw 68:857–860

Stafl A, Mattingly RF, Foley DV et al. (1974) Clinical diagnosis of vaginal adenosis. Obstet Gynecol 43:118–128

Stafl A, Wilkinson EJ, Mattingly RF (1977) Laser treatment of cervical and vaginal neoplasia. Am J Obstet Gynecol 128:128–136

Strauss JH, Lucas WE, Naftolin F et al. (1973) Vaginal adenosis diagnosed by plapation. N Engl J Med 288:525–526

Studdiford WE (1965) Vaginal lesions of adenomatous origin. Am J Obstet Gynecol 73:641–656

Tsukada Y, Hewitt WJ, Barlow JJ (1972) Clear cell adenocarcinoma (mesonephroma) of the vagina. Three caes associated with maternal synthetic nonsteroid estrogen therapy. Cancer 29:1208–1214

Veridiano NP, Weiner EA, Tancer ML (1976) Squamous cell carcinoma of the vagina associated with vaginal adenosis. Obstet Gynecol 47:689–692

von Preuschen (1877) Über Cystenbildung in der Vagina. Virchows Arch 70:111–128

Vooijs PG, Ng ABP, Wentz WB (1973) The detection of vaginal adenosis and clear cell carcinoma. Acta Cytol (Baltimore) 17:59–63

Welch WR, Robboy SJ, Townsend DE et al. (1978) Comparison of histologic and colposcopic findings in DES exposed females. Obstet Gynecol 52:454–461

Zermer J, Fu Y-S, Taxiarchis LW (1980) A clinical pathologic study of vagina and cervix in DES exposed progeny. Diagn Gynecol Obstet 2:245–256

Clear Cell Carcinoma

Chambers J, Rogers LW, Julian CG (1978) Minute clear cell carcinoma of the vagina with early metastasis to pelvic nodes. Am J Obstet Gynecol 131:223–225

Fu Y-S, Regan JW, Richart RM et al. (1979) Nuclear DNA and histologic studies of genital lesions in diethylstilbestrol exposed progeny. II Intraepithelial glandular abnormalities. Am J Clin Pathol 72:515–520

Herbst AL, Anderson D (1979) Clinical correlations and management of vaginal and cervical clear cell adenocarcinoma: In Herbst AL, Bern HA (eds) Development effects of diethylstilbestrol (DES) in pregnancy. Thieme/Stratton, New York, pp 71–80

Herbst AL, Kurman RJ, Scully RE et al. (1972) Clear cell adenocarcinoma of the genital tract in young females. N Engl J Med 287:1259–1264

Herbst AL, Robboy SJ, Scully RE et al. (1974) Clear cell adenocarcinoma of the vagina and cervix in girls: analysis of 170 registry cases. Am J Obstet Gynecol 119:713–724

Herbst AL, Cole P, Colton T et al. (1977) Age incidence and risk of diethylstilbestrol-related clear cell adenocarcinoma of the vagina and cervix. Am J Obstet Gynecol 128:43–50

Herbst AL, Cole P, Norusis MJ et al. (1979a) Epidemiologic aspects and factors related to survival in 384 registry cases of clear cell adenocarcinoma of the vagina and cervix. Am J Obstet Gynecol 135:876–886

Herbst AL, Norusis MJ, Rosenow PJ et al. (1979b) An analysis of 346 cases of clear cell adenocarcinoma of the vagina and cervix with emphasis on recurrence and survival. Gynecol Oncol 7:111–122

Holt LH, Herbst AL (1982) DES related female genital changes. Semin Oncol 9:341–348

Jefferies JA, Robboy SJ, O'Brient PC et al. (1984) Structural anomalies of the cervix and vagina in women enrolled in the diethylstilbestrol adenosis (DESAD) project. Am J Obstet Gynecol 148:59–66

Jones WB, Koulos JP, Saigo PE et al. (1987) Clear cell adenocarcinoma of the lower genital tract: Memorial Hospital 1974–1984. Obstet Gynecol 70:573–577

Lewis JL Jr, Nordqvist SRB, Richart RM (1973) Studies of nuclear DNA in vaginal adenosis and clear cell adenocarcinoma. Am J Obstet Gynecol 115:737–750

Melnick S, Cole P, Anderson D et al. (1987) Rates and risks of diethylstilbestrol related clear cell adenocarcinomas of the vagina and cervix. An update. N Engl J Med 316:514–516

Robboy SJ, Herbst AL, Scully RE (1974) Clear cell adenocarcinoma of the vagina and cervix in young females: analysis of 37 tumors that persisted or recurred after primary therapy. Cancer 34:606–614

Robboy SJ, Scully RE, Herbst AL (1975) Pathology of vaginal and cervical abnormalities associated with prenatal exposure to diethylstilbestrol (DES). J Reprod Med 15:13–18

Scully RE, Robboy SJ, Herbst AL (1974) Vaginal and cervical abnormalities including clear cell adenocarcinomas related to prenatal exposure to stilbestrol. Ann Clin Lab Sci 4:222–233

Silverberg SG, DeGiorgi LS (1972) Clear cell carcinoma of the vagina: a clinical, pathologic and electron microscopic study. Cancer 29:1680–1690

Welch WR, Prat J, Robboy SJ et al. (1978) Pathology of prenatal diethylstilbestrol exposure. Pathol Annu 13 (pt 1):201–216

Adenocarcinoma Not Related to DES

Addison WA, Hammond CB, Parker RT (1979) The occurrence of adenocarcinoma in endometriosis of the rectovaginal septum during progestational therapy. Gynecol Oncol 8:193–197

Andryjowicz E, Qizilbash AH, De Petrillo AD et al. (1985) Adenocarcinoma in coecal neovagina – complication of irradiation: report of a case and review of literature. Gynecol Oncol 21:235–239

Ballon S, Lagasse L, Chung N et al. (1979) Primary carcinoma of the vagina. Surg Gynecol Obstet 149:233–237

Bamford DS (1967) Primary adenocarcinoma of the vagina. Proc R Soc Med 60:999–1000

Barbosa E (1956) Primary adenocarcinoma of the vagina. Am J Surg 91:839–841

Blaikley J, Deshurt C, Ferrira H et al. (1971) Vaginal adenosis: clinical and pathological features with special reference to malignant change. Br J Obstet Gynaecol 78:1115–1122

Brooks JJ, Wheeler JE (1977) Malignancy arising in extragonadal endometriosis: a case report and summary of the world literature. Cancer 40:3065–3073

Davis PC, Franklin EW III (1975) Cancer of the vagina. South Med J 68:1239–1242

Daw E (1971) Primary carcinoma of the vagina. J Obstet Gynaecol Br Commenw 78:853–856

Dockerty MB, Pratt JH, Decker DG (1954) Primary adenocarcinoma of the rectovaginal septum probably arising from endometriosis. Cancer 7:893–898

Ferreira HP, Clayton SG (1958) Three cases of malignant changes in endometriosis, including two cases arising in the rectovaginal septum. J Obstet Gynaecol Br Emp 65:41–44

Frick HC, Jacox HW, Taylor HC Jr (1968) Primary carcinoma of the vagina. Am J Obstet Gynecol 101:695–703

Fukushima M, Twigg LB, Okagaki T (1986) Mixed intestinal adenocarcinoma-argentaffin carcinoma of the vagina. Gynecol Oncol 23:387–394

Goldberg MI, Ng ABP, Belinson JL et al. (1978) Clear cell adenocarcinoma arising in endometriosis of the rectovaginal septum. Obstet Gynecol 51 [Suppl]:38–40

Granai CO, Walters MD, Safaii H et al. (1984) Malignant transformation of vaginal endometriosis. Obstet Gynecol 64:592–595

Hayman MP (1977) Extraovarian endometrioid carcinoma: review of literature and report of two cases with unusual features. Am J Clin Pathol 68:522–527

Kapp DS, Merino M, LiVolsi V (1982) Adenocarcinoma of the vagina arising in endometriosis. Long term survival following radiation therapy. Gynecol Oncol 14:271–278

Kurman RJ, Scully RE (1974) The incidence and histogensis of vaginal adenosis. Hum Pathol 5:265–276

Lash SR, Rubenstone AI (1959) Adenocarcinoma of the rectovaginal septum probably arising in endometriosis. Am J Obstet Gynecol 78:299–302

Ledward RS (1972) Primary carcinoma of the vagina. Proc R Soc Med 65:95–97

Lewis GC Jr, Brady L (1967) Carcinoma of the vagina. Clin Obstet Gynecol 10:655–663

Livingston R (1950) Primary carcinoma of the vagina. Thomas, Springfield, p 33

Marcus S (1960) Primary carcinoma of the vagina. Obstet Gynecol 15:673–689

Mawad RM, Latour JPA (1974) Primary adenocarcinoma of the vagina. Obstet Gynecol 44:889–893

Mostoufizadeh M, Scully RE (1980) Malignant tumours arising in endometriosis. Clin Obstet Gynecol 23:951–963

Palumbo L Jr, Shingleton HM, Fishburne JI Jr et al. (1969) Primary carcinoma of the vagina. South Med J 62:1048–1053

Plaut A, Dreyfuss ML (1940) Adenosis vagina and its relation to primary adenocarcinoma of vagina. Surg Gynecol Obstet 71:756–765

Ray J, Ireland K (1985) Non clear cell adenocarcinoma arising in vaginal adenosis. Arch Pathol Lab Med 109;781–783

Rhatigan RM, Majodidi Q (1973) Adenosquamous carcinomas of the vulva and vagina. Am J Clin Pathol 60:208–217

Ritchie RN (1929) Primary csyrcinoma of the vagina following Baldwin reconstruction operation for congenital absence of the vagina. Am J Obstet Gynecol 18:794–799
Sampson JA (1925) Endometrial carcinoma of the ovary arising in endometrial tissue in that organ. Arch Surg 10:1–72
Samsuddin AKM, Villa Santa U, Tank C-K et al. (1979) Adenocarcinoma arising from extragonadal endometriosis 14 years after total hysterectomy and bilateral salpingo-oopherectomy: report of a case with ultrastructural studies. Am J Obsstet Gynecol 133:858–586
Sandberg EC, Danielson RW, Cawet RW et al. (1965) Adenosis vaginae. Am J Obstet Gynecol 93:209–222
Scott RB (1959) Malignant changes in endometriosis. Obstet Gynecol 2:283–289
Strachan GI (1932) Adenocarcinoma of the vagina. J Obstet Gynaecol Br Emp 39:566–572
Wade-Evans T (1976) The etiology and pathology of cancer of the vagina. Clin Obstet Gynecol 3:229–241
Way S (1948) Primary carcinoma of the vagina. J Obstet Gynaecol Br Emp 55:739–755
Young EA, Gamble CN (1969) Primary adenocarcinoma of the rectovaginal septum arising from endometriosis. Cancer 24:597–601

22.3 Naevi and Melanoma

22.3.1 Naevi

Naevi are uncommen in the vagina and are often diagnosed clinically as malignant melanoma. Most of the benign pigmented lesions of the female genital tract have been reported from the vulva and cervix. The vaginal pigmented lesions comprise melanosis (Norris and Taylor 1966; Tsukada 1976), lentigo (Norris and Taylor 1966; Lee et al. 1984), pigmented naevi (Nicholson 1936) and blue naevi (Rodriguez and Ackerman 1968; Tobon and Murphy 1977).

Melanosis occurs as a blue patch and is characterised histologically by pigmentation of the basal layer of the squamous epithelium and scattered melanocytes among the squamous epithelial cells.

22.3.1.1 Blue Naevi

Blue naevi occur commonly in the skin over the wrists, buttocks and shoulders. In the female genital tract, the cervix seems to be the more frequent site (Goldman and Friedman 1967; Rodriguez and Ackerman 1968; Qizilbash 1968). They are only occasionally seen in the vagina. The genital lesion can be associated with naevi at other parts of the body (Rodriguez and Ackerman 1968).

Grossly, blue naevi are generally well-circumscribed, raised, pink-blue nodules of average diameter 0.5 cm.

Microscopically, they are composed of irregular bundles of elongated, spindle-shaped melanocytes with dendritic processes, arranged parallel to the base of the epidermis. Melanin can be demonstrated by Fontana-Masson stain as granular deposits in the cells. Occasionally, melanin pigments may be so densely distributed in the naevus cells and macrophages that individual cells cannot be distinctly identified. Fontana stain, immunoperoxidase study for S-100 protein and ultrastructural study in such circumstances can help in establishing the diagnosis. There is usually a non-pigmented zone of fibro-collagenous tissue separating the naevi and epidermis.

Treatment is by excision.

(For other types of naevi see Vulva.)

22.3.2 Melanoma

Melanocytes are found only in 1%–3% of adult vaginas (Nigogosyan et al. 1964), but primary vaginal melanomas are still rarer, constituting about 0.3% of all melanomas of the body (Ariel 1981) and 2.8% of all vaginal tumours (Chung et al. 1980).

22.3.2.1 Clinical Features

The age of the patients ranges between 28 (Mino et al. 1948) and 83 years old (Daw 1972), the peak incidence occurring in the late 50s and 60s. The most common symptoms are vaginal bleeding and discharge. The patient may also complain of vaginal irritation, soreness, dysuria and vaginal mass.

22.3.2.2 Gross Appearance

Melanomas vary in shape and size from a small flat plaque or small elevated nodule of 0.5 cm in diameter to a large tumour filling the whole vagina. The average size is about 1.5–2.0 cm. The tumour may be nodular, polypoid, papillary, fungating or ulcerated. The colour varies from brown, red-brown to black. Melanomas can occur anywhere in the vagina (Collantes et al. 1967) but commonly involve the anterior or posterior wall of the lower half (Ragni and Tobon 1974).

22.3.2.3 Microscopical Appearance

While melanomas can occur de novo in the vagina, secondary lesions from the vulva, cervix and urethra are far more common, as these parts of the genital system closely share a common lymphatic system (Abeshouse 1958). Primary malignant melanoma can arise in atypical melanocytic hyperplasia (Bottles et al. 1984), lentigo and melanosis (Norris and Taylor 1966; Lee et al. 1984). All pigmented lesions of the vagina should, therefore, be considered potentially malignant and excised (Norris and Taylor 1966) and submitted for histopathological examination. Like other mucosal melanomas, the vaginal melanomas tend to show lateral junctional spread (Takagi et al. 1974), and the presence of junctional changes adjacent to the malignant melanoma is considered diagnostic of a primary vaginal lesion (Batsakis and Dito 1962; Genton et al. 1981).

The vaginal melanomas are mostly of the nodular type, which is followed in incidence by the superficial spreading type of Clark et al. (1969) and McGovern (1970). The nodular melanoma is uniformly invasive from the onset. The nodule is formed by focal proliferation of atypical and anaplastic melanocytes and rapidly assumes a vertical growth phase. Initially, the atypical melanocytes form small nests which aggregate into a large nodule. The overlying epithelium is either attenuated or becomes ulcerated. The superficial spreading melanoma is characterised by the presence of pagetoid melanocytes in the epidermis in the pre-invasive phase and in the dermis in the invasive phase. The malignant cells may be epithelioid with abundant cytoplasm, large nuclei and prominent nucleoli. Cytoplasmic melanin is finely granular.

Although several cell types – polygonal, epithelioid and spindle – are seen in invasive melanomas of the skin, the vaginal melanomas tend to be composed of anaplastic and pleomorphic cells (Hasumi et al. 1978) with the spindle cells predominating in 50% of patients. These lesions are often mistaken for undifferentiated sarcomas, rhabdomyosarcomas and anaplastic carcinomas, more so, when melanin pigments are not identified (Fig. 22.12). Small cell melanoms may likewise be misdiagnosed as small cell carcinoma of the vagina (Jentys et al. 1975). Sometime the spindle cell lesions, like other mucosal melanomas, may also resemble lentiginous melanomas.

Like the vulval and labial mucosa, the vaginal mucosa lacks a well-defined paillary dermis. Staging of these lesions according to Clark's staging system cannot therefore be done with accuracy. The FIGO staging system used exclusively for squamous cell carcinoma is, according to many workers (Bouma et al. 1982; Jaramillo et al. 1985), inadequate for melanomas. Direct measurement from the surface to the deepest point of invasion has been used by serveral workers in cutaneous (Breslow 1975) and vaginal melanomas (Chung et al. 1980; Beller et al. 1986) and found to be a good predictor of prognosis. Chung et al. (1975) proposed the following staging system:

Level 1 – Tumour is confined to the epithelium
Level 2 – Superficial penetration of the tumour into the dermis or lamina propria to a depth of 1 mm or less, as measured from the granular layer or its estimated position in the epidermis or from the otuermost epithelial layer in the mucos
Level 3 – Penetration of 1–2 mm deep into the sub-epithelial tissue
Level 4 – Invasion beyond 2 mm into the fibrous and fibromuscular tissue but not the fat
Level 5 – Extension to underlying fat

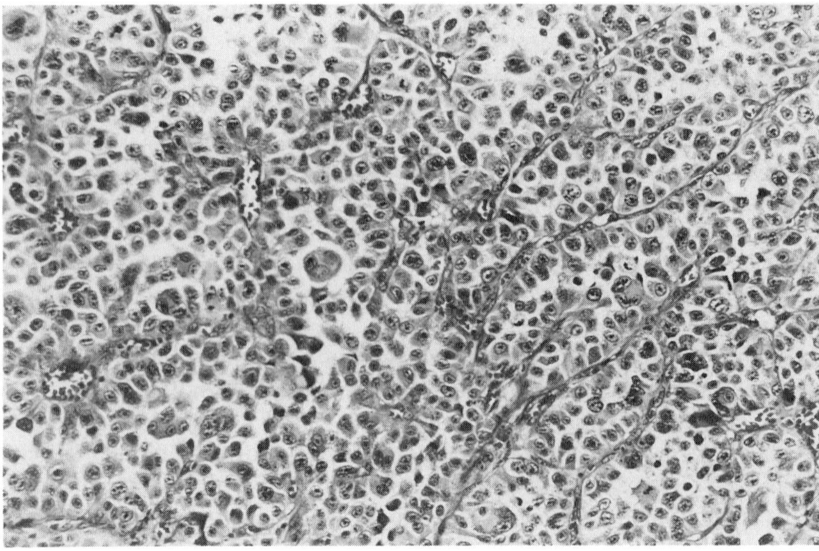

Fig. 22.12. Melanoma: alveolar arrangement may be mistaken for rhabdomyosarcoma

22.3.2.4 Prognosis

The prognosis of vaginal melanoma is generally poor (Collantes et al. 1967; Fenn and Abell 1973; Ragni and Tobon 1974; Pomante 1975). The level of invasion (Chung et al. 1980) and tumour volume (Beller et al. 1986) are considered important prognostic parameters.

22.3.2.5 Metastases

Metastasis to the regional lymph nodes occurs in about 10%–15% of vaginal melanomas (Norris and Taylor 1966; Morrow and DiSaia 1976) and satellite lesions in one-third of all patients (Morroy and DiSaia 1976). According to Deutsch et al. (1974), the incidence of early regional node metastases from a vaginal melanoma is not higher than that form a vaginal carcinoma. Ariel (1981) on the other hand noted that 20% of patients had distant metastases when first seen.

22.3.2.6 Treatment

The treatment of vaginal melanoma has remained problematic. It has varied from wide local excision (Freund et al. 1959) to vulvectomy and vaginectomy with bilateral superficial and deep node dissection (Collantes et al. 1967). Chemotherapy and radiation (Ragni and Tobon 1974) have also been tried. It is generally considered that radical surgery is the method of choice for vaginal melanomas (Ariel 1981). Das Gupta and D'Urso (1964) advocated a similar management to that in vulval melanoma when the lower third of vagina is affected. The lesion occurring above the middle third on the lateral wall should be treated by complete vaginectomy, vulvectomy and bilateral groin dissection. Partial and subtotal vaginectomy may be unsafe as microscopic foci of melanoma may extend beyond the macroscopic limit.

Anterior or posterior exenteration may be considered when the lesion has involved the urinary bladder or rectum, and when there is no distant metastasis (Ariel 1981).

The role of radiotherapy is uncertain. Melanomas are thought to be tumours of low radiosensitivity although some workers (Jentys et al. 1975) achieved remission in some patients. Radiation may be useful for patients who are unsuitable for surgery or refuse surgical treatment (Ariel 1981). Radiation may also be tried in combination with surgery to control the disease in the pelvis (Deutsch et al. 1974).

References

Naevi

Goldman RL, Friedman NB (1967) Blue nevus of the uterine cervix. Cancer 20:210–214

Lee RB, Buttoni L Jr, Dhru K et al. (1984) Malignant melanoma of the vagina: a case report of progression from pre-existing melanosis. Gynecol Oncol 19:238–245

Nicholson GW (1936) Epidermal heteromorphosis of vaginal vault. J Pathol Bacteriol 43:209–221

Norris HJ, Taylor HB (1966) Melanomas of the vagina. Am J Clin Pathol 46:420–426

Qizilbash AH (1973) Blue nevus of the uterine cervix: report of a case. Am J Clin Pathol 59:803–806

Rodriguez HA, Ackerman LV (1968) Cellular blue nevus: clinicopathologic study of forty-five cases. Cancer 21:393–405

Tobon H, Murphy AI (1977) Benign blue nevus of the vagina. Cancer 40:3174–3176

Tsukada Y (1976) Benign melanosis of the vagina and cervix. Am J Obstet Gynecol 124:211–212

Melanoma

Abeshouse BS (1958) Primary and secondary melanomas of the genitourinary tract. South Med J 51:994–1006

Ariel IM (1981) Malignant melanoma of the female genital system: a report of 48 patients and review of the literature. J Surg Oncol 16:371–383

Batsakis JG, Dito WR (1962) Primary malignant melanoma of vagina. Obstet Gynecol 20:109–111

Beller U, Demopoulos RI, Beckman EM (1986) Vulvovaginal melanoma: a clinicopathologic study. J Reprod Med 31:315–319

Bottles K, Lacey GG, Miller TR (1984) Atypical melanocytic hyperplasia of the vagina. Gynecol Oncol 19:226–230

Bouma J, Weening JJ, Elders A (1982) Malignant melanoma of the vulva: report of 18 cases. Eur J Obstet Gynecol Reprod Biol 13:237–251

Breslow A (1975) Tumor thickness, level of invasion and node dissection in stage 1 cutaneous melanoma. Ann Surg 182:572–575

Chung AF, Woodruff JM, Lewis JL Jr (1975) Malignant melanoma of the vulva: a report of 44 cases. Obstet Gynecol 45:638–646

Chung AF, Casey MJ, Flannery JT et al. (1980) Malignant melanoma of the vagina – report of 19 cases. Obstet Gynecol 55:720–727

Clark WH Jr, From L, Bernardino EA et al. (1969) The histogenesis and biological behavior of primary human malignant melanoma of the skin. Cancer Res 29:705–726
Collantes TM, Pratt JH, Dockerty MB (1967) Primary malignant melanoma of the vagina. Obstet Gynecol 29:508–514
Das Gupta T, D'Urso J (1964) Melanoma of female genitalia. Surg Gynecol Obstet 119:1074–1078
Daw E (1972) Primary melanoma of the vagina. Am J Obstet Gynecol 112:307–308
Detsch M, Fried AB, Parsons JA et al. (1974) Primary malignant melanoma of the vagina. Oncology 30:509–516
Fenn ME, Abell MR (1973) Melanoma of vulva and vagina. Obstet Gynecol 41:902–911
Freund DR, Kegal EE, Dugger JH (1959) Primary malignant melanoma of the vagina. Am J Obstet Gynecol 78:290–294
Genton CY, Kunz J, Schreiner WE (1981) Primary malignant melanoma of the vagina and cervix uteri: report of a case with ultrastructural study. Virchows Arch [A] 393:245–250
Hasumi K, Sakamoto G, Sugano H et al. (1978) Primary malignant melanoma of the vagina: study of four autopsy cases with ultrastructural findings. Cancer 42:2675–2686
Jaramillo BA, Ganjei P, Averette HE et al. (1985) Malignant melanoma of the vulva. Obstet Gynecol 66:398–401
Jentys W, Sikorowa L, Mokrzanowski A (1975) Primary melanoma of the vagina: clinico-pathologic study of 7 cases. Oncology 31:83–91
Lee RB, Buttoni L Jr, Dhru K et al. (1984) Malignant melanoma of the vagina: a case report of progression from pre-existing melanosis. Gynecol Oncol 19:238–245
McGovern VJ (1970) The classification of melanoma and its relationship with prognosis. Pathology 2:85–98
Mino RA, Mino VH, Livingstone RG (1948) Primary melanoma of the vagina with a review of the literature. Am J Obstet Gynecol 56:325–334
Morrow CP, DiSaia PJ (1976) Malignant melanoma of the female genitalia: a clinical analysis. Obstet Gynecol Surv 31:233–271
Nigogosyan G, Pava SDL, Piekern JW (1964) Melanoblasts in vaginal mucosa: origin for primary malignant melanoma. Cancer 17:912–913
Norris HJ, Taylor HB (1966) Melanomas of the vagina. Am J Clin Pathol 46:420–426
Pomante RG (1975) Malignant melanoma primary in the vagina. Gynecol Oncol 3:15–20
Ragni MV, Tobon H (1974) Primary malignant melanoma of the vulva. Obstet Gynecol 43:658–664
Takagi M, Ishikawa G, Mori W (1974) Primary malignant melanoma of the oral cavity in Japan: with special reference to mucosal melanosis. Cancer 34:358–370

22.4 Mesenchymal Origin

22.4.1 Benign

22.4.1.1 Leiomyoma

22.4.1.1.1 Incidence

Smooth muscle tumours are the most common mesenchymal tumours of the adult vagina (Kaufman and Gardner 1964). According to one report (Bennett and Ehrlich 1941), nine samples of vaginal leiomyoma could be found among more than 50 000 gynaecological specimens.

22.4.1.1.2 Clinical Features

Vaginal leiomyomas have been reported in patients from puberty to 71 years of age (Nurnberger 1930) but most frequently in the age range between 38 and 48 years (Farell and Abrams 1956). A leiomyoma of average size between 3 and 4 cm is usually asymptomatic. The patients may complain of a mass protruding from the vagina, lump in the vagina, vaginal discomfort and discharge and dyspareunia. Sub-urethral tumours may cause urinary symptoms (Adduci 1965; Sered et al. 1956). Large tumours can cause difficult labour (Moghissi 1960; Schonberg et al. 1963); recurrence of the tumour has occasionally been reported during pregnancy (Rywlin et al. 1969). Leiomyomas can arise at any point in the vagina (Bennett and Ehrlich 1941), but according to some series (Berman 1938; Shanahan 1942; Quan and Birnbaum 1961; Marcus 1966), the anterior vaginal wall is the predominent site. This was followed by the posterior and lateral walls. Leiomyomas of the vagina are commonly single, sessile tumours covered by intact vaginal epithelium. Ulceration may occasionally complicate them and may cause vaginal bleeding and purulent discharge. A vaginal tumour can co-exist with the uterine leiomyoma, but such an occurrence is considered simply coincidental (Farell and Abrams 1956; Ingemanson and Alfredsson 1970).

22.4.1.1.3 Gross Appearance

The size of the tumour varies from 1.5 cm (Ingemanson and Alfredsson 1970) to 16 cm (Rywlin et al. 1969), but the majority of them are between 1.5 and 3 cm in diameter. The tumours are well-encapsulated, firm to rubbery in consistency and grey to light pink in colour. The cut surface presents a typical whorled appearance.

22.4.1.1.4 Microscopical Appearance

The tumours are composed of interlacing bundles of smooth muscle fibres which traverse in all directions (Fig. 22.13), forming distinctive whorls. The individual muscle fibres are elongated cells possessing abundant eosinophilic cytoplasm with an indistinct cell border and plump nuclei with rounded blunt ends. The tumours are not in general mitotically active. A correlation has been noted between tumour recurrences and the presence of 5 or more mitoses per 10 high power fields as well as with cellular atypia (Tavassoli and Norris 1979). Tumours with infiltrating margins are aggressive and more likely to be sarcomas (Tavassoli and Norris 1979). Oedema, haemorrhage, hyaline and other degenerative changes are not uncommon. Rywlin et al. (1969) observed increased cellularity, nuclear atypia, mitotic activity and hypervascularity in a recurrent tumour during pregnancy. The tumour became smaller and changes disappeared after delivery. The authors considered these signs as proof of hormone dependency. Tavassoli and Norris noted epitheloid leiomyoma and leiomyoblastomas in their series (Tavassoli and Norris 1979). The epithelioid leiomyomas consisted mainly of round and polygonal cells with abundant eosinophilic cytoplasm and large round or oval nuclei displaying an organoid arrangement. The leiomyoblastomas consist of round and polygonal cells

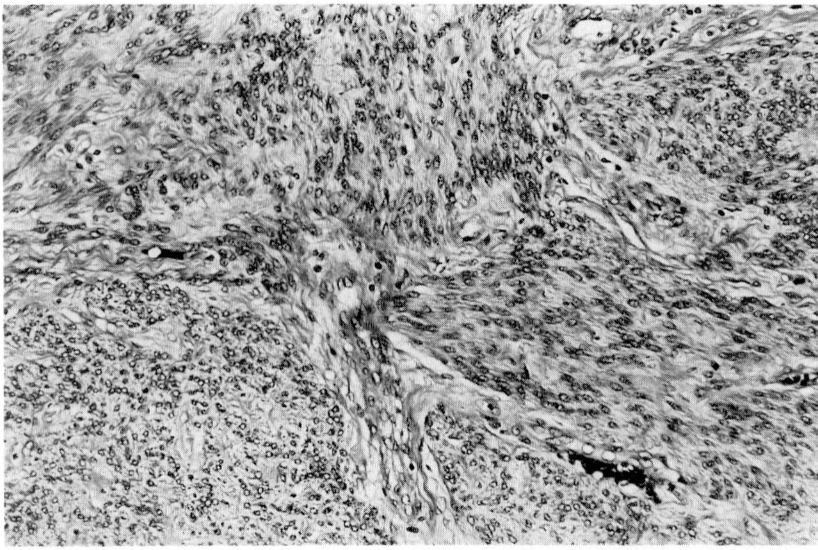

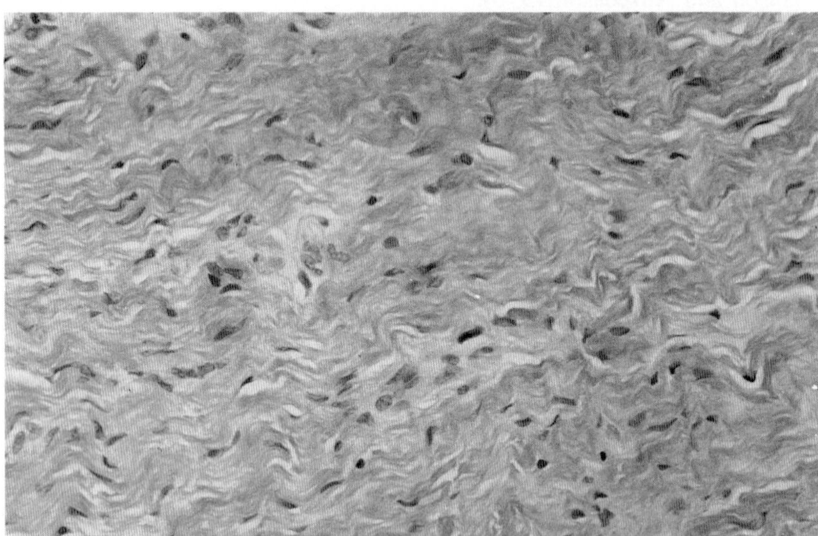

Fig. 22.13. Leiomyoma: composed of interlacing bundles of smooth muscle fibres

Fig. 22.14. Neurofibroma: diffuse proliferation of nerve sheath elements

with prominent perinuclear vacuolations. They can occur in the uterus as well as at extra-uterine sites such as the stomach and small intestine.

22.4.1.1.5 Treatment
The treatment is local excision.

22.4.1.2 Neurofibroma

There are a few reported cases of neurofibromatosis involving the urinary bladder and vagina (Gold 1972), but the primary solitary neurofibroma of the vagina is rare. Tavassoli and Norris (1979) mentioned 5 neurofibromas while reporting on 60 smooth muscle tumours of the vagina. The neurofibromas, which according to many authors are hamartomas, can occur anywhere in the vagina. Depending on their size and degree of degeneration, symptoms may vary; dyspareunia, bloody and purulent discharge and frequency or urgency of micturition can be the main complaints. When the tumour is large, it may complicate labour. The café-au-lait spots of the skin which are seen in neurofibromatosis can also be found in patients with vaginal lesions (Gold 1972).

22.4.1.2.1 Gross Appearance
The average size of the tumour is 4–6 cm, but it may grow up to 12 cm (Norris and Cooper 1950). The tumours are unencapsulated, slightly lobulated, firm masses, which on a cut surface present a homogeneous, greyish-white appearance. Cystic and mucoid changes are not infrequent on the cut surface.

22.4.1.2.2 Microscopical Appearance
Neurofibromas consist of localised or diffuse proliferations of neurites and elements of the nerve sheath with Schwann's cells commonly predominating (Fig. 22.14). The nerve bundles are distorted and show irregular and haphazard arrangements often merging imperceptibly with the proliferating Schwann's cell component. The overall texture of the tumour may be loose due to the oedematous separation of spindle-shaped Schwann's cells and collagen bundles. In some areas, the spindle cells may be arranged in prominent wavy or tortuous configurations and in others, compact parallel bands. Occasionally, whorls and organoid structures reminiscent of Wagner-Meissner bodies may be seen. Mitotic figures are rare. Azzopardi et al. (1983) reported a neurofibroma with rhabdomyomatous differentiation (triton tumour) in the vagina which was designated by the authors as benign triton tumour, in contrast to the malignant tumours which display rhabdomyosarcomatous differentation. Malignant changes in neurofibromatosis have been reported in about 13% of patients (Hosoi 1931). Such changes in the small neurofibromas arising in the superficial peripheral nerves are, however, very rare.

22.4.1.2.3 Treatment
The treatment is complete surgical excision.

22.4.1.3 Rhabdomyoma

Rhabdomyomas, the benign tumours of striated muscles which are known to occur at different anatomical sites, namely, the heart, pharynx, nose, larynx, tongue, stomach and skeletal muscles, are infrequent in the female genital tract. Although rhabdomyosarcomas are common sarcomas of the infant vagina, rhabdomyomas are distinctly uncommon in this age group.

22.4.1.3.1 Clinical Features
Extra-genital rhabdomyomas have been reported in patients between 8 weeks (Pendle 1897) and 81 years (Tsukuda and Pickern 1965) of age, but patients with vaginal rhabdomyomas are usually between 34 (Ceremsak 1969) and 56 years old (Dehner et al. 1972), with the peak incidence occurring in the 4th decade. The tumours are often asymptomatic and discovered incidentally during gynaecological examination. Vaginal heaviness, cyst in the vagina (Ceremsak 1969) and occasionally vaginal discharge may be the main complaints.

22.4.1.3.2 Pathological Features
Rhabdomyomas are generally classified according to their location, such as cardiac and extra-cardiac. The cardiac rhabdomyomas are commonly associated with hamartoma complex, comprising sebaceous adenoma, tuberous sclerosis and hamartomas of other organs (Moran and Enterline 1964). The extra-cardiac rhabdomyomas have been further subdivided into adult and fetal types. The adult type occurs almost exclusively in the head and neck region of adults (Di Sant Agnese and Knowles 1980). The less recognised group is the fetal type, which occurs commonly in the head and neck region of infants and young children, with a particular predilection for the post-auricular region (Dehner et al. 1972).

The tumours vary in size from 1 to 5 cm, are well circumscribed and encapsulated and display mild surface lobulations. Cut sections present a light tan to grey appearance.

22.4.1.3.3 Microscopical Appearance
The tumours consist of large round and polygonal cells with abundant acidophilic granular cytoplasm, a large nucleus and a prominent nucleolus. Some of these cells may reveal cross-striations. The others show a focal collection of crystal-like particles which are arranged in a jack-straw pattern and are stained intensely by phosphotungstic acid-haematoxylin (Moran and Enterline 1964). The fetal rhabdomyomas are made up of haphazardly arranged small, oval to spindle-shaped, mesenchymal cells containing little cytoplasm and small, oval to spindle-shaped nuclei and immature skeletal muscle fibres in varying stages of differentiation.

Some of the cells of the latter type are strap-shaped with abundant acidophilic cytoplasm and dark, round to vesicular nuclei. Cross-striations and myofibrils may be noticed in some larger strap cells. The connective tissue stroma is usually scant, oedematous and myxoid. The genital lesions are also grouped as fetal type (Ceremsak 1969; Gold and Bosson 1976) and are different in light and electron microscopic features from the extra-genital lesions (Gad and Eusebi 1975). The genital rhabdomyomas contain abundant stromal connective tissue and larger and more mature muscle cells (Gold and Bossen 1976). The peripheral cytoplasmic vacuoles and rod-like crystalline bodies representing hypertrophied Z lines (Dehner et al. 1972) that are present in tumour cells of extra-genital rhabdomyomas are not seen in the genital tumours (Cad and Eusebi 1975; Gold and Bossen 1976). The squamous epithelium covering the tumour is usually intact.

Recently, Di Sant Agnese and Knowles (1980) have sub-classified them into fetal myxoid and fetal cellular types. The histological appearances of myxoid varient do not differ much from those of classic rhabdomyomas. The cellular variant is composed of interlacing bundles of spindle cells with areas of herring-bone pattern, nuclear palisading and occasional ribbon or strap cells (Di Sant Agnese and Knowles 1980). Ultrastructurally, the rhabdomyoblasts contain well-organised myofibrils with Z bands, poorly formed desmosomes, cytoplasmic bodies and sacs of sarcoplasmic reticulum containing junctional granules. There are occasional aggregates of myoblastic cells within a common basement membrane (Cornog and Gontas 1967; Leoni and Taylor 1973; Gold and Bossen 1976).

The benign fetal rhabdomyomas are differentiated from the embryonal rhabdomyosarcomas by the absence of mitoses, cambium layer and infiltrative growth pattern of the latter. The embryonal rhabdomyosarcomas occur in much younger patients and have a rapid growth rate. The common benign vaginal polyp does not contain striated muscle fibres and is made of loose connective tissue which may occasionally display atypical changes. Also, patients with a polyp are older than patients with the common fetal type of rhabdomyoma.

22.4.1.3.4 Treatment

The treatment is local excision.

22.4.1.4 Glomus Tumour

Glomus tumours, which are infrequent, soft tissue tumours, arise from the cells of the arterio-venous anastomosis or glomus body, a thermo-regulatory body normally present in the dermis. The glomus cells are thought to be of myoneural origin, and their ultrastructural features closely resemble those of smooth muscle cells (Venkatachalam and Greally 1969). The tumours commonly arise in the sub-ungual region, and more than 70% occur in the upper extremities (Shugart et al. 1963) of adults. Unusual locations such as stomach, eyelids, patella and nose, where glomus bodies are usually absent, have also been reported (Appleberg and Teasley 1968). In the female genital tract, these tumours are extremely rare; less than half a dozen patients have been reported in the English medical literature (Banner and Winkelmann 1957; Spitzer et al. 1985). The patients are in their 3rd and 4th decades and present with vaginal tenderness, bleeding and dyspareunia. Clinically, these tumours are to be differentiated from endometriosis, melanoma and, when they arise in the anterior vaginal wall, from the inflammatory and neoplastic conditions of the urethra.

A glomus tumour is a well-circumscribed and lobulated, blue-tan mass 1–4 cm in average size. The cut surfaces are pink and homogeneous.

22.4.1.4.1 Microscopical Appearance

These tumours are composed characteristically of many layers of uniform glomus cells around endothelium-lined, irregular, vascular spaces (Fig. 22.15). These cells are fusiform, polygonal and round, with abundant clear or faintly eosinophilic cytoplasm and round small nuclei. Mitoses are rare. The stromal connective tissue, which may be thin or thick, hyalinised and myxoid, separates the sheet of glomus cells. The stroma may be inconspicuous within the cell mass, although silver stain may show reticulin fibres around the individual cell.

22.4.1.4.2 Treatment

These tumours are benign and cured by complete surgical excision.

22.4.2 Malignant

22.4.2.1 Sarcoma Botryoides

Botryoides in Greek means "like a bunch of grapes", and sarcoma botryoides is so named because of its grape-like appearance. It is a highly malignant, mesenchymal tumour which occurs in the vagina and cervix of infants and young girls. It also occurs at other anatomical areas like the head and neck region (Donaldson et al. 1973), urinary bladder, prostate (Grosfield et al. 1972) and common bile duct (Farinacci et al. 1956). Occasionally, sarcoma botryoides has been noticed in elderly women (Spademan et al. 1953), but it is predominantly a disease of the first 2 decades of life (Crawford 1959). The tumour may be congenital and noticed in the vagina of a newborn in the delivery room (Ober et al. 1958; Kaufman and Stout 1965). Sarcoma botryoides is a rare gynaecological tumour, and only very few gynaecologists see one during their professional life (Duncan and Fahmy 1953). Although the rhabdomyosarcomas constitute only 10%–20% of soft tissue sarcomas (Bizer 1969), sarcoma botryoides, a variant of rhabdomyosarcoma, has generated considerable interest, particularly during the past 2 decades.

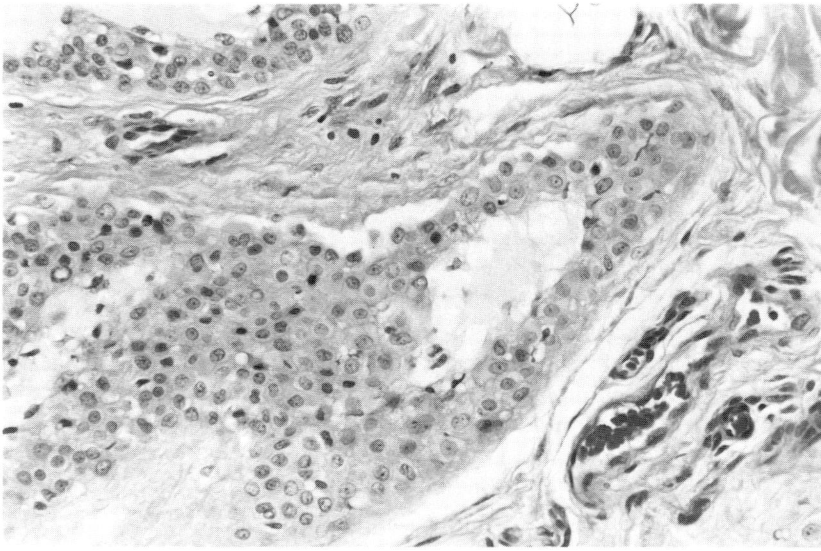

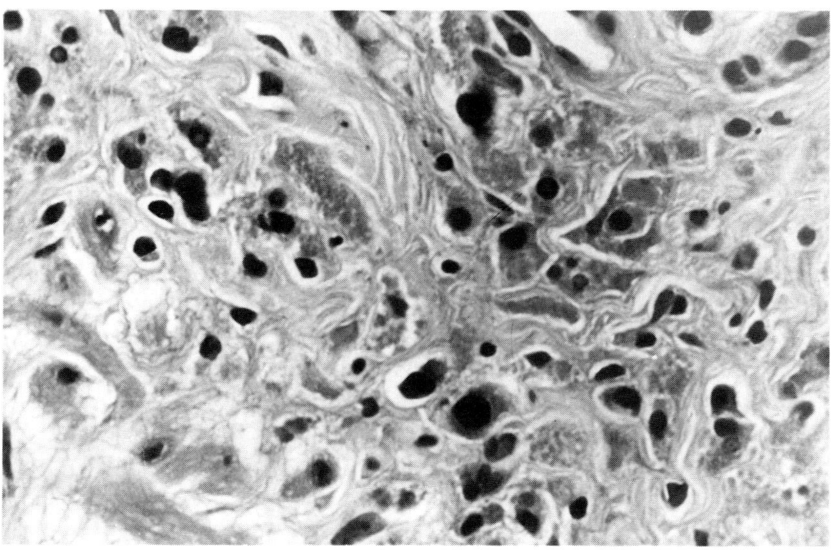

Fig. 22.15. Glomus tumour: irregular vascular spaces containing glomus cells in the wall

Fig. 22.16. Sarcoma botryoides: round and elongated rhabdomyoblasts arranged haphazardly. Strap cells can be seen in one area (*lower left*)

22.4.2.1.1 Clinical Features

Vaginal bleeding, vaginal mass protruding through the introitus and vaginal discharge are the major clinical manifestatiaons. In the advanced stage of the disease, urinary symptoms like dysuria and urinary obstruction and lower bowel symptoms may develop. Pain is not an initial symptom, but in the later stage, patients may experience vaginal and abdominal pain. Vaginal and rectal examinations under anaesthesia reveal a polypoid, grape-like mass arising from a localised or a wide area of the vaginal wall. The tumour may fill and distend the entire vagina and protrude through the introitus. It does not show any predilection for a particular site in the vagina and involves indiscriminately the vaults, anterior, posterior and lateral walls. The vagina may also be secondarily involved due to extension from the primary cervical botryoid tumour. The parametrium and whole of the pelvic cavity may be infiltrated due to the direct extension of the vaginal tumour.

Several clinical staging systems have been used in the past by several workers (Pratt et al. 1972; Donaldson et al. 1973; Holton et al. 1973; Ehrlich et al. 1971; Hilgers 1975; Rivard et al. 1975) for assessing the treatment results and prognosis. Although much information was gained from these classifications, because of their different approaches in formulation they were not accepted uniformly. In 1975, the Intergroup Rhabdomyosarcoma Study (National Istitutes of Health 1975) introduced a clinical staging system based on the extent of the disease and the type of surgery performed:

Group I – Patients had localised desease completely resected (regional nodes not involved)
(a) Confined to muscle or organ of origin
(b) Infiltrations outside this structure, as through fascial planes

Group II – (a) Grossly resected tumour with microscopic residual disease (nodes negative)
(b) Regional disease, completely resected (nodes positive or negative)
(c) Regional disease with involved nodes, grossly resected, but with evidence of microscopic residual disease.

Group III – Incomplete resection or biopsy with gross residual disease

Group IV – Metastatic disease present at onset

22.4.2.1.2 Gross Appearance

The tumour appears as small papillae of 1–3 mm in size or as small nodules in the initial stage (Hilgers et al. 1970). The nodules grow to the shape of a large bunch of grapes or a lobulated cauliflower-like mass (Hilgers et al. 1973). Multiple polypoid tumours are frequent, although single tumours can be seen. The tumours may be sessile as well as pedunculated. The polypoid tumours are pink, shiny, translucent and soft to firm in consistency. The cut surface is usually smooth and intact but may be haemorrhagic, ulcerated and granular; it is oedematous and myxomatous or pinkish-grey with small areas of haemorrhage.

22.4.2.1.3 Microscopical Appearance

Botryoid sarcomas are composed of diffuse proliferations of two basic cell types – round or polygonal and spindle cells (Fig. 22.16). The round cells are small and densely packed and contain scanty cytoplasm and hyperchromatic nuclei. The spindle cells have elongated nuclei and a variable amount of cytoplasm and may possess numerous anastomosing processes. Both types of cells represent undifferentiated neoplastic rhabdomyoblasts (Hilgers et al. 1970). In some tumours or in some parts of the tumour, the spindle cells may predominate and be arranged in interlacing and anastomosing bands. More commonly, the cells are loosely arranged with a myxoid background. Distinct rhabdomyoblastic strap cells, racquet-shaped and bizarre, multinucleate, polyhedral, giant cells containing abundant eosinophilic cytoplasm may be seen scattered among these undifferentiated elements. Some of these cells show well-formed cross-striations, which, however, are not invariably present in all tumours (Weichert et al. 1976).

Beneath the layer of squamous epithelium which covers the tumour nodules, one may find a compact, multilayered band of neoplastic cells arranged parallel to the surface. This "cambium layer of Nicholson", when present, is of diagnostic help (Horn and Enterline 1958). Below this layer, the neoplastic cells are sparse and loosely structured. The tumour shows a very active growth pattern which is reflected in the numerous mitotic figures. The tumour cells may be set in a myxoid stroma which becomes particularly prominent at the central part. In others, the stroma may be fairly compact and fibrous. With the proliferation of neoplastic cells and as the tumour becomes more invasive, the myxomatous areas gradually disappear (Rigby 1966). Haemorrhage and necrosis may be seen but are not common features. After Stout's first detailed histopathological description of rhabdomyosarcoma (1946) which is greatly responsible for the characterisation of this tumour, several histological variants, namely, pleomorphic, alveolar, embryonal and botryoid, have subsequently been described (Stobbe and Dargeon 1950; Horn and Enterline 1958), but their distriction is not always clear cut (Gonzalez-Crussi 1979). Despite a difference in gross appearance, botryoid sarcoma is considered a sub-variant of embryonal rhabdomyosarcoma which assumes a botryoid appearance when it originates in the sub-mucous tissue of the hollow cavity (Daniel et al. 1959).

Several theories have been postulated as to the nature of these tumours: (i) dysontogenetic, mixed tumours (McFarland 1935; Ober and Edgcomb 1954), (ii) malignant, mixed, müllerian tumour (Dorgan 1953; Duncan and Fahmy 1953; Duckett et al. 1957) and (iii) mesenchymal tumours (Ober et al. 1958).

Histogenetically, these tumours have been thought to arise from the sub-mucosal undifferentiated mesenchyme (Sirsat 1953; Crawford 1959; Cywes and Louw 1961; Rigby 1966) and rhabdomyoblasts (Daniel et al. 1959; Patton and Horn 1962). Nakamura et al. (1981) reported a sarcoma botryoides involving the vagina and urinary bladder in association with bilateral nephroblastomas and multiple congenital malformations in a 1-year-old child and suggested that an oncogenic stimulus might have acted on the mesenchyme of both the vagina and urinary tract.

22.4.2.1.4 Clinical Behaviour

Embryonal rhabdomyosarcomas are rapidly growing tumours which spread locally as well as by the lymphatics and blood stream. After infiltration of the vagina, the tumours invade the neighbouring lymphatics and metastasise to the regional lymph nodes (Hilgers et al. 1970). Rhabdomyosarcomas of the genitourinary tract have a higher incidence of lymphatic metastases than those of other areas (Lawrence et al. 1977). Local recurrences are common and have been attributed commonly to treatment failure (Rutledge and Sullivan 1967). Embryonal and alveolar rhabdomyosarcomas tend to metastasise frequently to the soft tissues (73%), serosal surface (64%), lymph nodes (64%) and lungs (55%) (de la Monte et al. 1986). Distant metastases are usually late (Rutledge and Sullivan 1967), and when they occur, the lungs are the most common site.

22.4.2.1.5 Treatment

Early diagnosis is the hallmark for a successful outcome of treatment (Hilgers et al. 1970). Equally important is the assessment of the stage of the disease at operation for the purpose of selection of an optimal treatment plan (Hilgers et al. 1973). Such assessment should include both the clinical and microscopical extent of the lesion. In the earlier literature, surgery with or without radiotherapy had been the conventional modality of treatment. The surgical procedures included both local excision and more radical exenterative surgery. Initial radical extirpation has been considered to be the only definitive and recommended mode of therapy for rhabdomyosarcoma of the urogenital tract (Horn and Enterline 1958; Hilgers et al. 1970; Tank et al. 1972; Exelby 1974). Limited surgery in these patients has been followed by recurrences and metastases (Tefft and Jaffe 1973). Radiotherapy alone (Nelson 1968; Ehrlich et al. 1971) or in combination with surgery or chemotherapy has been used. In some reports, the result of therapy with surgery or radiation has not been encouraging (Grosfield et al. 1969; Holton et al. 1973). Rhabdomyosarcomas have been variously found to be radiosensitive (Lederman 1956), radiocurable in selective cases (Conte and Segerman 1971) and temporarily radiosensitive (Duncan and Fahmy 1953; Hilgers et al. 1970). Two patients were treated with radiotherapy only and survived for 25 years (El-Mahdi et al. 1974; Shirkey and Saenger 1978). Some authors expressed concern about the large dose of radiation (about 6000 rads) needed to destroy the tumour cells (Edland 1965). Such a large dose is not without hazard to the normal tissue and bony pelvis and risk to the bladder and bowel functions (Tefft and Jaffe 1973). Various success rates have been claimed with combined chemotherapy and radiotherapy (Flamant et al. 1979), intensive chemotherapy prior to surgery or radiation (Rivard et al. 1975) and surgery and chemotherapy (Copeland et al. 1985). The adjunct of chemotherapy to the conventional treatment regimen during the past decade has made a substantial impact on the overall improvement of prognosis of rhabdomyosarcoma. In this multidisciplinary approach, surgery is still the most important mode to eradicate or reduce the tumour bulk (Ghavimi et al. 1973). Using surgery, radiotherapy and multiagent chemotherapy, the survival rate of the patients have become much better than the survival rate of the patients treated by a single mode of therapy (Pratt et al. 1972; Donaldson et al. 1973; Ghavimi et al. 1973; Heyen et al. 1974). The preliminary report of the Intergroup Rhabdomyosarcoma Study (Maurer et al. 1977; Tefft et al. 1977) indicated substantial improvement in the prognosis of these patients by following its treatment design formulated in 1972. The group I disease (completely resected) was treated by vincristine, actinomycin and cyclophosphamide (VAC), group II (microscopic residual/nodal involvement) by post-operative radiotherapy plus VAC, group III (localised disease, not treated by gross total resection) and group IV (metastases present at onset) both with initial intensive chemotherapy followed by radiotehrapy. The recommendation of the Intergroup Rhabdomyosarcoma Study III regarding the management of pelvic rhabdomyosarcoma resulted in a 72% disease-free rate in patients with bladder and prostatic primaries (Lacey et al. 1986). Following the Intergroup Rhabdomyosarcoma study protocols of initial multiagent chemotherapy and subsequent hysterectomy and/or partial vvaginectoma, Hays et al. (1988) achieved a 6-year, relapse-free period in 19 of 26 patients. The overall outlook appears to be promising, and cure of the condition in earlier stages appears to be within achievable reach.

22.4.2.2 Leiomyosarcoma

Leiomysarcomas are rare in the vagina, yet they are the most common sarcomas occurring in adult women. Leiomyosarcomas represent 2% of all malignant lesions of the vagina (Akhtar et al. 1978). About 50 cases have so far been reported in the English literature.

22.4.2.2.1 Clinical Features

The age of the patients ranges from 22 to 70 years (Peters et al. 1985), peak incidence being in the mid-50s. Patients usually present with a painless mass in the vagina, vaginal discharge and bleeding and vaginal tenderness. Pain may be the only presenting symptom in some. More than one-third of patients with vaginal leiomyosarcoma have a history of previous irradiation to the pelvis either for cervical cancer or artificial induction of menopause (Malkasian et al. 1963; Peters et al. 1985). The tumours do not appear to have any preferential site (Brown et al. 1960), although the upper part is more favoured according to another report (Davos and Abell 1976).

22.4.2.2.2 Gross Appearance

Leiomyosarcoma occurs as firm to indurated, single, unencapsulated mass measuring from 0.8 to 10 cm in size. The tumours may be nodular, bulky and spherical with grey and light tan appearances on the cut surface, which may show areas of haemorrhage and cystic changes. Infiltrations to the para-vaginal and recto-vaginal soft tissues may be the cause of an irregular outer surface when the lesion is removed at surgery. The vaginal mucosa overlying the tumour may be ulcerated.

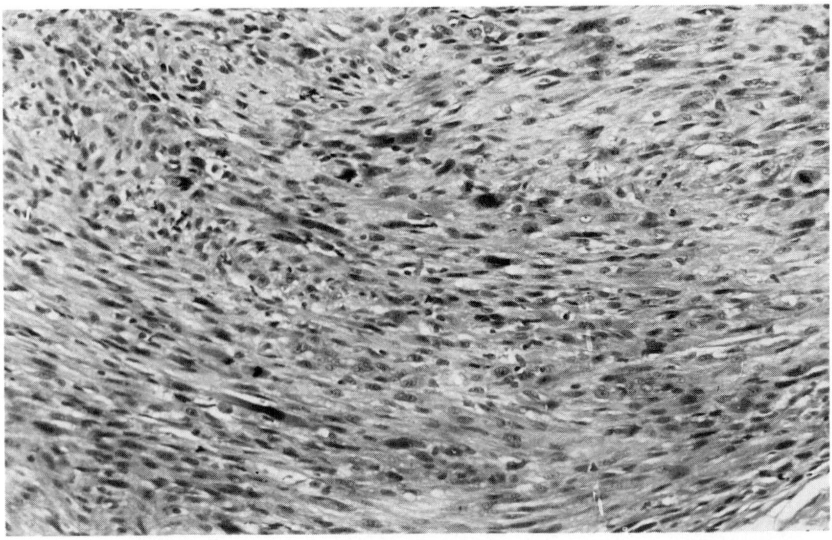

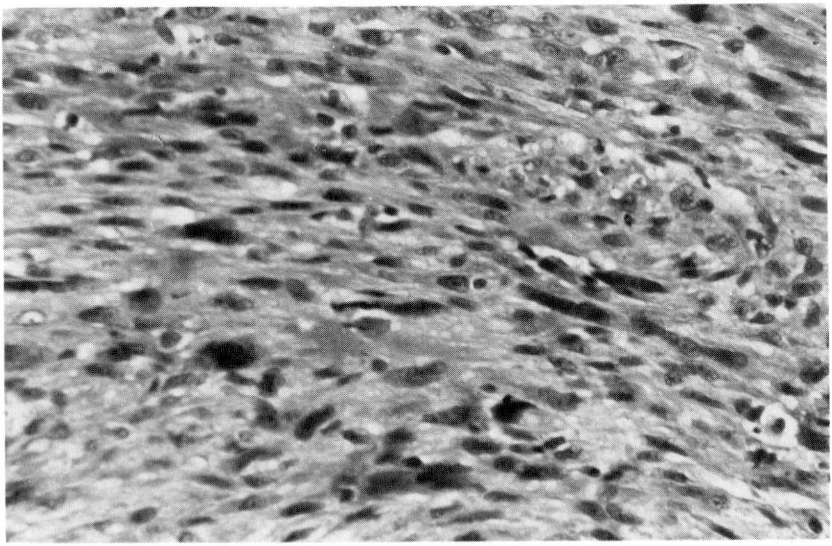

Fig. 22.17. Leiomyosarcoma: pleomorphic spindle and fusiform cells forming intersecting fascicles

Fig. 22.18. Leiomyosarcoma: mitosis and pleomorphism

22.4.2.2.3 Microscopical Appearance

The tumour is composed of interlacing bundles of spindle and fusiform cells, often intersecting each other at wide angles, or forming various-sized vague and well-formed whorls (Figs. 22.17, 22.18). The muscle bundles may traverse in all directions with a haphazard arrangement (Schram 1958). The constituent cells possess moderate to abundant eosinophilic cytoplasm and centrally placed, blunt-ended, hyperchromatic nuclei with prominent nucleoli. The parallel longitudinal myofibrils, which are numerous in the cytoplasm of a relatively well-differentiated tumour, may be absent in a less differentiated one. A variable amount of glycogen can often be demonstrated in the cytoplasm, which appears vacuolated. Bizarre-shaped nuclei and multinuclear giant cells may be quite frequent in some tumours or in some areas of the tumour. In aggressive tumours, irregular columns of malignant cells infiltrating the adjacent tissue may be seen at the periphery. The presence of cellular atypia and number of mitotic figures vary in different tumours, and both features have been related to tumoral behaviour and prognosis. A tumour tends to recur when the mitotic figures exceed 4 per 10 high power fields or when there is moderate atypia in the tumour cells (Tavassoli and Norris 1979). Using a grading system of 1 to 4 based on the cellularity, cellular atypia, mitotic figures and differentiation of the tumour, Rastogi et al. (1984) noticed a poor prognosis with high grade tumours.

Degenerative changes in a leiomyoma sometimes causes bizarre cellular changes, comprising smudginess of the nuclear mass, loss of definition of chromatin and blurring of the nuclear and cytoplasmic outlines. These changes should not be mistaken for malignancy, which is characterised by nuclear atypia, hyperchromasia, mitoses and giant cell formation.

The pericytoma-like vascular pattern and neurilemmoma-like nuclear regimentation that are present in some leiomyomas can also occur in the leiomyosarcoma. Areas of hyaline and myxomatous changes are also common features.

The excision margins of the tumour should be carefully examined for extension into the neighbouring structures. Local recurrences are attributed to incomplete excisions.

Ultrastructurally, the tumour cells contain elongated nuclei with grooved nuclear membranes, abundant, well-defined myofilaments and prominent dense bodies in the cytoplasm. Mitochondria usually conglomerate at the nuclear poles. The cells display marginal pinocytic vesicles and are covered by the basal lamina (Tobon et al. 1973).

22.4.2.2.4 Behaviour

Despite frequent recurrences and a high risk of haematagenous spread (Malkasian et al. 1963), the outlook with vaginal leiomyosarcoma is not invariably grave (Davos and Abell 1978). Survival with this tumour has been variable (Malkasian et al. 1963) and depends largely on the initial extent of the lesion and type of surgical procedure (Davos and Abell 1978). Relations between the histological grades, size of the tumour and ultimate prognosis have been suggested but not firmly established.

22.4.2.2.5 Treatment

Because of the rarity of the lesions, a definite modality of treatment has not been worked out, and surgery appears to be the therapy of choice. Wide local excision (Rastogi et al. 1984), where feasible, vaginectomy or pelvic exenteration (Peters et al. 1985), depending on the degree of histological atypia, size and extent of the lesion, are performed (Davos and Abell 1978). Chemotherapy and radiotherapy have been found to be of very limited benefit.

22.4.2.3 Alveolar Soft Part Sarcoma

Alveolar soft part sarcoma, first described by Christopherson et al. (1952), is a rare tumour of uncertain histogenesis. The tumour is common in the extremities (Lieberman et al. 1966) and rare in the female genitalia (Kasai et al. 1980; Chapman et al. 1984). The two patients reported to have the tumour in the vagina were pregnant when the tumours were discovered by their attending gynaecologists. The patients were asymptomatic at the initial examination, but one patient developed pain 3 years later (Kasai et al. 1980). Another patient reported by O'Toole et al. (1985) was nulliparous and asymptomatic.

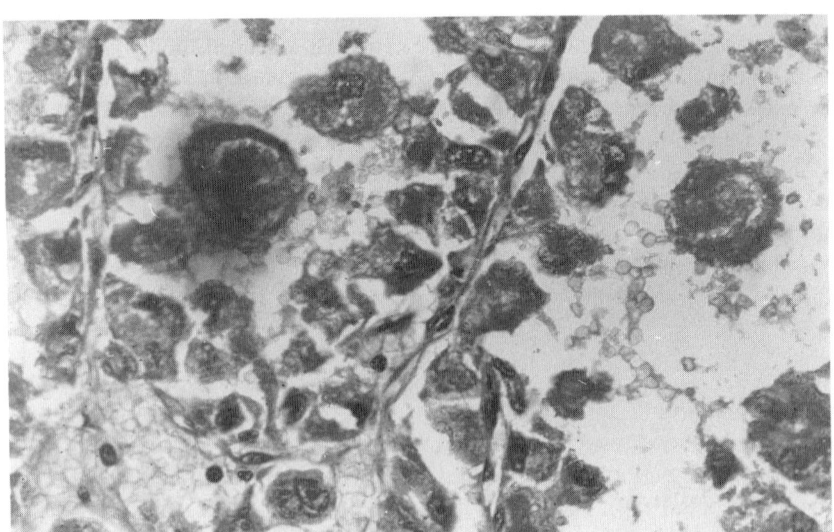

Fig. 22.19. Alveolar soft part sarcoma: alveolar arrangement of polyhedral cells

22.4.2.3.1 Gross Appearance

The alveolar soft part sarcomas are well circumscribed and encapsulated tumours varying in size from 1.5 to 10 cm. The tumours are firm in consistency, and the cut surface is yellow-white to buffy-grey in appearance.

22.4.2.3.2 Microscopical Appearance

The tumours are composed of a characteristic alveolar, pseudo-alveolar or organoid arrangement of cells which are large, round and polyhedral with vacuolated or granular eosinophilic cytoplasm and oval, vasicular nuclei with irregular rims (Fig. 22.19). The nucleoli are small but may be prominent. Occasional binucleate cells can be seen within the tumour, but mitoses are rare. The cytoplasm of the tumour cells contains diastase-resistant, PAS-positive crystalline material which has been suggested by ultrastructural studies to be aggregates of secretion granules and protein in nature (Kasai et al. 1980). The crystals are bounded by a limiting membrane, a characteristic feature differentiating them from the crystals found in rhabdomyoma (Welsh et al. 1972). The individual alveolus or organoid nest of cells is bounded by distinct basal lamina and separated from one another by thin-walled vascular channels. Irregular bands of fibrous tissue are often seen to course through the tumour, separating these alveoli and nests into numerous groupings. Fisher and Reibord (1971) have suggested a myogenous origin of the tumour, thus making it a unique type of rhabdomyosarcoma, while Deschryver-Kieskemiti et al. (1982) thought that it derives from renal juxtaglomerular cells.

22.4.2.3.3 Behaviour

Vascular invasion by the tumour cells is common, and metastasis occurs early. The tumours may recur locally in 25% of patients (Lieberman et al. 1966). Occasional patients survive up to 20 years, but the overall 5-year survival rate is about 59% (Lieberman et al. 1966). The most common sites of metastasis are the lungs, bones and brain.

22.4.2.3.4 Treatment

Radical resection and adjuvant chemotherapy and/or immunotherapy have been recommended by Shen et al. (1982). These tumours are only moderately radiosensitive (Asvall et al. 1969). For tumours with local recurrences after an excision with wide margin, local radiation may be indicated (Chapman et al. 1984). Chemotherapy does not seem to be effective, although thiotepa has been beneficial in two patients (Asvall et al. 1969). A few reports found local excision, radiotherapy and chemotherapy ineffective (Ruberfield 1971; Blumberg and Chang 1976).

22.4.2.4 Vaginal Haemanigopericytoma

The tumour haemangiopericytoma, originally described by Stout and Murray (1942), is uncommon in the female genital tract, in which the majority have been reported in the myometrium. In a series of 106 patients described by Enzinger and Smith (1976), the lower extremities were found to be the most common sites, followed by the retroperitoneium and pelvis. There are only two reported cases of vaginal haemangiopericytomas in the English literature (Buscema et al. 1985; Hiura et al. 1985).

22.4.2.4.1 Clinical Features

One of the patients with a vaginal tumour was 50 years old and presented with vaginal bleeding. The tumour was 5 cm in diameter and located in the recto-vaginal septum. The other patient was 20 years old and presented with a 5 cm mass protruding from the vaginal orifice. Her main complaints were a gradually increasing painful mass and vaginal bleeding.

The tumours, particularly those of retroperitoneal location, can be associated with paraneoplastic hypoglycaemia and autoimmune haemolytic anaemia (Wilbanks et al. 1975).

22.4.2.4.2 Gross Appearance

Haemangiopericytomas are well-circumscribed tumours which vary in size from less than 1–20 cm; the average is about 5 cm. They have been described as meaty, friable, firm and rubbery, with colour ranging from grey to tan. Cystic changes and haemorrhages are often present.

22.4.2.4.3 Microscopical Appearance

The tumours are composed of densely packed, elongated and oval cells with a moderate amount of eosinophilic cytoplasm and round to oval, vesicular to hyperchromatic nuclei arranged in various-sized, numerous, vascular channels. The cytoplasmic borders of the cells are often indistinct, and nuclear outlines are irregular. The nucleoli are generally absent and when present are inconspicuous. The number of mitotic figures varies, and 2–3 figures per 10 high power fields may be noticed. Tumours displaying 4 or more mitotic figures per 10 high power fields, pleomorphism and increased cellularity tend to be aggressive with a rapid growth potential and distant metastasis (Enzinger and Weiss 1983). Histological criteria on the other hand have been considered unreliable in classifying these tumours into benign and malignant forms (Backwinkel and Diddams 1970). The blood vessels are thin and lined by a single layer of flattened endothelial cells. Areas of haemorrhage and necrosis may be present in the aggressive tumours. Myxoid changes may also occur. With silver preparation the individual tumour cell is seen to be surrounded by reticulin fibres.

The tumour is of uncertain histogenesis but generally believed to arise from the pericytes, the cells first described by Zimmermann (1923) as specialised, elongated and contractile mesenchymal cells which surround the endothelial-lined blood vessels.

The tumour cells are ultrastructurally oval to elongated in shape, arranged in nests in close association with the blood vessels (Buscema et al. 1985; Hiura et al. 1985; Hahn et al. 1973; Eimoto 1977; Newland et al. 1978). The cell cytoplasm contains numerous free fibrosomes, sparse endoplasmic reticulum, a few large mitochondria and bundles of microfilaments with polymorphic dense spots. The cytoplasmic processes are broad and show interdigitations in places. The cell junctions are generally poorly developed. These appearances have been stated to be consistent with the pericytic origin of the tumour cells.

22.4.2.4.4 Behaviour

The haemangiopericytomas are known to be aggressive, with a tendency to recurrence and metastases. Late recurrences (after 5 years) are not uncommon, and metastases can appear in up to 50% of patients (Cook et al. 1974). The uterine tumours on the other hand appear to bear a better prognosis (Wilbanks et al. 1975) and are relatively less aggressive than the tumours of other sites (Harris 1972). The tumours showing more than 4 mitotic figures per 10 high power fields hypercellularity and pleomorphism are more likely to behave aggressively.

22.4.2.4.5 Treatment

Wide surgical excision of the tumours should be the optimum treatment. With surgery the cure rate is about 53%, whereas with radiotherapy it is only about 13% (Backwinkel and Diddams 1970). The incompletely excised tumours should be treated with adequate doses of radiotherapy. For metastatic and recurrent disease, additional surgery, irradiation and chemotherapy have been advocated (Wilbanks et al. 1975).

22.4.2.5 Malignant Fibrous Histiocytoma

Malignant fibrous histiocytoma (MFH) is one of the most common sarcomas of soft tissue (Kearney et al. 1980) (see also Vulva). According to O'Brien and Stout (1964), it is of histiocytic origin. The tumour occurs usually in middle to late adult life (Limacher et al. 1978). The common sites are the extremities, followed by the trunk and retroperitoneal area (Kearney et al. 1980). The tumours are rare in the female genital tract, and only about half a dozen cases have been reported from the vulva and vagina. Webb et al. (1974) described an asymptomatic, 31-year-old patient with a vaginal lesion consisting of four nodules; the largest one was 2 cm in diameter. The tumour was located in the left posterolateral wall of the vagina, 4 cm from the introitus, and at and around the site of a previous operation. She had a nodule in the posterior vaginal wall removed 3 years earlier. Upon further review, the lesion was found to be a malignant fibrous histiocytoma. Microscopically, the nodule was composed predominantly of spindle cells with a vague storiform pattern, intercellular collagen and mitotic figures (Webb et al. 1974). The patient was treated by abdominal total hysterectomy, with removal of the left upper third of the vagina and a wedge of perineal tissue. There was no further recurrence at 16 months when the patient came for follow-up.

Generally, these tumours can be superficial in the subcutaneous tissue or deep within the muscle.

22.4.2.5.1 Gross Appearance

MFH occurs as nodules of various sizes, which on their cut surfaces are firm in consistency and grey to pink-white and yellowish in appearance.

22.4.2.5.2 Microscopical Appearance

The tumours are composed of spindle and round cells organised in a storiform pattern, benign and malignant giant cells and a variable number of inflammatory cells (Weiss and Enzinger 1978). The tumour also contains many foam cells (Limacher et al. 1978). Several histological sub-types have been described, namely fibrous, giant cell, myxoid and inflammatory (Kearney et al. 1980). The tumours display frequent mitotic figures.

22.4.2.5.3 Behaviour

MFH tends to recur and metastasise with rates of 44% and 42%, respectively (Weiss and Enzinger 1978). Metastases occur by the haematogenous and lymphatic routes. The deeper tumours carry a worse prognosis than the superficial ones (Kearney et al. 1980).

22.4.2.5.4 Treatment

Early surgical removal of the tumour is indicated (Weiss and Enzinger 1978), with a wide margin (Kearney et al. 1980). Post-surgical radiotherapy and chemotherapy should be considered according to the extent and stage of the lesion (Kearney et al. 1980).

22.4.2.6 Angiosarcoma

Malignant tumours arising from the endothelial cells of a blood vessel have been so rarely reported in the vagina (Marck et al. 1953; Prempree et al. 1983) that their incidence, behaviour and treatment are difficult to evaluate.

Generally, angiosarcomas occur commonly in the skin, soft tissue and less commonly in the deeper organs. In the female genital organs, except the breast, the uterus appears to be the most common site. The patient with a vaginal tumour may present with irregular menstruation or post-coital bleeding (Marck et al. 1953) or may be asymptomatic (Prempree et al. 1983).

22.4.2.6.1 Gross Appearance
The tumours are 1–5 cm in size, reddish, polypoid and soft and tend to be ulcerated.

22.4.2.6.2 Microscopical Appearance
The tumours are composed of intercommunicating vascular channels lined by irregular and hyperchromatic endothelial cells displaying mitoses. Endothelial cell-lined, short, papillary structures can be seen in the irregular vascular spaces. There are also areas of spindle-shaped and epithelial-like cells arranged in a solid pattern. Silver stains outline the vascular channels. In the immunoperoxidase reactions, the tumour cells are seen to be positive for factor VIII antigen.

22.4.2.6.3 Behaviour
Angiosarcomas tend to recur and ultimately to metastasise by the blood stream.

22.4.2.6.4 Treatment
Prempree et al. (1983) advocated combined external and intra-cavitary brachytherapy after excision of the tumour.

22.4.2.7 Myxosarcoma

Reports on myxosarcoma of the female genital tract are scanty. Christie (1945) mentioned one occurring in the vagina of a 39-year-old woman. The tumour was an unencapsulated nodule of rubbery consistency with myxomatous stroma. The tumour had an infiltrating margin and was treated by surgical excision followed by radiotherapy. The patient was well at the 5-year follow-up. From the histological description, the exact nature of the tumour is difficult to ascertain, but it could be an adult-type rhabdomyoma or leiomyoma with myxoid changes. Other cases reported as myxosarcoma are probably heterogenous sarcomas with myxoid changes (Diehl and Haught 1946; Amolseh 1939). Some authors (Sponsel et al. 1952) believe that myxosarcoma as a separate entity does exist and can metastasise.

22.4.2.8 Aggressive Angiomyxoma

See under Vulva.

22.4.3 Tumour-like Conditions

22.4.3.1 Angiomyolipoma of the Vagina

Angiomyolipoma is a hamartomatous growth commonly occurring in the renal parenchyma of patients with tuberous sclerosis complex. Occurrence in the normal population is rare. The other stigmata of the complex are focal thickening of the astrocytic fibrils in the brain, retinal phacomas, cutaneous adenoma sebaceum, subungual nodules, cardiac glycogen-filled nodules, pulmonary fibrosis and bronchial hamartomas. It is an autosomally dominant disease. Expression of the complex varies from multiple organ involvement to the solitary lesion in the kidney (Farrow et al. 1968). Some 68% of patients with tuberous sclerosis may have renal angiolipomas (Walker et al. 1976). In non-tuberous lesions the renal lesion is unilateral and solitary (McCullogh et al. 1971). Rarely, angiomyolipoma occurs at other sites (Busch et al. 1976; Brody and Lipshutz 1955), including the female genital tract. The rare lipoleiomyoma of the uterus bears close similarities to angiolipoma (Demopoulos et al. 1973). The condition has also been reported in the vagina (Peh and Sivanesaratnam 1988). The patient was a 46-year-old woman who presented with progressive lower abdominal swelling for 3 months. On exploration, the lesion was found to arise from the sub-mucosa of the vaginal wall. Rare adipocytic metaplasia, which has been reported in the vaginal wall (Honore 1980), should not be confused with angiomyolipoma.

22.4.3.1.1 Gross Appearance

The renal angiomyolipomas vary in size from a few to many centimeters (Hajdu and Foote 1969). The vaginal mass was 20 cm in diameter. The lesion is a circumscribed, unencapsulated mass, grey to grey-yellow in colour. The cut surface may show haemorrhage and necrosis.

22.4.3.1.2 Microscopical Appearance

Angiomyolipomas are composed of fat, smooth muscles and blood vessels. The fat cells are mature, with large cytoplasmic vacuoles and peripheral nuclei. The smooth muscle cells may be arranged haphazardly or in bundles displaying an occasional mitosis. In some areas they may appear to be streaming from the wall of the blood vessels. The blood vessels are of small and medium-sized arteries with thickened walls and an eccentric lumen. Any of the components, lipomatous, leimyomatous or angiomatous, may predominte. Many of the angiomyomas show a bizarre histological picture with nuclear hyperchromasia and pleomorphism (Hajdu and Foote 1969).

22.4.3.1.3 Treatment

Angiomyolipomas are benign. Renal lesions are usually treated by partial nephrectomy if possible. The vaginal tumour was removed surgically via the abdominal route (Peh and Sivanesaratnam 1988).

22.4.3.2 Reactive Fibrohistiocytic Proliferation Simulating Histiocytoma

Several fibrohistiocytic proliferative lesions occurring in response to surgical trauma and foreign bodies have recently been reported under headings such as reactive fibrohistiocytic lesion simulating histiocytoma, spindle cell nodules, etc. (Weiss et al. 1978; Snover et al. 1981; Proppe et al. 1984). The importance of recognition of these lesions lies in their histological similarity to some benign and malignant mesenchymal tumours for which they may be mistaken. The lesions grow as ill-defined nodules to an average size of 3 cm over a period of weeks or months. Histologically, they are composed of bundles of spindle cells arranged either in a storiform pattern (Snover et al. 1981) or intersecting fascicles of spindle cells (Proppe et al. 1984). Some lesions may display a mild degree of cellular pleomorphism and mitotic figures. The overall appearances are, however, bland. Inflammatory cells – lymphocytes, histiocytes, plasma cells and polymorphs – in variable numbers are always present in these reactive lesions. Some lesions contain foreign body-type giant cells.

Ultrastructurally, the cells display lipid droplets, phagolysosomes, microfilaments with dense bodies and basal lamina suggesting a myofibroblastic nature.

They are nonneoplastic and of limited growth potential. Although most of the reported lesions have been reactive, they may occasionally arise spontaneously (Ro et al. 1986).

22.4.3.2.1 Treatment

Adequate excision of the lesion is curative.

References

Leiomyoma

Adduci J (1965) Leiomyoma of the anterior vaginal wall in a suburethral location causing stress incontinence: report of a case. J Urol 96:255–257

Bennett HG, Ehrlich MM (1941) Myoma of the vagina. Am J Obstet Gynecol 42:314–320

Berman W (1938) Myoma of the vagina. J Miss State Med Assoc 35:215–216

Farell DM, Abrams J (1956) Myoma of the vagina. Am J Obstet Gynecol 72:455–456

Ingemanson C-A, Alfredsson J (1970) Recurrent fibromyoma of the vagina: a case report. Acta Obstet Gynecol Scand 49:271–273

Kaufman RH, Gardner HL (1964) Tumors of the vulva and vagina benign mesodermal tumors. Clin Obstet Gynecol 8:953–981

Marcus JL (1966) Fibromyoma of vagina. J Obstet Gynaecol Br Commonw 73:1013–1015

Moghissi K (1960) Myoma of the vagina: report of a case and review of literature. Obstet Gynecol 15:235–236

Nurnberger L (1930) Handbuch der Gynäkologie, 3rd edn. Veit-Stoeckel, Munich, p 489

Quan A, Birnbaum SJ (1961) Vaginal leiomyoma: report of a case and review of literature. Obstet Gynecol 18:360–362

Rywlin AM, Simmonds RJ, Robinson MJ (1969) Leiomyoma of vagina recurrent in pregnancy. South Med J 62:1449–1451

Schonberg LA, Oliver R, Burks N et al. (1963) Giant fibromyoma of the vagina complicating pregnancy: report of a case. Obstet Gynecol 22:234–236

Sered H, Philipp EA, Foss HG (1956) Suburethral fibromas. Am J Obstet Gynecol 71:1362–1365

Shanahan TH (1942) Large tumor of vagina. Am J Surg 56:513

Tavassoli FA, Norris HJ (1979) Smooth muscle tumors of the vagina. Obstet Gynecol 53:689–693

Neurofibroma

Azzopardi JG, Eusebi V, Tison V et al. (1983) Neurofibroma with rhabdomyomatous differentiation: benign 'Triton' tumour of the vagina. Histopathology 7:561–572

Gold BM (1972) Neurofibromatosis of the bladder and vagina. Am J Obstet Gynecol 113:1055–1056

Hosoi K (1951) Multiple neurofibromatosis (von Recklinghausen's disease) with special references to malignant transformation. Arch Surg 22:258–281

Norris JW, Cooper JR (1950) Primary neurofibroma of the vagina: a case report. J Kans Med Soc 51:128–130

Tavassoli FA, Norris HJ (1979) Smooth muscle tumors of the vagina. Obstet Gynecol 53:689–693

Rhabdomyoma

Ceremasak RJ (1969) Benign rhabdomyoma of the vagina. Am J Clin Pathol 52:604–606

Cornog JL Jr, Gontas LK (1967) Ultrastructure of rhabdomyoma. J Ultrastruct Res 20:433–450

Dehner LP, Enzinger FM, Font RL (1972) Fetal rhabdomyoma – an analysis of nine cases. Cancer 30:160–166

Di Sant Agnese PA, Knowles DM II (1980) Extracardiact rhabdomyoma: a clinicopathologic study and review of the literature. Cancer 46:780–789

Gad A, Eusebi V (1975) Rhabdomyoma of the vagina. J Pathol 115:179–181

Gold JH, Bossen EH (1976) Benign vaginal rhabdomyoma a light and electron microscopic study. Cancer 37:2283–2284

Leoni PG, Taylor HB (1973) Ultrastructure of benign polypoid rhabdomyoma of the vagina. Cancer 31:1414–1417

Moran JJ, Enterline HT (1964) Benign rhabdomyoma of the pharynx: a case report: review of the literature and comparison with cardiac rhabdomyoma. Am J Clin Pathol 42:174–181

Pendl F (1897) Über ein congenitales Rhabdomyom der Zunge. Z Heilkunde 18:457–468

Tsukuda Y, Pickern JW (1965) Rhabdomyoma of sublingual region – a report of a case. Oral Surg 20:640–644

Glomus Tumour

Appleberg DB, Teasley JL (1968) Unusual locations and manifestations of glomus tumors (glomangiomas). Am J Surg 116:62–64

Banner EA, Winkelman RK (1957) Glomus tumor of the vagina: report of a case. Obstet Gynecol 9:326–328

Shugart RR, Soule EH, Johnson EW Jr (1963) Glomus tumor. Surg Gynecol Obstet 117:334-340

Spitzer M, Molho L, Seltzer VL (1985) Vaginal glomus tumor: case presentation and ultrastructural findings. Obstet Gynecol 66 [Suppl]:86–88

Venkatachalam MA, Greally JG (1969) Fine structure of glomus tumor: similarity of glomus cells to smooth muscle. Cancer 23:1176–1184

Sarcoma Botryoides

Bizer LS (1969) Rhabdomyosarcoma. Am J Surg 118:453–458

Conte PJ, Segerman RH (1971) Embyronal rhabdomyosarcoma of the middle ear with long term survival. N Engl J Med 284:92–93

Copeland LJ, Gershenson DM, Saul PB et al. (1985) Sarcoma botryoides of the female genital tract. Obstet Gynecol 66:262–266
Crawford EJ (1959) Sarcoma botryoides: a case report. Am J Obstet Gynecol 78:618–620
Cywes S, Louw JH (1961) Sarcoma botryoides of the vagina: a report of two cases. S Afr Med J 35:911-917
Daniel WW, Koss LG, Brunschwig A (1959) Sarcoma botryoides of the vagina. Cancer 12:74–84
De la Monte SM, Hutchins GM, Moore GW (1986) Metastatic behavior of rhabdomyosarcoma. Pathol Res Pract 181:148–152
Donaldson SS, Castro JR, Wilbur JR et al. (1973) Rhabdomyosarcoma of head and neck in children: combination treatment by surgery, irradiation and chemotherapy. Cancer 31:26–35
Dorgan LT (1953) Sarcoma botryoides: a case report. Obstet Gynecol 2:127–132
Duckett HC, Davis CD, McCall JB (1957) Sarcoma botryoides, a clinical and pathological review and report of four new cases. Obstet Gynecol 9:517–522
Duncan AS, Fahmy EC (1953) Sarcoma botryoides of the vagina and cervix in chidlren: a report of 2 cases and a plea for early diagnosis. J Obstet Gynaecol Br Commonw 60:87–91
Edland RW (1965) Embryonal rhabdomyosarcoma. Am J Roentgenol Radium Ther Nucl Med 93:671–685
Ehrlich FE, Haas JE, Kieswetter WB (1971) Rhabdomyosarcomas in infants and children: factors affecting long term survival. J Pediatr Surg 6:571–577
El-Mahdi AM, Marks RM Jr, Thornton WN et al. (1974) Twenty five year survival of sarcoma botryoides treated by irradiation. Cancer 33:653–656
Exelby PR (1974) Management of embryonal rhabdomyosarcoma in children. Surg Clin North Am 54:849–857
Farinacci CJ, Fairchild JP, Sulak MH et al. (1956) Sarcoma botryoides (form of embryonal rhabdomyosarcoma) of common bile duct: report of 2 cases. Cancer 9:408–417
Flamant F, Chassagne D, Cosset J-M et al. (1979) Embryonal rhabdomyosarcoma of the vagina in children: conservative treatment with curietherapy and chemotherapy. Eur J Cancer 15:527–533
Ghavimi F, Exelby PR, D'Angio GJ (1973) Combination therapy of urogenital embryonal rhabdomyosarcoma in children. Cancer 32:1178–1185
Gonzalez-Crussi F (1979) Rhabdomyosarcoma of infancy and childhood. Am J Surg Pathol 3:157–170
Grosfield JL, Cartworthy HW Jr, Newton WA Jr (1969) Combined therapy in childhood rhabdomyosarcoma: an analysis of 42 cases. J Pediatr Surg 4:637–645
Grosfield JL, Smith JP, Cartworthy HW Jr (1972) Pelvic rhabdomyosarcoma in infants and children. J Urol 107:673–675
Hays D, Shimada H, Raney RB et al. (1988) Clinical staging and treatment results in rhabdomyosarcoma of the female genital tract among children and adolescents. Cancer 61:1893–1903
Heyen RM, Holland R, Newton WA et al. (1974) The role of combined chemotherapy in the treatment of rhabdomyosarcoma in children. Cancer 34:2128–2142
Hilgers RD (1975) Pelvic exenteration for vaginal embryonal carcinoma. Obstet Gynecol 45:175–180
Hilgers RD, Malkasian GD Jr, Soule EH (1970) Embryonal rhabdomyosarcoma (botryoid type) of the vagina: a clinicopathologic review. Am J Obstet Gynecol 107:484–502
Hilgers RD, Ghavimi F, D'Angio GJ et al. (1973) Memorial hospital experience with pelvic exenteration and embryonal rhabdomyosarcoma of the vagina. Gynecol Oncol 1:262–270
Holton CP, Chapman KE, Lackey RW et al. (1973) Extended combination therapy of childhood rhabdomyosarcoma. Cancer 32:1310–1316
Horn RC Jr, Enterline HT (1958) Rhabdomyosarcoma: a clinicopathological study and classification of 39 cases. Cancer 11:181–199
Kaufman SL, Stout AP (1965) Congenital mesenchymal tumors. Cancer 18:460–476

Lacey SR, Jewett TC Jr, Karp MP et al. (1986) Advances in the treatment of rhabdomyosarcoma. Semin Surg Oncol 2:139–146

Lawrence W Jr, Hays DM, Moon TE (1977) Lymphatic metastases with childhood rhabdomyosarcomas. Cancer 39:556–559

Lederman M (1956) Radiotherapy in the treatment of orbital tumours: Br J Ophthalmol 40:592–610

Maurer HM, Moon T, Donaldson M et al. (1977) The intergroup rhabdomyosarcoma study. Cancer 40:2015–2026

McFarland J (1935) Dysontogenetic and mixed tumours of urogenital region: with report of new case: sarcoma botryoides vaginae in child and comments upon nature of sarcoma. Surg Gynecol Obstet 61:42–57

Nakamura Y, Nakashima T, Nakashima H et al. (1981) Bilateral cystic nephroblastomas and botryoid sarcoma involving vagina and urinary bladder in a child with microcephaly, archinecephaly and bilateral cataracts. Cancer 48:1012–1015

National Institute of Health (1975) Intergroup rhabdomyosarcoma study. Objectives and clinical staging, classification. Pediatr Surg 10:977–978

Nelson AJ III (1968) Embryonal rhabdomysarcoma: report of twenty four cases and study of the effectiveness of radiation therapy upon the primary tumour. Cancer 22:64–68

Ober WB, Edgcomb JH (1954) Sarcoma botryoides in female genital tract. Cancer 7:75–91

Ober WB, Smith JA, Rouilard FC (1958) Congenital sarcoma botryoides of the vagina: report of 2 cases. Cancer 11:620–623

Patton RB, Horn RC Jr (1962) Rhabdomysarcoma: clinical and pathological features and comparison with human fetal and embryonal skeletal muscle. Surgery 52:572–584

Pratt CB, Hustu HO, Fleming ID et al. (1972) Co-ordinated treatment of childhood rhabdomyosarcoma with surgery, radiotherapy and combinec chemotherapy. Cancer Res 32:606–610

Rigby C (1966) The pathology of rhabdomyosarcoma in children. Proc R Soc Med 59:411–412

Rivard G, Ortega J, Hittle R et al. (1975) Intensive chemotherapy as primary treatment for rhabdomyosarcoma of the pelvis. Cancer 36:1593–1597

Rutledge F, Sullivan MP (1967) Sarcoma botryoides. Ann NY Acad Sci 142:694–708

Shirkey HC, Saenger EL (1978) Sarcoma botryoides of the vagina in childhood, treated by irradiation and vaginal reconstruction. Am J Obstet Gynecol 132:339–340

Sirsat MV (1953) Sarcoma botryoides. Indian J Med Res 41:379–381

Spademan LC, Cohen ES, Girton FW (1953) Sarcoma botryoides. Am J Obstet Gynecol 65:203–207

Stobbe GD, Dargeon HW (1950) Embryonal rhabdomyosarcoma of head and neck in children and adolescents. Cancer 3:826–836

Stout AP (1946) Rhabdomyosarcoma of skeletal muscle. Ann Surg 123:447–472

Tank ES, Fellman SL, Wheeler ES et al. (1972) Treatment of urogenital tract rhabdomyosarcoma in infants and children. J Urol 107:324–328

Tefft M, Jaffe N (1973) Sarcoma of the bladder and prostate in children: rationale for the role of radiation therapy based on review of literature and report of 14 additional patients. Cancer 32:1161–1177

Tefft M, Fernandez CH, Moon TE (1977) Rhabdomyosarcoma response with chemotherapy prior to radiation in patients with gross residual disease. Cancer 39:665–670

Weichert KA, Bove KC, Aron BS et al. (1976) Rhabdomyosarcoma in children: a clinicopathological study of 35 patients. Am J Clin Pathol 66:692–701

Leiomyosarcoma

Akhtar M, Ahmeduddin J, Valencia M (1978) Primary leiomyosarcoma of the vagina: light and electron microscopic study of a case with review of literature. Tex Med 74:67–71

Brown KL, Segal AJ, Hurd GB (1960) Masses of the rectovaginal septum: a proposed classification review of the literature and report of a case of leiomyosarcoma. Am J Surg 99:309–315
Davos I, Abell MR (1976) Sarcomas of the vagina. Obstet Gynecol 47:342–350
Malkasian GD Jr, Welch JS, Soule EH (1963) Primary leiomyosarcoma of the vagina. Am J Obstet Gynecol 86:730–736
Peters WA III, Kumar NB, Andersen WA (1985) Primary sarcoma of the adult vagina: a clinicopathologic study. Obstet Gynecol 65:699–704
Rastogi BL, Bergman B, Angervall L (1984) Primary leiomyosarcoma of the vagina: a study of five cases. Gynecol Oncol 18:77–86
Schram M (1958) Leiomyoma of the vagina: report of a case and review of literature. Obstet Gynecol 12:195–198
Tavassoli FA, Norris HJ (1979) Smooth muscle tumours of the vagina. Obstet Gynecol 53:689–693
Tobon H, Murphy AI, Salazar H (1973) Primary leiomyosarcoma of the vagina: light and electron microscopic observations. Cancer 32:450–457

Alveolar Soft Part Sarcoma
Asvall JE, Hoeg K, Kleppe K et al. (1969) Alveolar soft part sarcoma. Clin Radiol 20:426–432
Blumberg MB, Chang CHJ (1976) Alveolar soft part sarcoma. South Med J 69:282–285
Chapman GW, Bendar J, Williams T (1984) Alveolar soft part sarcoma of the vagina. Gynecol Oncol 18:125–129
Christopherson WM, Foote FW Jr, Stewart FW (1952) Alveolar soft part sarcoma. Cancer 5:100–111
Deschryver-Kieskemiti K, Kraus FT, Engleman W et al. (1982) Alveolar soft part sarcoma – a malignant angioreninoma. Am J Surg Pathol 6:5–18
Fisher ER, Reibord H (1971) Electron microscopic evidence suggesting the myogenous derivation of the so-called alveolar soft part sarcoma. Cancer 27:150–159
Kasai K, Yoshidar Y, Okumura M (1980) Alveolar soft part sarcoma in the vagina: clinical features and morphology. Gynecol Oncol 9:227–236
Lieberman PH, Foote FW Jr, Stewart FW et al. (1966) Alveolar soft part sarcoma. JAMA 198:1047–1051
O'Toole RV, Tuttle SE, Lucas JG et al. (1985) Alveolar soft part sarcoma of the vagina: an immunochemical and electron microscopic study. Int J Gynecol Path 4:258–265
Ruberfeld S (1971) Radiation therapy in alveolar soft part sarcoma. Cancer 28:577–580
Shen J, D'Ablaing G, Morrow CP (1982) Alveolar soft part sarcoma of the vulva: report of the first case and review of the literature. Gynecol Oncol 13:120–128
Welsh RA, Bray DM III, Shipkey FH et al. (1972) Histogenesis of alveolar soft part sarcoma. Cancer 29:191–204

Haemangiopericytoma
Backwinkel K, Diddams JA (1970) Hemangiopericytoma: report of a case and comprehensive review of the literature. Cancer 25:896–901
Buscema J, Rosenshein NB, Taqi F et al. (1985) Vaginal hemangiopericytoma: a histopathologic and ultrastructural evaluation. Obstet Gynecol 66 [Suppl]:82–85
Cook C, Kakos GS, Roberts S (1974) Hemangiopericytoma: a case report and rationale for aggressive therapy. Cancer 34:1830–1833
Eimoto T (1977) Ultrastructure of an infantile hemangiopericytoma. Cancer 40:2161–2170
Enzinger FM, Smith BH (1976) Hemangiopericytoma: an analyse of 106 cases. Hum Pathol 7:61–82
Enzinger FM, Weiss SW (1983) Hemangiopericytoma in soft tissue tumors. Mosby, St Louis, pp 463–481

Hahn MJ, Dawson R, Esterly JE aet al. (1973) Hemangiopericytoma an ultrastructural study. Cancer 31:255–261

Harris HR (1972) Two cases of haemangiopericytoma arising in the uterus. J Clin Pathol 25:556-557

Hiura M, Nagawa T, Nagai N et al. (1985) Vaginal hemangiopericytoma: a light microscopic and ultrastructural study. Gynecol Oncol 21:374–384

Newland RC, Maxwell LE, Constance TJ et al. (1978) Malignant haemanigopericytoma: case report and ultrastructural study. Pathology 10:277–283

Stout AP, Murray MR (1942) Haemangiopericytoma: a vascular tumour featuring Zimmermann's pericytes. Ann Surg 116:26–33

Wilbanks GD, Szymanska Z, Miller AW (1975) Pelvic hemangiopericytoma: a report of 4 patients and review of the literature. Am J Obstet Gynecol 123:555–569

Zimmermann KW (1923) Der feinere Bau der Blutkapillaren. Z Anat Entwicklungsgesch 68:29–109

Malignant Fibrous Histiocytoma

Kearney MM, Soule EH, Ivins JC (1980) Malignant fibrous histiocytoma, a retrospective study of 167 cases. Cancer 45:167–178

Limacher J, Delage C, Lagace R (1978) Malignant fibrous histiocytoma. Am J Surg Pathol 2:265–274

O'Brien JE, Stout AP (1964) Malignant fibrous xanthoma. Cancer 17:1445–1455

Webb MJ, Symmonds RE, Weiland LH (1974) Malignant fibrous histiocytoma of the vagina. Am J Obstet Gynecol 119:190–192

Weiss SW, Enzinger FM (1978) Malignant fibrous histiocytoma. An analysis of 200 cases. Cancer 41:2250–2266

Angiosarcoma

Marck A, Wirthwein C, Melamed A (1953) Hemangioendothelioma of the vagina. Am J Obstet Gynecol 66:436–440

Prempree T, Tank C-K, Hatef A et al. (1983) Angiosarcoma of the vagina: a clinicopathologic report. Cancer 51:618–622

Myxosarcoma

Amolseh AL (1939) Mixed mesodermal tumours of the uterus and vagina. Am J Cancer 37:435–444

Christie GS (1945) Myosarcoma of the vagina associated with early pregnancy. Am J Obstet Gynecol 50:553–554

Diehl WK, Haught JS (1946) Sarcoma of the vagina. Am J Obstet Gynecol 52:302–310

Sponsel KH, McDonald JR, Ghormley PK (1952) Myxoma and myxosarcoma of the soft tissues of the extremities. J Bone Joint Surg [Am] 34:820–826

Angiomyolipoma

Brody H, Lipshutz H (1955) Concomitant intrarenal and pararenal angiomyolipomas. J Urol 74:741–746

Busch FM, Bark CJ, Clyde HR (1976) Benign renal angiolipoma with regional lymph node involvement. J Urol 116:715–717

Demopoulos RI, Denarvaez F, Kaji V (1973) Benign mesodermal of the uterus: a histogenetic study. Am J Clin Pathol 60:377–383

Farrow GM, Harrison EG Jr, Utz DC et al. (1968) Renal angiomyolipoma: a clinicopathologic study of 32 cases. Cancer 22:564–570

Hajdu SI, Foote FW Jr (1969) Angiomyolipoma of the kidney: report of 27 cases and review of the literature. J Urol 102:396–401

Honore LH (1980) Adipocytic metaplasia associated with idiopathic vaginal adinosis. Case report. Aust NZ J Obstet Gynaecol 20:129–131

McCullogh DL, Scott R Jr, Seybold HM (1971) Renal angiolipoma (hamartoma): review of the literature and report of 7 cases. J Urol 105:32–44

Peh SC, Sivanesaratnam V (1988) Angiomyolipoma of the vagina – an uncommon tumor. Case report. Br J Obstet Gynaecol 95:820–823

Walker DE, Barry JM, Hodges CV (1976) Angiomyolipoma: diagnosis and treatment. J Urol 116:712–714

Reactive Fibrohistiocytic Proliferation

Proppe KH, Scully RE, Rosai J (1984) Post operative spindle cell nodules of genitourinary tract resembling sarcoma. Am J Surg Pathol 8:101–108

Ro JY, Ayala AG, Ordonez NG et al. (1986) Pseudosarcomatous fibromyxoid tumour of the urinary bladder. Am J Clin Patahol 86:583–590

Snover DC, Phillips G, Dehner LP (1981) Reactive fibrohistiocytic proliferation simulating fibrous histiocytoma. Am J Clin Pathol 76:232–235

Weiss SW, Enzinger FM, Johnson FB (1978) Silica reaction simulating fibrous histiocytoma. Cancer 42:2738–2743

22.5 Lymphoma

Vaginal lymphomas are most often part of the systemic lesions and of non-Hodgkin's type lymphoma. The incidence of involvement of the female genital tract by lymphomas has been estimated to be about 30%, with vaginal involvement in 7% (Lathrop 1967). The primary lesion or initial manifestation in the female genital tract is very rare. Iliya et al. (1968) on analysis of autopsies of patients with reticulum cell sarcoma found only 4% arising in the female genital tract. The initial presentation of Hodgkin's disease is rarely extra-nodal (Lamb 1982). Patients with vaginal lymphomas are all elderly women (4th to 7th decades of age) who present with dyspareunia (Buchler and Kline 1972), abnormal vaginal bleeding (Chorlton et al. 1974), vaginal discharge or vaginal mass. There are several clinical staging systems of lymphoma. The Ann Arbor Clinical System (Carbone et al. 1971) for extra-nodal lymphomas can be used for staging the lymphomas of the female genital tract:

Stage I – Involvement of a single lymph node region (I) or of a single extra-lymphatic organ or site (IE)

Stage II – Involvement of two or more lymph node regions on the same side of the diaphragm (II) or localised involvement of an extra-lymphatic organ or site and of one or more lymph node regions on the same side of the diaphragm (IIE)

Stage III – Involvement of lymph node regions on both sides of the diaphragm (III) which may also be accompanied by localised involvement of the spleen (IIIS), extra-lamphatic site (IIIE) or both (IIISE)

Stage IV – Diffuse or disseminated involvement of one or more extra-lymphatic organs or tissue with or without associated lymph node enlargement

According to this system, the involvement of the uterus, cervix, vagina and/or parametrial tissues in contiguity should be included in stage IE and involvement of pelvic and/or abdominal nodes in stage IIE (Harris and Scully 1984).

The FIGO clinical classification can also be applied in the staging of malignant lymphomas and has been found to correlate fairly well with survival (Chorlton et al. 1979). About 50% of vaginal lymphomas are in the FIGO stage I when first discovered. The survival rate is better with this localised disease.

22.5.1 Gross Appearance

The vaginal lymphomas present as nodules of about 2–3 cm in size, occasionally as an ill-defined thickening or induration on the vaginal wall.

22.5.2 Microscopical Appearance

Diagnosis of lymphomas from vaginal biopsies is difficult unless one keeps in mind that the female genital tract can also be a rare primary site of lymphomas. Diagnosis such as chronic inflammation or anaplastic carcinoma are more common. The finding of a monomorphous rather than a polymorphous cellular composition of the lesion should raise a high suspicion of lymphoma. Ultrastructural and immunohistochemical studies are helpful in establishing the final diagnosis.

During the last 2 decades several histological classifications of the lymphomas have been put forward. Modifications of this classification have been introduced from time to time on the basis of newer knowledge gained by the morphological, functional, immunological and cytochemical studies. All these classifications have merits of high rate of reproducibility and have been claimed to be biological predictors of high accuracy. While all these classifications have also created considerable confusion, the histopathologists are inclined to follow the classification most suited to their own liking and satisfaction. The classification of the non-Hodgkin's lymphoma introduced by Rappaport 2 decades ago has been widely used (Rappaport 1966) and is still the favourite with many pathologists. This classification, which has been subsequently modified, is based on the morphology of the lymphoma cells and their geographical arrangement. One of the main objections to this classification has been that the group labelled as histiocytic lymphoma is a heterogeneous group and is most often not histiocytic in origin. The following is the modified Rappaport classification of non-Hodgkin's lymphoma (Byrne 1977):

Nodular lymphomas
- Poorly differentiated lymphocytic
- Mixed
- Histiocytic

Diffuse lymphomas
- Well-differentiated lymphocytic

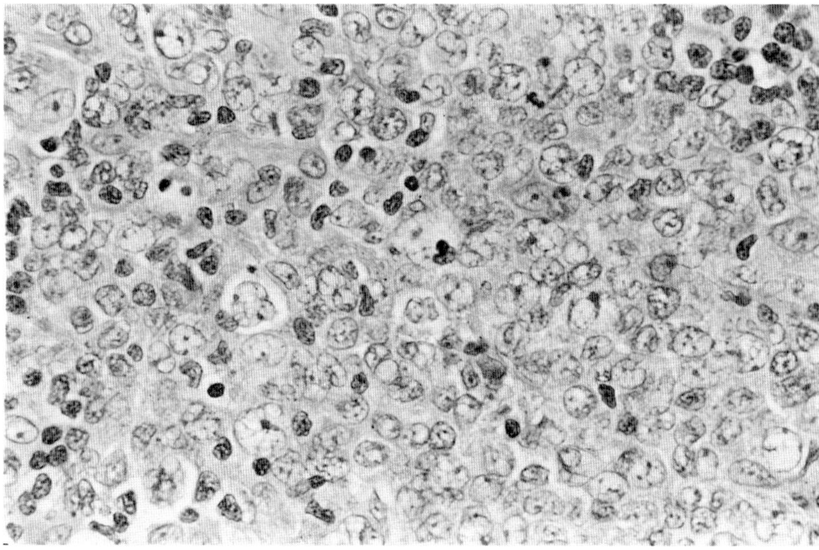

Fig. 22.20. Lymphoma: large cell variant

Poorly differentiated lymphocytic
Mixed
Histiocytic
Lymphoblastic
Undifferentiated (Burkitt and non-Burkitt)

It is probably because of the rarity of primary lymphomas in the female genital tract that application of any of the recent classifications has been very low (Chorlton et al. 1974; Castaldo et al. 1979; Crisp et al. 1982; Harris and Scully 1984). In 1982, the National Cancer Institute of the United States of America organised a multi-institutional study on the non-Hodgkin's lymphomas (NHL) and formulated a working system for clinical usage (NCI), dividing it into three major prognostic groups – low, intermediate and high grade – comprising different histological types of malignant lymphomas. The reader should refer to the NCI classification for further guidance.

The extra-nodal lymphomas, which are commonly diffuse histocytic type (Fig. 22.20), are also common lymphomas of the pelvis (Lathrop 1967). The diffuse histocytic lymphomas were labelled in the older classification as lymphoblastic lymphoma and reticulum cell sarcoma. Accordingly, the majority of vaginal lymphomas previously reported appear to belong to the histiocytic group (Epperson 1950; Weseley and Berrigan 1958; Buchler and Kline 1972; Castaldo et al. 1979). Well-differentiated lymphocytic lymphoma, mixed lymphocytic and histiocytic (Chorlton et al. 1974), nodular mixed (Harris and Scully 1984) and undifferentiated lymphomas (Calstaldo et al. 1979) can also occur at this site. Sclerotic changes with variable amounts of fibrous tissue separating individual or groups of cells have been found to be common features of vaginal and cervical lymphomas (Harris and Scully 1984).

The overall prognosis of vaginal lymphomas is good and similar to that of other extra-nodal lymphomas with about 70% five year survival rate (Freeman et al. 1972; Harris and Scully 1984). Nodular and well-differentiated lymphocytic lymphomas have a better prognosis than the diffuse lymphomas (Crisp et al. 1982), and diffuse, large cell, cleaved lymphomas have a more favourable outlook than the non-cleaved and immunoblastic type (Harris and Scully 1984).

22.5.3 Treatment

Careful evaluation of the patient is important. Localised disease is potentially curable by surgery and/or radiotherapy. With combination chemotherapy cyclophosphamide, vincristine and prednisolone (CVP) and cyclophosphamide, adriamycin and prednisolone (CHOP) in nodular and diffuse lymphomas, 70%–95% remission rates can be expected (Crisp et al. 1982). Nodular lymphomas have a prolonged course, and its long-term outlook is poor, whereas 35% of diffuse lymphomas have a good cure rate (Crisp et al. 1982).

References

Buchler DA, Kline JC (1972) Primary lymphoma of the vagina. Obstet Gynecol 40:235–237

Byrne GE Jr (1977) Rappaport classification of non-Hodgkin's lymphoma: histologic features and clinical significance. Cancer Treat Rep 61:935–944

Carbone PD, Kaplan HS, Musshoff K et al. (1971) Report of the committee on Hodgkin's disease staging classification. Cancer Res 31:1860–1861

Castaldo TW, Ballon SC, Lagasse LD et al. (1979) Reticuloendothelial neoplasia of the female genital tract. Obstet Gynecol 54:116–170

Chorlton I, Karnei RF Jr, King FM et al. (1974) Primary malignant reticuloendothelial disease involving, vagina, cervix and corpus uteri. Obstet Gynecol 44:735–748

Crisp WE, Surwit EA, Grogan TM et al. (1982) Malignant pelvic lymphoma. Am J Obstet Gynecol 143:69–74

Epperson JWW (1950) Case of the reticulum cell variety of lymphosarcoma involving the female genitalia. West J Surg Obstet Gynecol 58:701–703

Freeman C, Berg JW, Cutler SJ (1972) Occurrence and prognosis of extranodal lymphomas. Cancer 29:252–260

Harris NL, Scully RE (1984) Malignant lymphoma and granulocytic sarcoma of the uterus and vagina: a clinicopathologic analysis of 27 cases. Cancer 53:2530–2545

Iliya FA, Muggia, O'Leary JA et al. (1968) Gynecologic manifestation of reticulum cell sarcoma. Obstet Gynecol 31:266–269

Lamb EJ (1982) In discussion malignant pelvic lymphoma: Crisp EW et al. Am J Obstet Gynecol 143:69–74

Lathrop JC (1967) Malignant pelvic lymphomas: views and reviews. Obstet Gynecol 30:137–145

National Cancer Institute (1982) Sponsored study of classification of non-Hodgkin's lymphomas. Summary and description of working formulation for clinical usage. Cancer 49:2112–2135

Rappaport H (1966) Tumors of hemopoietic system. In: Atlas of tumour pathology, sect 3, fasc 8. Armed Forces Institute of Pathology, Washington, pp 270
Weseley AC, Berrigan MV (1958) Reticulum cell sarcoma of the vagina: report of a case. Obstet Gynecol 11:192–195

22.6 Plasmacytoma

Solitary or localised plasmacytomas are uncommon tumours and usually seen in the head and neck region (Gromer and Duvall 1973; Pohar 1977) and more particularly in the upper respiratory tract (Castro et al. 1973; Noorani 1975). They can, however, occur anywhere in the body including the soft tissues (Tong et al. 1980). The patients are usually between 50 and 70 years old; men are more affected than women.

Neoplastic proliferation of plasma cells has been classified by Dohlin and Dewar (1956) into multiple myeloma, solitary medullary myeloma, plasma cell leukemia and extra-medullary plasmacytoma. Multiple myeloma is the systemic form typically involving the bone marrow and represents neoplastic proliferation of single line plasma cells which produce monoclonal protein (Gorenstein et al. 1977). Localised plasmacytoma may be a variant of multiple myeloma (Oken 1984) and occasionally the first evidence of generalised dyscrasia (Gorenstein et al. 1977). The relationship of solitary plasmacytoma of soft tissue, extra-medullary plasmacytoma or solitary plasmacytoma of bone to multiple myeloma is not clear cut. While many solitary plasmacytomas of bone evolve ultimately to multiple myeloma (Wiltshaw 1976), there are also reports of patients who have survived more than 20 years (Wright 1961). In one series, only 2 of 12 patients with extra-medullary plasmacytoma developed multiple myeloma (Corwin and Lindberg 1979), suggesting a better prognosis for extra-medullary plasmacytoma.

Plasmacytoma of the female genital tract is undoubtedly a rare condition. Appleberg (1953) reported localised plasmcytoma in a 74-year-old patient whose main complaint was blood-stained vaginal discharge. The patient had 2 masses, each 1 cm in diameter, located on both the anterior and posterior wall of the vagina above the introitus. Biopsy revealed a plasmacytoma, and the patient was treated by radiotherapy. There was no recurrence at short-term follow-up.

When a histological diagnosis of extra-medullary plasmacytoma has been made, a thorough biochemical, haematological and radiological investigation should be done to exclude multiple myeloma.

Grossly, solitary plasmacytomas of the soft tissue are smooth in outline and soft to firm in consistency. Cut surfaces are greyish to grey-tan in colour.

22.6.1 Microscopical Appearance

Diffuse sheets of plasma cells with scanty, thin and incomplete fibrovascular stroma replace the soft tissue in which the tumour occurs. The tumour may be well differentiated and composed of plasma cells similar to the ones seen in inflammation (Fig. 22.21). Immature nuclei with a fine chromatin network and prominent nucleoli have been correlated to a higher risk for progression to multiple myeloma. (Meis et al. 1987).

Immunohistiochemically, the plasma cells may display monotypic kappa or lambda staining (Meis et al. 1987), although only very rarely is paraprotein detectable in the serum of patients with localised plasmacytoma.

22.6.2 Behaviour

Local recurrences are seen in almost one-third of patients with extra-medullary plasmacytoma (Wollersheim et al. 1984) and are seen usually within the first 5 years of treatment. Also about one-third develop regional node metastases (Knowling et al. 1983).

22.6.3 Treatment

Plasmacytomas are generally radiosensitive (Castro et al. 1973) and can be treated successfully by radiotherapy. When high dose radiotherapy is used, the risk of dissemination is greatly reduced (Mill and Griffith 1980). Some authors (Kirshenbaum and Rhone 1985) advocate local excision followed by radiotherapy, while

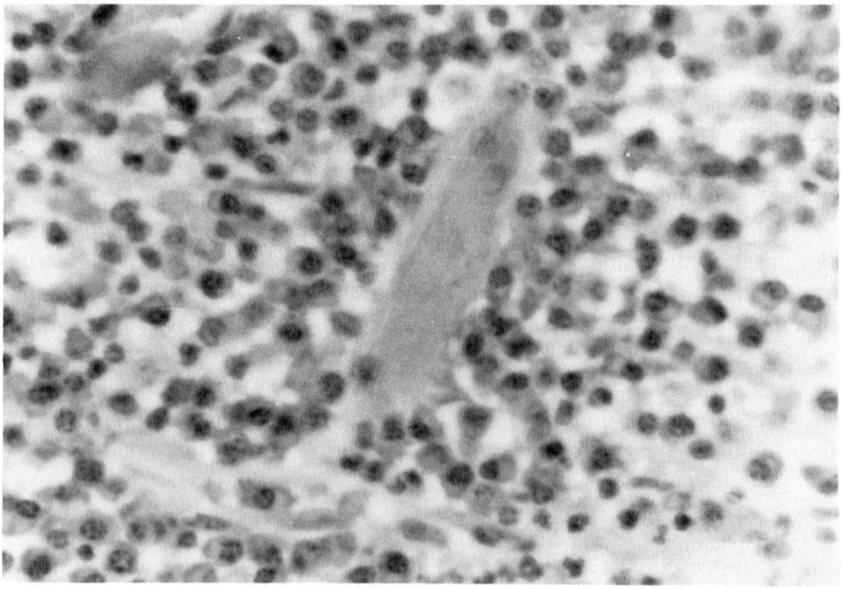

Fig. 22.21. Plasmacytoma: the tumour is composed of sheets of well-differentiated plasma cells and may mimic chronic inflammation

others (Kotner and Wang 1972) reserve surgery for reoccurrence. Radioresistant and recurrent cases can be treated by alkylating agent (Woodruff et al. 1979) with good results.

References

Appleberg G (1953) Plasmacytoma of the vagina. Case report. Acta Radiol 39:84–86

Castro EB, Lewis JS, Strong EW (1973) Plasmacytoma of the paranasal sinuses and nasal cavity. Arch Otolaryngol 97:326–329

Corwin J, Lindberg RD (1979) Solitary plasmacytoma of bone vs extramedullary plasmacytoma and their relationship to multiple myeloma. Cancer 43:1007–1013

Dohlin S, Dewar JP (1956) Extramedullary plasmàcytoma. Am J Pathol 32:83–103

Gorenstein A, Neel B III, Devine KD et al. (1977) Solitary extramedullary plasmacytoma of the larynx. Arch Otolaryngol 103:159–161

Gromer RC, Duvall AJ III (1973) Plasmacytoma of the head and neck. J Laryngol Otol 58:861–872

Kirshenbaum G, Rhone DP (1985) Solitary extramedullary plasmacytoma of the breast with serum monoclonal protein: a case report and review of the literature. Am J Clin Pathol 83:230–232

Knowling MA, Harwood AR, Berslagel DE (1983) Comparison of extramedullary plasmacytomas with solitary and multiple plasma cell tumors of bone. J Clin Oncol 1:255–262

Kotner LM, Wang CC (1972) Plasmacytoma of the upper air and food passages. Cancer 30:414–418

Meis JM, Butler JJ, Osborne BM et al. (1987) Solitary plasmacytoma of bone and extramedullary plasmacytomas: a clinicopathologic and immunohistiochemical study. Cancer 59:1475–1485

Mill WB, Griffith R (1980) The role of radiation therapy in the management of plasma cell tumors. Cancer 45:647–652

Noorani MA (1975) Plasmacytoma of middle ear and upper respiratory tract. J Laryngol Otol 98:105–113

Oken MM (1984) Multiple myeloma. Med Clin North Am 68:757–787

Pohar AL (1977) Extramedullary plasmacytoma of head and neck, parotid, submandibular salivary glands. J Laryngol Otol 91:241–258

Tong D, Griffin TW, Laramore GE et al. (1980) Solitary plasmacytoma of bone and soft tissue. Radiology 135:195–198

Wiltshaw E (1976) The natural history of extramedullary plasmacytoma and its relation to solitary myeloma of bone and myelomatosis. Medicine (Baltimore) 55:217–238

Wollersheim HCH, Holdrinet RSG, Haanen C (1984) Clinical course and survival in 16 patients with localised plasmacytoma. Scand J Haematol 32:423–428

Woodruff RK, Whittle JM, Malpas JS (1979) Solitary plasmacytoma. I Extramedullary soft tissue plasmacytoma. Cancer 43:2340–2343

Wright CJE (1961) Long survival in solitary plasmacytoma of bone. J Bone Joint Surg [Br] 43:767–771

22.7 Granulocytic Sarcoma

Granulocytic sarcomas or chloromas are the tumours of poorly differentiated myeloid cells occurring in extra-medullary sites. These tumours develop during the course of or as a presenting sign of myelogenous leukemia and occasionally precede peripheral or bone marrow manifestations of acute leukemia (Mason et al. 1973). The granulocytic sarcomas have been suggested to represent extramedullary foci of malignant granulopoiesis (Liu et al. 1973). Although the common location is the sub-periosteal region, the lesions can occur at other sites. The female genital tract is involved on rare occasions (Chorlton et al. 1974; Seo et al. 1977), and then the ovary is usually the most common site. The vaginal lesion is very rare and co-exists with lesions at other sites (Socinski et al. 1983). The patient complains of vaginal discharge or bleeding. Examination reveals a grey-white, haemorrhagic mass of 3–6 cm in size arising from the vaginal wall.

22.7.1 Microscopical Appearance

The tumour consists of sheets of immature cells containing pleomorphic and hyperchromatic nuclei with numerous mitotic figures. The cells are usually more immature than those in the peripheral blood. The nucleo-cytoplasmic ratio is low. Necrosis may be marked. Careful examination of an intact area reveals the presence of myelocytic and metamyelocytes, depending upon the degree of maturity, among the immature cells. The presence of granules in the eosinophilic cytoplasm and indented nuclei should immediately raise suspicions of granulocytic sarcoma in the absence of a clinical history of leukaemia. The naphthol-ASD chloracetate stain which can be done in formalin-fixed tissue helps in the identification of granulocytic precursors. Ultrastructural examination (Scott and Horn 1970) may show large red particles in the cytoplasm of some neoplastic cells (Hartford 1968).

22.7.2 Treatment

The survival in granulocytic sarcoma is similar to that in the acute leukaemia (Ross 1955). With modern chemotherapy using adriamycin and cytosine arabinoside, complete remission has been achieved (Krause 1979).

References

Chorlton I, Karnei RF Jr, Norris HJ (1974) Primary malignant reticuloendothelial disease involving vagina, cervix and corpus uteri. Obstet Gynecol 44:735–748

Hartford CE (1968) Bleeding from the uterus caused by chloroma. Obstet Gynecol 31:166–172

Krause JR (1979) Granulocytic sarcoma preceding acute leukemia: a report of 6 cases. Cancer 44:1017–1021

Liu PI, Ishimaru T, McGregor DE et al. (1973) Autopsy study of granulocytic sarcoma (chloroma) in patients with myclogenous leukemia, Hiroshima-Nagasaki 1949–1969. Cancer 31:948–955

Mason TE, Demaree RS Jr, Margolis CI (1973) Granulocytic sarcoma (chloroma) two years preceding myclogenous leukemia. Cancer 31:423–432

Ross RR (1955) Chloroma and chloroleukemia. Am J Med 18:671–676

Scott RG, Horn RG (1970) Ultrastructural aspects of neutrophil granulocyte development in human. Lab Invest 23:202–215
Seo IS, Hull MT, Park HY (1977) Granulocytic sarcoma of the cervix as a primary manifestation. Case without overt leukemia features for 26 months. Cancer 40:3030–3037
Socinski MA, Ershler WB, Belinson JL (1983) Co-existent breast and vaginal granulocytic sarcoma. Gynecol Oncol 16:299–304

22.8 Neuroectodermal Tumours

22.8.1 Paraganglioma

The ganglion and paraganglion cells are derived from the neural crest. The cells destined to be paraganglia migrate very close to the autonomic ganglia during embryonic life and form small masses of cells. From birth until puberty, these cells progressively involute. The chief cells of the paraganglia store neurotransmitter substance or norepinephrine in their cytoplasmic grannules. The largest collections of paraganglion cells occur in the adrenal medulla. The tumours arising from the extra-adrenal paraganglion cells are known as paraganglioma and those in the adrenal medulla, phaeochromocytoma. The carotid body and aortic body paragangliomas have chemoreceptors. It is believed that paragangliomas develop from cells which fail to involute during childhood (Fries and Chamberlain 1968). Although 10% of the phaeochromocytomas are seen in extra-adrenal sites, they have been known to occur in all possible areas where the autonomic nervous system is present. The tumours may be functional in occasional patients.

The female genital tract is a very uncommon site. Pezeshkpour (1981) reported a vaginal paraganglioma in a 22-year-old woman and mentioned another two in the vagina of a 66-year-old woman. In the first patient, the tumour was asymptomatic. The second presented with purulent vaginal discharge.

22.8.1.1 Gross Appearance

Generally, the size of the tumour varies from 1.5 to 20 cm. The vaginal tumour reported (Pezeshkpour 1981) was 3 cm in size. The gross appearance of tumour usually depends on its site of origin. It is usually well circumscribed but unencapsulated or partially capsulated. The cut surfaces may vary from greyish-white or greyish-tan to purple with focal areas of haemorrhage and necrosis.

22.8.1.2 Microscopical Appearance

The characteristic microscopical feature of these tumours is an organoid arrangement of cells in solid nests surrounded by vascular fibrous stroma (Fig. 22.22). Two types of cells are usually seen. The predominant cells are chief cells which are large and polygonal, containing abundant clear or homogeneous eosinophilic cytoplasm and vesicular nuclei. The less numerous cells are small and round, with finely granular or clear cytoplasm and hyperchromatic, round to oval nuclei. When the

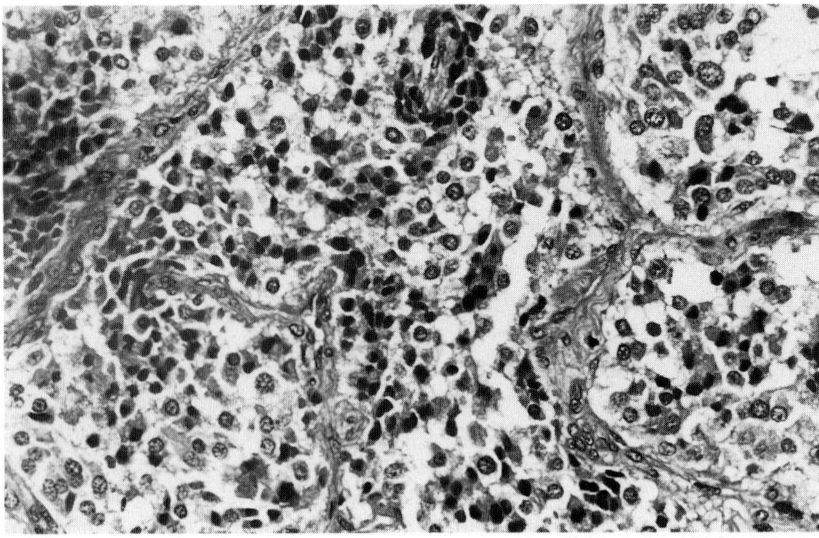

Fig. 22.22. Paraganglioma: solid nests of tumour cells surrounded by fibrous stroma

cells with clear cytoplasm predominate, the tumour may be mistaken for metastatic clear cell carcinoma (Makinen and Nickels 1979). Occasionally, the tumour cells are fusiform and arranged in peritheliomatous sheets mimicking a haemangiopericytoma. Scattered large cells with hyperchromatic nuclei may also be noticed in the tumour. Mitoses are only rarely seen. Thick bands of fibrous stroma traverse the tumour mass and divide it into irregular compartments. The argentaffin and argyrophil reactions of the tumour cells are variable with commonly used Fontana-Masson stains, but Barroso-Moguel and Costero (1962) consistently demonstrated argentaffin and argyrophil cells by del Rio Hortega techniques. Ultrastructually, the tumour cells contain neurosecretory granules.

These tumours are generally benign. Only 10% of these tumours are malignant; they infiltrate locally or metastasise by the lymphatic channels or haematogenously.

22.8.1.3 Treatment

The treatment is surgical exsision.

22.8.2 Neuroepithelioma

Neuroepithelioma is an exceedingly rare, malignant tumour of the peripheral nerve. Only a very few cases have been reported in the literature and only one tumour from the female genital tract. The tumour occurred in the recto-vaginal septum of a 31-year-old woman whose main complaint was lump in the rectum, dysuria, dysmenorrhoea and constipation (Solomons and Dockeray 1949).

Grossly, these tumours are round or fusiform in shape with an average size about 4 cm. The cut surfaces are lobulated and grey in colour (Harper et al. 1981).

Microscopically, the characteristic cellular components are closely packed, polyhedral cells arranged in rosettes and clusters. The nuclei are pleomorphic and hyperchromatic, displaying many mitotic figures. The tumour cells do not possess neurofibrils. The case reported in the recto-vaginal septum by Solomons and Dockeray (1949) displayed, in addition, numerous corpora amylacea-like bodies scattered in the tumour tissue.

The histogenesis of these tumours is debatable. Schwann cell, ependymal cell and neural crest origins have been suggested (Harper et al. 1981). These are malignant tumours and can recur and metastasise.

22.8.2.1 Treatment

Surgery, radiotherapy and chemotherapy have been used. Only a very few cases have been reported, and experience in treating these tumours is therefore exceedingly limited.

References

Paraganglioma

Barroso-Moguel R, Costero I (1962) Argentaffin cells of the carotid body tumor. Am J Pathol 41:389–402

Fries JG, Chamberlain JA (1968) Pheochromocytoma: literature review and report of a cervical pheochromocytoma. Surgery 63:269–279

Makinen J, Nickels J (1979) Paraganglion cells mimicking metastatic clear cell carcinoma. Histopathology 3:459–465

Pezeshkpour G (1981) Solitary paraganglioma of the vagina: report of a case. Am J Obstet Gynecol 139:219–221

Neuroepithelioma

Harper PG, Pringle J, Souhami RL (1981) Neuroepithelioma – a rare malignant periphal nerve tumour of primitive origin: report of two new cases and review of literature. Cancer 48:2282–2287

Solomons B, Dockeray G (1949) A case of neuoepithelioma of the rectovaginal septum. J Obstet Gynaecol Br Emp 56:875–876

22.9 Germ Cell Tumours

22.9.1 Benign Teratoma

Teratoma of the vagina is rare. Only about half a dozen cases have been reported in the literature. These are cystic lesions of 2–8 cm in size occurring mostly at the upper part of the vagina. The cyst contains skin, hair follicles and sebaceous materials (Curtis 1913), sweat glands and teeth (Furtado 1950), mucinous glands, neural tissue and smooth muscle (Harle 1937). The presence of thyroid and parathyroid tissues in dermoid cyst of the vagina has also been reported (Kurman and Prabha 1973).

The tumour is benign and surgical excision is adequate.

22.9.2 Endodermal Sinus Tumour

In the female genital tract, endodermal sinus tumours are most commonly encountered in the ovaries. The vagina is an uncommon site. The tumours at the extragonadal sites are said to originate in aberrant germ cells or germ cells arrested during their embryonic migration. These tumours are distributed mostly along the midline and seen in the pineal, mediastinal and retroperitoneal areas. The occurrence of these tumours in the vagina has been explained by the close proximity of the upper part of the vagina to the sacral region (Rezaizadeh and Woodruff 1978), which is a recognised location for teratomatous tumours. According to other views, they are a mesonephric carcinoma (Siegel et al. 1970; Norris et al. 1970).

22.9.2.1 Clinical Features

All the reported patients were 2 years old or less and presented with vaginal bleeding or discharge, Vaginal examination under anaesthesia or rectal examination revealed a mass in the vagina.

22.9.2.2 Gross Appearance

The endodermal sinus tumours are polypoid, grey-pink to yellow coloured, solid masses of average 3–5 cm in diameters. The consistency is firm to rubbery. The external surface is usually smooth but may be ulcerated.

22.9.2.3 Microscopical Appearance

The tumours are composed of a reticular arrangement of channels and tubules lined by cuboidal cells with a moderate amount of vacuolated or pale eosinophilic cytoplasm and hyperchromatic, round to oval nuclei. Epithelial papillae supported on thin-walled blood vessels (Schiller-Duval bodies) are usually seen in these areas (Fig. 22.23). In some areas, the tubules and channels display an intercommunicating and anastomosing arrangement (festoon arrangement). The lumina of the tubules and channels are usually devoid of any secretions but may contain desquamated cells and granular material. The tumour cells, in general, are set in a loose background, and only occasionally are tightly packed solid small sheets seen. Mitotic figures can alsways be demonstrated in the tumours. In an occasional tumour, the neoplastic cells are polygonal, possessing abundant eosinophilic cytoplasm vesicular nuclei and prominent nucleoli, and arranged in solid sheets resembling hepatocytes (Prat et al. 1982).

Diastase-resistant, PAS-positive, intra- and extra-cellular hyaline bodies as well as abundant intra-cytoplasmic glycogen can be demonstrated in the tumour cells (Copeland et al. 1985). The tumour cells stained by immunoperoxidase techniques show positive reactions for alpha-fetoprotein. Some tumours are also positive for α_1-antitrypsin (Copeland et al. 1985). Patients' sera usually contain elevated levels of alpha-fetoprotein. In one patient, alpha-fetoprotein could also be demonstrated in the vaginal fluid (Norgaard-Pedersen et al. 1976). Serial estimations of alpha-fetoprotein in the patients' serum can be used to monitor the post-operative behaviour of the tumour (Kohorn et al. 1985).

There is little difficulty in differentiating the tumour from sarcoma botryoides. The tumour is to be differentiated from clear cell carcinoma of the vagina, which occurs in older children (Allyn et al. 1971) and adults. Histologically, clear cell carcinoma consists of tubules and cystic spaces lined by clear cells rich in glycogen and hobnail cells (Herbst and Scully 1970).

22.9.2.4 Prognosis and Treatment

Local recurrences are common (Liebhart 1986). Endodermal sinus tumours spread via the lymphatics and bloodstream (Kohorn et al. 1985). They were considered in the past to be one of the most aggressive tumours with a very poor prognosis (Huntington and Bullock 1970; Allyn et al. 1971). In recent years, the outlook has improved significantly due to the use of multiagent chemotherapy such as vincristine, actinomycin D and cyclophosphamide (VAC). The tumours are now considered curable in most cases (Young and Scully 1984). With this modality of treatment, the necessity for mutilating surgery has been greatly reduced. Good results have indeed been achieved with chemotherapy followed by local surgery (Kohorn et al. 1985). Radiotherapy has not been found particularly useful (Allyn et al. 1971) and may, in fact, have an adverse affect on the growing pelvic bones (Dewhurst and Ferriera 1981).

22.9.3 Carcinoma of the Infant Vagina (Embryonal Carcinoma)

Embryonal carcinoma in the infant vagina is rare. Vawter (1965) reported primary embryonal carcinoma in two infants 16 and 14 months old, who presented with episodic and continuous vaginal bleeding.

Grossly, the embryonal carcinomas are variable in size, friable, polypoid and yellowish-tan in colour. In the gonads, they may occur either as a pure form or as a component of other malignant germ cell tumours.

Microscopically, the tumours are composed of large polyhedral cells with a distinct cell outline, clear or granular cytoplasm, distinct nuclei and one or more nucleoli (Fig. 22.24). The cells tend to arrange around spaces, in papillary fashion or in large aggregates. Intracellular hyaline bodies, glycogen and fat globules as well as extracellular mucin-like materials can also be present. Glomeruloid-like structures are occasionally noticed. The stroma is vascular.

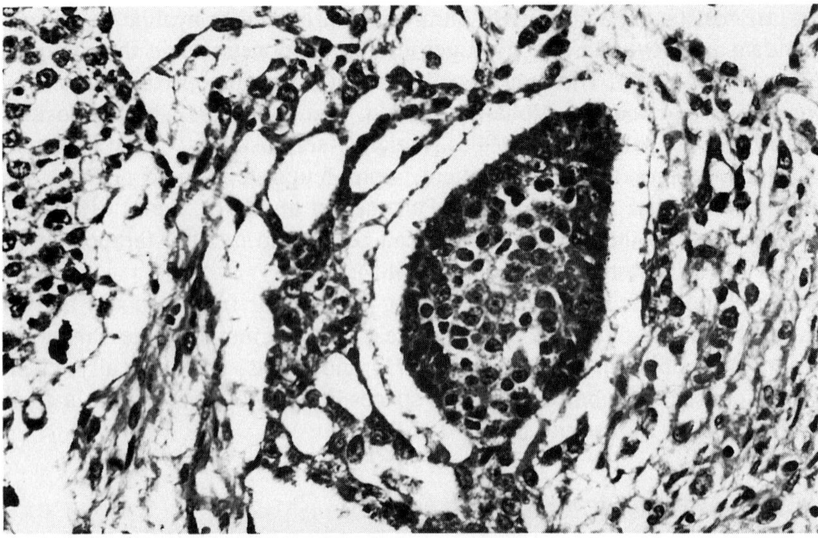

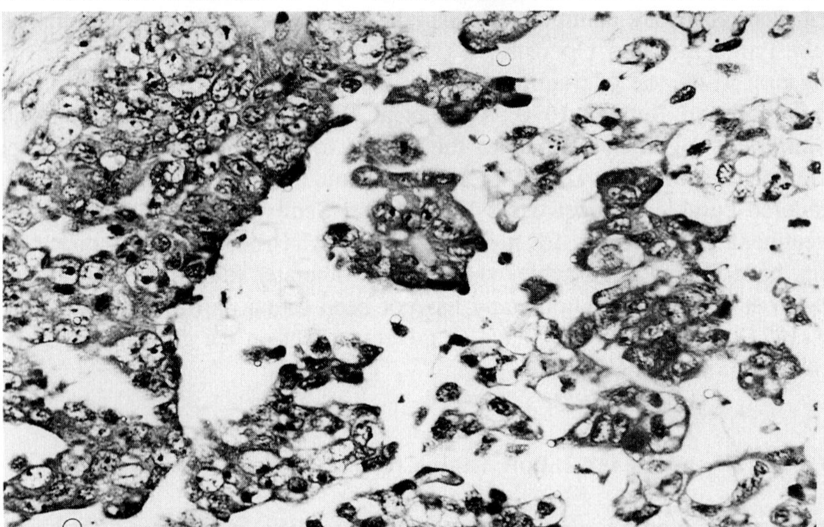

Fig. 22.23. Endodermal sinus tumour: reticular area with a Schiller-Duval body

Fig. 22.24. Carcinoma of the infant vagina: sheet of large polyhedral cells and fragment of a papilla

The histogenesis of these tumours is controversial. They are histologically similar to the embryonal carcinoma of the infant testes, containing an endodermal sinus pattern. Norris et al. (1970), who reported six similar cases, considered them to be distinct tumours most likely of mesonephric remnant origin. Gibson (1973) saw three cases of carcinoma of the infant vagina, and because of their close similarities to the endodermal sinus tumour he concluded that these tumours were extra-gonadal germ cell tumours. The patients reported by Norris et al. (1970) were treated by surgery (simple or radical vaginectomy), post-operative radiotherapy and in one case actinomycin D. Two of the patients were alive 3 and 6 years post-operatively. Four patients died of metastatic disease.

22.9.3.1 Treatment

Both infants reported by Vawter (1965) were treated by surgery, actinomycin D and radiation but died of metastatic disease within 18 months of initial diagnosis. The tumour reported by Hoge and Benn (1943) was probably a similar tumour. The report, however, lacks the histological details. These authors also mentioned another patient described by Lovegren (1931). She was a 17-month-old infant with a papillary epithelial tumour of the vagina.

References

Benign Teratoma

Curtis AH (1913) Transaction of societies: Chicago Gynecological Society. Surg Gynecol Obstet 16:715

Furtado AH (1950) Solid vaginal teratoma. Rev Ginecol Obstet 2:520

Harle F (1937) Deremoidzapfen in der Scheide. Zentralbl Gynakol 61:1488–1489

Kurman RJ, Prabha C (1973) Thyroid and parathyroid gland tissue in the vaginal wall. Am J Clin Pathol 59:503–507

Endodermal Sinus Tumours

Allyn DL, Silverberg SG, Sulzbert AM (1971) Endodermal sinus tumour of the vagina. Cancer 27:1231–1238

Dewhurst SJ, Ferriera HP (1981) An endodermal sinus tumour of the vagina in an infant with seven year survival. Br J Obstet Gynaecol 88:859–862

Herbst AL, Scully RE (1970) Adenocarcinoma of the vagina in adolescence: a report of 7 cases including 6 clear cell carcinomas (so called mesonephromas). Cancer 25:745–757

Huntington RW Jr, Bullock WK (1970) Yolk sac tumors of the ovary. Cancer 25:1354–1367

Kohorn EI, McIntosh S, Lytton B et al. (1985) Endodermal sinus tumor of the infant vagina. Gynecol Oncol 20:196–203

Liebhart M (1986) Histopathological diagnosis of vaginal endodermal sinus tumors in infants. Int J Gynecol Pathol 5:217–222

Norgaard-Pedersen B, Lundborg CJ, Laursen AM (1976) Infantile vaginal tumour with alpha-fetoprotein synthesis. Acta Pathol Microbiol Scand [A] 87:223–226

Norris HJ, Bageley GP, Taylor HB (1970) Carcinoma of the infant vagina: a distinctive tumor. Arch Pathol 90:473–479

Prat J, Bhan AK, Dickersin GR et al. (1982) Hepatoid yolksac tumor of the ovary. Cancer 50:2355–2368

Rezaizadeh MM, Woodruff JD (1978) Endodermal sinus tumor of the vagina. Gynecol Oncol 6:459–463
Siegel HA, Sagerman R, Berdon WE et al. (1970) Mesonephric adenocarcinoma of the vagina in a 7 month old infant simulating sarcoma botryoides: sucessful control with supravoltage radiotherapy. J Pediatr Surg 5:468–470
Young RH, Scully RE (1984) Endodermal sinus tumor of the vagina: report of nine cases and review of the literature. Gynecol Oncol 18:380–392

Carcinoma Infant Vagina
Gibson AAM (1973) Embryonal carcinoma of vagina in infancy. Arch Dis Child 48:163
Hoge RH, Benn VA (1943) Carcinoma of the vulva and vagina in infancy. Am J Obstet Gynecol 46:286–290
Lovegren E (1931) Carcinoma vaginae im zweiten Lebensjahr. Acta Paediatr (Upsala) 10:371–378
Norris HJ, Bagley GP, Taylor HB et al. (1970) Carcinoma of the infant vagina. Arch Pathol 90:473–479
Vawter GF (1965) Carcinoma of the vagina in infancy. Cancer 18:1479–1484

22.10 Tumours of Meso- and Paramesonephric Duct Origin

22.10.1 Benign

22.10.1.1 Mesonephric Papilloma

The type of papillary tumours which have been labelled as mesonephric papilloma (Novak et al. 1954; Janovski and Kasdon 1963) are seen more commonly in the uterine cervix (James 1951; Selzer and Nelson 1962). Theoretically, they can occur anywhere along the course of the mesonephric ducts. Ulbright et al. (1981) reported one patient and considered these tumours to be of müllerian origin.

22.10.1.1.1 Clinical Features

These tumours occur in young children under 6 years of age. The main presenting symptoms are vaginal bleeding or discharge. Both the anterior and posterior walls, mostly of the upper part of the vagina, are involved.

22.10.1.1.2 Gross Appearance

Mesonephric papillomas are commonly seen as polypoid masses 1–5 cm in size projecting into the vaginal canal. They can occasionally be intra-mural (Ulbright et al. 1981). They are described as polypoid, solid and friable.

22.10.1.1.3 Microscopical Appearance

The tumours consist of various sized papillary fronds lined by cuboidal to columnar cells supported on fibrovascular cores. Formation of scattered small gland lumina and solid clusters by the tumour cells is not unusual (Ulbright et al. 1981). The luminal surface of epithelium show diastase-resistant, PAS-positive secretions, but intracellular mucin is not seen. Eosinophilic hyaline globules, also diastase-resistant and

PAS-positive, are randomly scattered within the solid clusters of tumour cells (Ulbright et al. 1981). Part of the papillary and glandular lining may occasionally be formed by squamous cells (Janovski and Kasdon 1963). The supporting stroma is myxomatous (Selzer and Nelson 1962) or hyalinised and may show diposition of calcium aggregates with the formation of psammoma body-like structures (Janovski and Kasdon 1963). Osseous metaplasia (Ulbright et al. 1918) may also be seen. The cellular and stroma components are uniform and bland in appearance. Mitoses and pleomorphism are not seen. The stroma does not contain any cells suggestive of myoblast with cytoplasmic myofibrils. Ulbright et al. (1981) demonstrated the presence of microvilli, perinuclear arrays of microfilaments, prominent lysosomes and features of squamous metaplasia on ultrastructural studies and suggested that the tumour was of müllerian origin.

These tumours are to be differentiated from sarcoma botryoides which shows sarcomatous stroma, mitoses and neoplastic rhabdomyoblasts.

22.10.1.1.4 Treatment

These tumours are benign, and recurrences after excision have not been reported.

22.10.1.2 Brenner Tumour

Chen (1981) reported a polypoid tumour 1.5 cm in size incidentally removed from the vagina of a 67-year-old woman, which was found to be a Brenner tumour. The tumour was composed of nests of epithelial cells which are transitional in appearance with pink, clear or granular cytoplasm and grooved nuclei (Fig. 22.25). Thick bands of fibroblastic tissue separated the nests. Some of the nests contained spaces lined by mucinous epithelium. The histological appearance of the tumour with both epithelial cell nests and connective tissue stroma bears close similarities of a Brenner tumour. The tumour reported as mixed tumour of the vagina (Buntine et al. 1979) probably also belongs to the same histogenetic group.

Brenner tumours, which are recognised as tumours of müllerian origin, occur commonly in the ovaries. They are also known to arise occasionally in extra-ovarian sites such as the uterus and broad ligament (Robinson 1950; Arhelger and Bocian 1976). The occurrence of such tumours in the vagina, a müllerian organ, is therefore not improbable.

22.10.1.2.1 Treatment

These tumours are benign, and surgical excision is adequate.

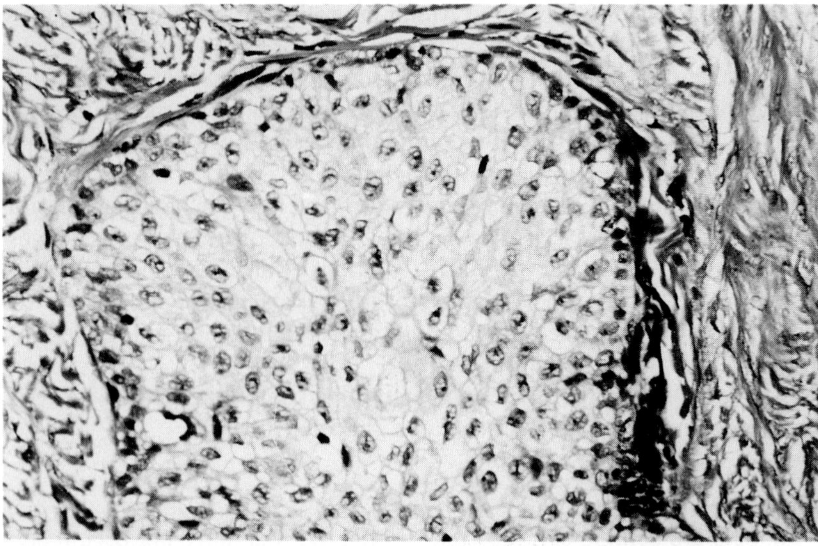

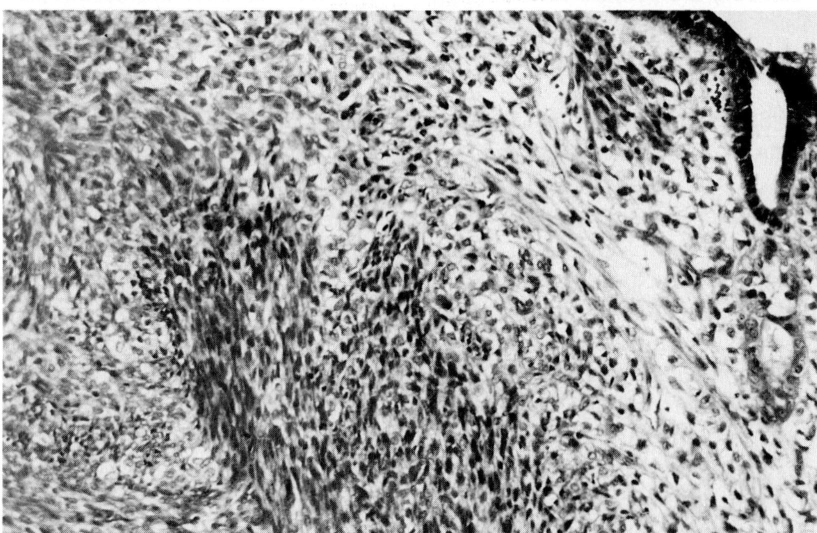

Fig. 22.25. Brenner tumour: nests of epithelial cells surrounded by dense fibrous stroma

Fig. 22.26. Malignant mixed mesodermal tumour: predominant spindle cell sarcoma with adenocarcinomatous component

22.10.2 Malignant

22.10.2.1 Malignant Mixed Mesodermal Tumour

Mesodermal mixed tumours (MMT) occur extremely rarely in the vagina. In one recent review on adult vaginal sarcoma by Peters et al. (1985), only three patients with mixed mesodermal tumour were mentioned.

Embryologically, the upper vagina develops from the lower part of the fused müllerian ducts, and one can expect to notice similar propensities of the vaginal tissue as of the uterus to develop malignant mixed müllerian tumours. They are, however, surprisingly rare at this site. In the earlier literature, variations in the diagnostic criteria led to the inclusion of a number of cases of sarcomasa botryoides in this category (Murphy and Dushane 1948; Amolsch 1939). The exact incidence of MMT in the vagina is difficult to estimate.

The majority of vaginal mixed mesodermal sarcomas are polypoid extensions of uterine or cervical sarcomas. Rutledge (1967) noted only one patient with vaginal mixed müllerian sarcoma amongst 101 patients with vaginal carcinoma but did not provide any specific details. The anatomical location of the tumour was at the middle part of the vagina. The case reported by Davis and Franklin (1975) appeared to arise in the upper vagina.

Malignant mesodermal mixed tumours are tumours of post-menopausal age. The patients complain of irregular vaginal bleeding and passing of necrotic tissue. In some patients, there is a history of previous pelvic irradiation.

Grossly, these tumours tend to be polypoid and bulky and are frequently haemorrhagic with areas of necrosis. Extension to neighbouring structures occurs quite early.

Microscopically, MMT are composed of both sarcomatous and carcinomatous elements. The sarcomatous elements frequently predominate and may be the major component of the tumour (Fig. 22.26). The carcinomatous components, which also vary in proportion, may comprise typical adenocaricnoma, serous papillary carcinoma, mucinous cystadenocarcinoma, clear cell carcinoma and occasionally squamous cell carcinoma. The sarcomatous component displays a wide range of appearances, namely, myxomatous, leiomyosarcomatous and fibrosarcomatous with areas of bizarre giant cells. Mitotic figures are usually frequent. Some authors prefer to differentiate MMT into homologous and heterologous sub-types histologically (Symmonds and Dockerty 1955). In the heterologous sub-type, mesenchymal elements consist of islands of malignant cartilage, bones and rhabdomyoblasts. The homologous carcinosarcomas are intimate mixtures of simple adenocarcinoma and spindle cell sarcoma. This sub-division has been considered useful in assessing the prognosis: some authors observed a significantly better prognosis for homologous mesodermal malignant tumours (Norris 1966; Schaepman-van Geuns 1970). Others (Chuang et al. 1970) did not find any difference between these two groups with regard to the clinical course and survival rates.

MMT are aggressive tumours that spread via the lymphatics and intraperitoneal routes. Metastatic spread occurs to the lungs, liver and bones through the blood stream. The metastatic deposits may be sarcomatous, carcinomatous or both. Prognosis depends on the stage of the disease at initial surgical exploration.

22.10.2.1.1 Treatment

Depending on the stage of the tumour, wide excision, vaginectomy or radical surgery when feasible should be attempted. Radiation and chemotherapy have not been found to improve the ultimate outcome significantly.

22.10.2.2 Endometrial Stromal Sarcoma

Berkowitz et al. (1978) reported an 8-cm cystic mass of endometrial stromal sarcoma arising at the vaginal apex 15 years after hysterectomy and left salpingo-oopherectomy for ovarian endometriosis. The patient had been on oestrogen therapy for the previous 11 years.

Endometrial stromal sarcomas are neoplasms most commonly of the uterus, infrequently of the ovaries and rarely of other sites. The patients' age ranges from 16 to 69 years with a median age of 43 years (Hart and Yoonessi 1977). The presenting symptom is abnormal vaginal bleeding when the tumour arises in the uterus or vagina.

Based on the number of mitoses, endometrial stromal sarcomas have been classified as of low or high grade malignancy. The low grade tumours, also known as endometrial stromal myosis, have less than 10 mitoses per 10 high power fields (Norris and Taylor 1966), whereas the stromal sarcomas exhibit more than 10 mitoses per 10 high power fields. The cellular atypia are more pronounced in the high

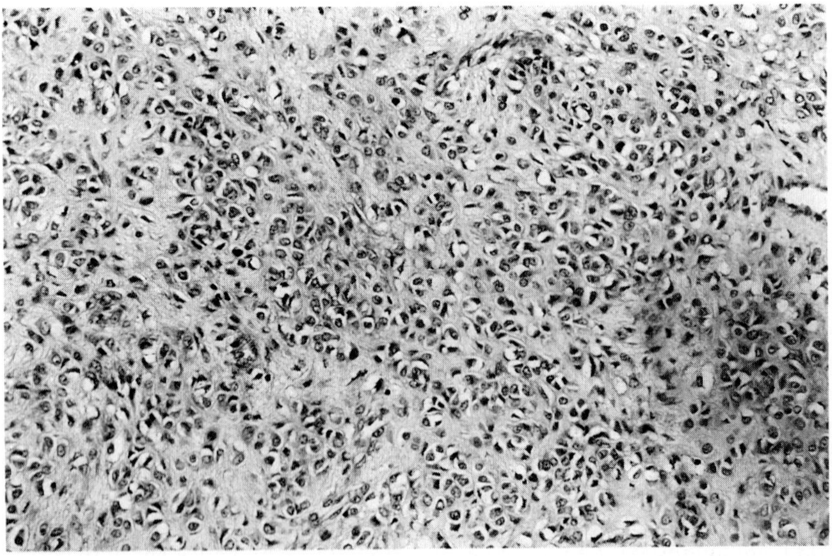

Fig. 22.27. Stromal sarcoma: tumour is composed of diffuse sheets of pleomorphic stromal cells

grade sarcomas. The tumours are composed of round and oval cells with scanty cytoplasm and oval or round nuclei with inconspicuous nucleoli (Fig. 22.27). The cells are mostly arranged in diffuse sheets but may occasionally be arranged in whorls, cords or nests. As seen in the silver preparation, the tumour is rich in reticulin fibres which surround individual or groups of cells. The tumours are vascular, and many, well-formed, small blood vessels can be seen scattered in almost every microscopic field.

Biologically, the low grade sarcomas are slowly growing, tend to infiltrate and recur. The high grade sarcomas have a rapid growth pattern and metastasise early. Recurrences have been noted in low grade stromal sarcomas 18–25 years after initial therapy (Koss et al. 1965).

22.10.2.2.1 Treatment

Radical surgery followed by radiotherapy appears to be the main mode of treatment for uterine tumours (Norris and Taylor 1966). Endometrial stromal sarcoma in the vagina is very rare and experiences of treating a large number of patients is not available. Berkowitz et al. (1978) treated their patient by partial vaginectomy with excision of the paravaginal and parametrial tissue followed by post-operative radiotherapy. The patient had already had total hysterectomy and bilateral salpingo-oopherectomy 15 years earlier. Although the role of progesterone, chemotherapy and radiotherapy as isolated forms of treatment is not clear, they may be tried in treating the recurrent and metastatic disease (Young et al. 1984).

22.10.2.3 Gartner's Duct Carcinoma

In adults, the remnants of Gartner's ducts are occasionally noticed in the lateral part of the cervix and rarely in the vaginal wall. Cysts are known to occur in these remnants along their course extending from the meso-ovarium to the outer third of the vagina. Several reports also suggest that benign and malignant tumours arise in the vaginal portion of the ducts and present as vaginal, paravaginal and adnexal masses (Wahlen and Gynning 1955; Kariminejad and Scully 1973; Taxy and Battifora 1976; Sivathondan et al. 1979; Hinchey et al. 1983).

Grossly, these tumours are solid and rubbery in consistency. The cut surfaces present a lobulated appearance with or without evidence of haemorrhage and necrosis.

Microscopically, the tumours are composed of tubular and papillary structures lined by cuboidal, columnar and flattened epithelium. Some of the tubules are dilated and cystic, being filled with colloid-like secretions (Wahlen and Glynning 1955). Between the tubular structures, the tumour may be composed of solid sheets of round, oval, elongated and small round cells with hyperchromatic nuclei. A variable number of mitotic figures is always noticed.

The tumours tend to infiltrate the surrounding tissue and can metastasise (Hinchey et al. 1983).

22.10.2.3.1 Treatment

The tumours should be treated by radical surgery and radiotherapy depending on the extent of the lesion. The excision margins should be carefully examined for microscopical extension to the surrounding tissue. The patient should be followed up regularly.

References

Mesonephric Papilloma

James T (1951) A benign polypoid tumour of the cervix uteri in a girl three years old. J Obstet Gynaecol Br Emp 58:762–763

Janovski MA, Kasdon EJ (1963) Benign mesonephric papillary and polypoid tumor of the cervix in childhood. J Pediatr 63:211–216

Novak E, Woodruff JD, Novak ER (1954) Probable mesonephric origin of certain female genital tumors. Am J Obstet Gynecol 68:1222–1242

Selzer I, Nelson HM (1962) Benign papilloma (polypoid tumor) of the cervix uteri in children: report of 2 cases. Am J Obstet Gynecol 84:165–169

Ulbright TM, Alexander RW, Kraus FT (1981) Intramural papilloma of the vagina evidence of mullerian histogenesis. Cancer 48:2260–2266

Brenner Tumours

Arhelger RB, Bocian JJ (1976) Brenner tumor of the uterus. Cancer 38:1741–1943

Buntine DW, Henderson PR, Biggs JSG (1979) Benign mullerian mixed tumor of the vagina. Gynecol Oncol 8:21–26

Chen KTK (1981) Brenner tumor of the vagina. Diagn Gynecol Obstet 3:255–258

Robinson TG (1950) Extraovarian Brenner tumour. J Obstet Gynaecol Br Commonw 57:890–891

Malignant Mixed Mesodermal Tumour

Amolsch AL (1939) Mixed mesodermal tumours of the uterus and vagina. Am J Cancer 37:435–444

Chuang JT, van Velden DJJ, Graham JB (1970) Carcinosarcoma and mixed mesodermal tumour of the uterine corpus. Obstet Gynecol 35:769–780

Davis PC, Franklin EW (1975) Cancer of the vagina. South Med J 68:1239–1242

Murphy GH, Dushane JW (1948) Mesodermal mixed tumour of the vagina: report of a case. Am J Obstet Gynecol 55:527–532

Norris HJ (1966) Clinical and pathologic study of 31 carcinosarcomas. Cancer 19:1459–1465

Peters WA III, Kumar NB, Andersen WA et al. (1985) Primary sarcoma of the adult vagina; a clinicopathologic study. Obstet Gynecol 65:699–704

Rutledge F (1967) Cancer of the vagina. Am J Obstet Gynecol 97:635–655

Schaepman-van Geuns EJ (1970) Mixed tumors and carcinosarcomas of the uterus evaluated five years after treatment. Cancer 25:72–74

Symmonds RE, Dockerty MB (1955) Sarcoma like proliferations of endometrial stroma. I clinicopathologic study of 19 mesodermal mixed tumors. Surg Gynecol Obstet 100:232–240

Endometrial Stromal Sarcoma

Berkowitz RS, Ehrman RL, Knapp RC (1978) Endometrial stromal sarcoma arising from vaginal endometriosis. Obstet Gynecol 51 [Suppl]:34–37

Hart WR, Yoonessi M (1977) Endometrial stromatosis of the uterus. Obstet Gynecol 49:393–403

Koss LG, Spiro RH, Brunschwig A (1965) Endometrial stromal sarcoma. Surg Gynecol Obstet 121:531–537
Norris HJ, Taylor HB (1966) Mesenchymal tumors of the tuerus: I A clinical and pathological study of 53 endometrial stromal tumors. Cancer 19:755–766
Young RH, Prat J, Scully RE (1984) Endometrial stromal sarcomas of the ovary: a clinicopathologic analysis of 23 cases. Cancer 53:1143–1155

Gartner's Duct Carcinoma
Hinchey WW, Silva EG, Guarda LA et al. (1983) Paravaginal wolffian duct (mesonephros) adenocarcinoma: a light and electron microscopic study. Am J Clin Pathol 80:539–544
Kariminejad MH, Scully RE (1973) Female adenxal tumour of probable wolffian origin: a distinctive pathologic entity. Cancer 31:671–677
Sivathondan Y, Solm R, Hughesdon PE et al. (1979) Female adnexal tumor of probable wolffian origin. J Clin Pathol 32:616
Taxy JB, Battifora H (1976) Female adnexal tumor of probable wolffian origin: evidence of low grade malignancy. Cancer 37:2349–2354
Wahlen T, Gynning I (1955) Carcinoma of Gartner's duct (a vaginal case). Acta Obstet Gynecol Scand 34:120–130

22.11 Tumours of Uncertain Histogenesis

22.11.1 Malignant Tumours Resembling Synovial Sarcoma

A 3-cm mass occurring at the upper and lateral aspect of the vagina of a 24-year-old woman was reported by Okagaki et al. (1976). The tumour consisted predominantly of flattened and epithelioid cells arranged in acinar and tubular fashions. Diastase-resistant, PAS-positive, proteinaceous material was occasionally seen within the acinar lumen. The tumour displayed peripheral infiltrating borders which were formed of spindle cells resembling those of fibrosarcoma. Mitoses were infrequent. Some of these spindle cells were also positive for mucin. Ultrastructurally, the tumour cells around the lumina showed large cytoplasmic vacuoles, occasional perinuclear intracytoplasmic filaments and slender long microvilli projecting into the lumina. The authors tentatively labelled this as "synovial tumour of the vagina". Shevchuk et al. (1978) reported a similar tumour occurring in the upper vagina of a 33-year-old woman who presented with post-coital bleeding. Ultrastructural features of the tumour, particularly the presence of prominant telolysosomes in the epithelial cells, were considered to be those of transitional epithelial differentiation.

Although the exact histogenesis of the tumours is uncertain, their histological appearance conforms closely to that of synovial sarcoma. Synovial sarcoma can occur in the pelvis, and infiltration of the vagina or surrounding structures may not be unusual.

The lesion should be treated radically as a synovial sarcoma.

A long-term follow-up of this lesion has not yet been reported, and its natural history is not known.

22.11.2 Mixed Tumour

This is also a tumour of uncertain histogenesis which has been reported to occur in the vagina of women between 20 and 53 years of age (Sirota et al. 1981). About a dozen cases have so far been reported in the literature (Brown 1953; Hertig and Gore 1960; Whelton 1962; Buntine et al. 1979; Chen 1981; Fowler et al. 1981; Sirota et al. 1981).

22.11.2.1 Clinical Features

Patients may be asymptomatic and the tumour may be detected incidentally during routine pelvic examination by a gynaecologist. Sometimes the patient may complain of a slowly growing, painless, vaginal mass. The majority of the reported tumours are located close to the hymenal ring (Sirota et al. 1981), but they can also rise from the vaginal vault (Buntine et al. 1979) and introitus (Chen 1981). The paravestibular tumour reported by Fowler et al. (1981) belongs to this group.

The müllerian mesenchyme is known to possess potentialities of diverse differentiation, and these tumours have been suggested to arise from the embryonic müllerian rests.

22.11.2.2 Gross Appearance

These tumours occur as single, submucosal nodules of 1–5 cm in size and are smooth-surfaced, discrete and unencapsulated. On their cut surface, they are grey to tan in colour and soft to firm in consistency.

22.11.2.3 Microscopical Appearance

The tumours are composed of fibrous tissue as well as epithelial cells. The connective tissue component consists of short spindle cells with uniform spindle and oval nuclei, which are arranged in interconnecting fascicles and whorls. In some areas they are tightly packed, and in others the pattern is relatively acellular, with hyaline material interposed between the fascicles. The tumours contain a variable amount of reticulin and collagen fibres. Mitoses are not seen. The other conspicuous component of the tumour is composed of nests, islands and cords of squamous cells. They are well delineated from the surrounding connective tissue and contain well-glycogenated keratinocytes with vacuolated cytoplasm and pyknotic nuclei. Keratin cysts can occasionally be seen within the tumour. Tubular structures lined by mucinous epithelium may also be present. The tubules may show papillary foldings (Sirota and Scully 1980).

22.11.2.4 Treatment

Surgical excision is curative, and none of the reported tumours has recurred after surgery.

References

Tumours Resembling Synovial Sarcoma

Okagaki T, Ishida T, Hilders RD (1976) A malignant tumor of the vagina resembling synovial sarcoma. Cancer 57:2306–2320

Schevchuk MM, Fenoglio CM, Lattes R et al. (1978) Malignant mixed tumor of the vagina probably arising in mesonephric rests. Cancer 42:214–223

Mixed Tumours

Brown CE (1953) Mixed epithelial tumor of the vagina. Am J Clin Pathol 23:237–240

Buntine DW, Henderson PR, Biggs JSG (1979) Benign mullerian tumor of the vagina. Gynecol Oncol 8:21–26

Chen KTK (1981) Benign mixed tumor of the vagina. Obstet Gynecol 57 [Suppl]:89–90

Fowler WC Jr, Lawrence H, Edelman DA (1981) Paravestibular tumor of the female genital tract. Am J Obstet Gynecol 139:109–111

Hertig AT, Gore H (1960) Tumors of the female sex organs. Armed Forces Institute of Pathology, Washington, pp 68–69

Sirota RL, Scully RE (1980) Mixed tumors of the vagina. Lab Invest 42:152

Sirota RL, Dickersin GR, Scully RE (1981) Mixed tumors of the vagina: A clinicopathological analysis of eight cases. Am J Surg Pathol 5:413–422

Whelton JA (1962) Mixed tumor arising in the vagina. Obstet Gynecol 19:803–805

22.12 Secondary Tumours

The vagina can be infiltrated by the direct extension of carcinomas from the cervix and vulva. Metastatic deposits occur predominantly from endometrial carcinoma (Fig. 22.28), the incidence of which has varied from 2% to 24% (Price et al. 1965; Glassburn 1981). Ovarian carcinoma can also metastasise to the vagina (Evans 1952; Tamaya et al. 1986) and may present initially as a vaginal lesion (Lifshitz et al. 1978). The lymphatic system of all parts of the lower genital tract communicates freely, so the vagina may be affected by a malignant tumour of any part of the genital tract (Fig. 22.29). Of the primaries of the distant extra-genital organs, renal cell carcinoma is by far the most commonly reported primary metastasising to the vagina (Sogani and Whitmore 1979; Nocks and Sacknoff 1980; O'Reilly et al. 1984). Retrograde venous metastasis via the ovarian vein and utero-vaginal venous plexus is the likely mode of spread to the vagina. Local clear cell carcinoma should be differentiated from metastatic renal cell carcinoma by careful clinical and radiological investigation of the kidney. Ultrastructural demonstration of lipid and the long slender microvilli in renal cell carcinoma are helpful parameters in establishing the diagnosis (Tannenbaum 1971).

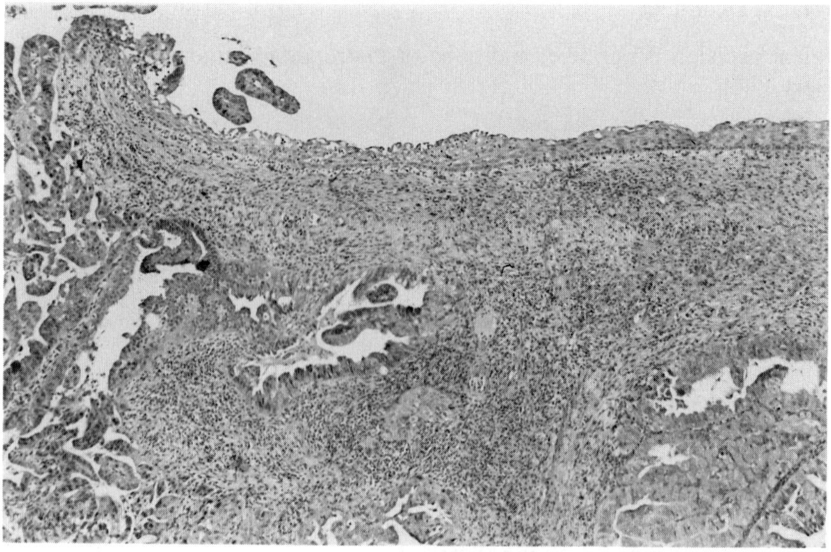

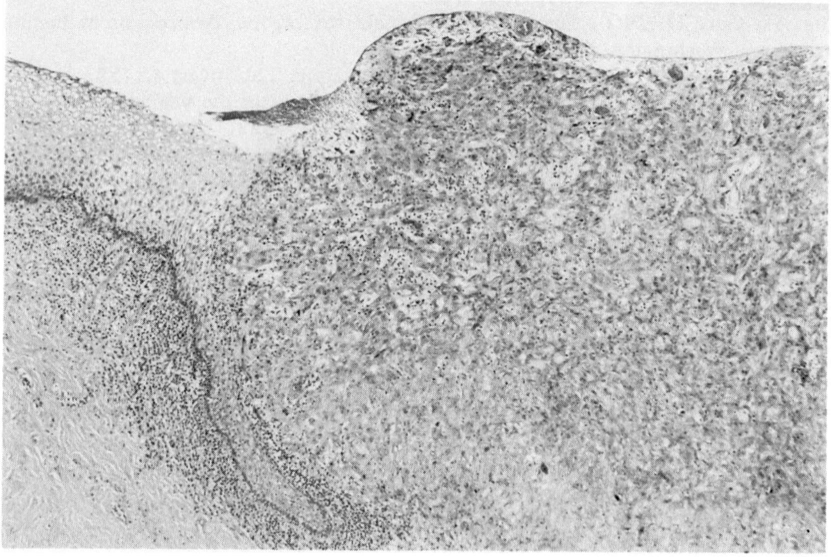

Fig. 22.28. Secondary deposit from an endometrial adenocarcinoma

Fig. 22.29. Secondary deposit from malignant melanoma of the uterine cervix

Colon (Raider 1966) and breast carcinoma can also metastasise to the vagina (Pineda and Sall 1978; Jacobs et al. 1983). They are, however, very uncommon.

References

Evans GM (1952) Vaginal metastases from the carcinoma of the ovary. J Obstet Gynaecol Br Emp 59:82–84

Glassburn JR (1981) Carcinoma of the endometrium. Cancer 48:575–581

Jacobs AJ, Deppe G, Kessinger A et al. (1983) Breast carcinoma metastatic to the vagina. Acta Obstet Gynecol Scand 62:83–85

Lifshitz S, Newland WH, Dolan TE et al. (1978) Ovarian carcinoma presenting as a vaginal lesion. JAMA 239:1788–1791

Nocks BN, Sacknoff EJ (1980) Vaginal metastasis of renal cell carcinoma without renal vein involvement. J Urol 52:327

O'Reilly AP, McLeod F, Craft I (1984) Hypernephroma presenting as a vaginal metastasis. Case report. Br J Obstet Gynaecol 91:812–815

Pineda A, Sall S (1978) Metastasis to the vagina from carcinoma of the breast. J Reprod Med 20:243–245

Price JJ, Hahn GA, Rominger CJ (1965) Vaginal involvement in endometrial carcinoma. Am J Obstet Gynecol 91:1060–1065

Raider L (1966) Remote vaginal metaseses from carcinoma of the colon. Am J Rad Ther Nucl Med 97:944–950

Sogani PC, Whitmore WF Jr (1979) Solitary vaginal metastasis from unsuspected renal cell carcinoma. J Urol 121:95–97

Tamaya T, Ito M, Fujimoto J et al. (1986) Ovarian squamous cell carcinoma derived from a dermoid cyst presenting as vaginal metastasis and implication of its steroid receptor levels – two case reports. Gynecol Oncol 23:44–50

Tannenbaum M (1971) Ultrastructural pathology of human renal cell tumors. Pathol Annu 6:249–278

23 Inflammatory Conditions That May Simulate Tumours

Almost all of the inflammatory conditions which affect the vulva may also involve the vagina (Van der Walt et al. 1973). Gross and histopathological features vary little. Biopsy, microbiological and serological investigations should be undertaken to establish the diagnosis. Only a few uncommon conditions are described here. The reader may refer to Chap. 16 for inflammatory conditions of the vulva.

23.1 Specific

Regarding syphilis and lymphogranulomas see "Vulva".

23.2 Nonspecific

23.2.1 Spindle Cell Nodules

Benign spindle cell nodules following vaginal hysterectomy have occasionally been reported (Proppe et al. 1984). The nodules are composed of interlacing fascicles of spindle cells, delicate small blood vessels, and chronic inflammatory cells. The spindle cells may infiltrate and destroy the surrounding smooth muscle bundles. The lesion may recur if incompletely excised (Proppe et al. 1984).

Reactive fibrohistiocytic proliferation, reported by Snover et al. (1981), is probably a similar lesion.

23.2.2 Xanthogranulomatous Tumour

Xanthogranuloma is an inflammatory pseudotumour which has been reported to occur in the kidney, retroperitoneum, ovary and other areas. Different types of microorganisms including staphylococci, proteus and *Escherichia coli* have been attributed as causative agents, but the mechanism of formation of the granuloma remains unclear. Persistent tissue destruction with liberation of lipid material which eventually accumulates within the macrophages may play an important role. Several other conditions such as malakoplakias and Whipple's disease have been included in the category of xanthogranulomatous lesions, a common feature in all these conditions being the collection of foam cells.

The patients with vaginal lesions may present for dyspareunia due to paravaginal mass, ulceration of the vaginal mucosa and bleeding (Gidwani et al. 1979) or with recurrent, bleeding, vaginal polyp (Strate et al. 1983). The size of the lesions vary from 3 to 10 cm.

Microscopically, the lesion consists of sheets of large, lipid-filled macrophages with abundant foamy or faintly eosinophilic cytoplasm and round pyknotic nuclei. Lymphocytes, plasma cells and neutrophils can be seen in variable numbers either intermixed with or surrounding by clusters of foamy macrophages. Capillaries, fibroblasts and occasionally multinucleate giant cells are also present. These lesions should be differentiated from metastatic renal cell carcinoma both clinically and histologically. The cells of renal carcinoma may display pleomorphism, mitoses and a tubular arrangement, but these are not constant features. Ultrastructural study (Strate et al. 1983) may be helpful in the identification of extra- and intra-cellular microorganisms within the macrophages.

The presence of intra-cytoplasmic, fine, eosinophilic granules may occasionally be misleading, suggesting a diagnosis of granular cell tumour (Strate et al. 1983), the cells of which are PAS-positive and ultrastructurally display numerous cytosegresomes (Moscovic and Azar 1967).

23.2.2.1 Treatment

Excision is curative. Radiation alone or in combination with surgery depending on the site, size and extent of the lesion can be used (Gidwani et al. 1979).

23.2.3 Malakoplakia

Malakoplakia is also an unusual, chronic, inflammatory process which can produce a tumour-like mass in the vaginal wall. The patients are usually women between 30 (Chalvardjian et al. 1980) and 74 years of age (Cremar and Bussany-Caspari 1979) and most commonly present with vaginal bleeding.

23.2.3.1 Gross Appearance

The lesion is similar to xanthogranuloma and can affect any part of the vagina. Occasionally, a structure develops, or the lesion appears as a yellowish-brown, papillary, necrotic mass mimicking a malignant tumour.

23.2.3.2 Microscopical Appearance

The histological picture is essentially similar to that of xanthogranuloma. The diagnostic hallmark of malakoplakia, however, is the presence of Michaelis-Gutmann bodies which are scattered among the inflammatory cells in variable numbers. These are intra- and extra-cellular, concentrically laminated bodies 1–20 μm in diameter which stain positively for calcium, iron and neutral mucopolysaccharides. Bacilli can be demonstrated in the cytoplasm of histiocytes called von Hansmann histiocytes. Several bacilli including *Proteus* and *E. coli* have been incriminated. Defective phagocytic functions of the monocytes to destroy ingested bacteria have been suggested to be the main factor in the genesis of the lesion.

23.2.3.3 Treatment

Antibiotics and excisions are adequate. Some lesions may recur which can also be treated surgically.

23.2.4 Vaginal Mass Due to Chlamydial Proctitis (Lymphogranuloma Venereum)

Schuch et al. (1984) reported a vaginal mass in a 36-year-old woman who had multiple partners and presented with dyspareunia and vaginal lump. A biopsy taken during drainage of the lump showed inflammatory changes and the presence of *Chlamydia trachomatis* on immunoperoxidase studies. Treatment with antibiotics (doxycycline) led to resolution of the mass.

23.2.5 Fistulous Lesions

Fustulous communications with neighbouring organs result from carcinomatous infiltrations, abscess, radiation and trauma. Of the inflammatory conditions, diverticular disease of the colon and Crohn's disease of the ileum are two common causes of fistulous tract opening into the vagina. Zeigerman et al. (1964) noticed that 9 patients developed sigmoido-vaginal fistula in a series of 327 patients with sigmoidal diverticulitis. The ilio-vaginal fistula is, on the other hand, much less common. Kyle and Sinclair (1969) found in the literature only 11 cases occurring due to Crohn's disease. Malignancy has been attributed to be the major cause of entero-vaginal fistula, with irradiation injury the second most important (Piver and Lele 1976).

References

Chalvardjian A, Picard L, Shaw R et al. (1980) Malakoplakia of female genital tract. Am J Obstet Gynecol 138:391–394

Cremar H, Busanny-Caspari W (1979) Die Malakoplakie der Scheide eine seltene Ursache einer vaginalen Blutung. Geburtshilfe Frauenheilkd 39:214–216

Gidwani GP, Ballard LA Jr, Jelden GL et al. (1979) Xanthogranuloma of the vagina. Cleve Clin Q 46:163–166

Kyle J, Sinclair WY (1969) Ileovaginal fistula complicating regional enteritis. Br J Surg 56:474–475

Moscovic EA, Azar HA (1967) Multiple granular cell tumours (myoblastomas): case reports with electron microscopic observations and review of literature. Cancer 20:2032–2041

Piver MS, Lelle S (1976) Enterovaginal and enterocutaneous fistulae in women with gynecologic malignancies. Obstet Gynecol 48:560–563

Proppe KH, Scully RE, Rosai J (1984) Postoperative spindle cell nodules of genitourinary tract resembling sarcoma: a report of eight cases. Am J Surg Pathol 8:101–108

Schuch RJ, Muisch JR, Nelson RL (1984) Chlamydial proctitis – unusual presentation as a symptomatic vaginal mass. Obstet gynecol 63:132–134

Snover DC, Phillips G, Dehner LP (1981) Reactive fibrohistocytic proliferation resembling fibrous histocytoma. Am J Clin Pathol 76:232–235

Strate SM, Taylor WE, Forney JP et al. (1983) Xanthogranulomatous pseudotumour of the vagina: evidence of a local response to an unusual bacterium (mucoid Esch Coli). Am J Clin Pathol 79:637–643

Van der Walt JJ, Marcus PB, De Wet JJ et al. (1973) Malakoplakia of vagina: first case report. S Afr Med J 47:1342–1344

Zeigerman JH, Stahlgren L, Tulsky EG (1964) Sigmoidovaginal fistula: review of the literature and report of a case. Am J Obstet Gynecol 89:1003–1008

References

Part III: Cysts, Tumours and Tumour-like Conditions of the Female Urethra

24 Classification of Cysts, Tumours and Tumour-like Conditions of the Female Urethra

I. Skene's duct cyst

II. Urethral diverticulum

III. Urethral caruncle

IV. Urethral tumours

Benign

Malignant

Carcinoma
Melanoma
Sarcoma

25 Cysts (Skene's Duct Cyst)

25.1 Cysts: Skene's Duct Cyst

The female urethra develops from the urogenital sinus which is surrounded by cuboidal cell-lined glands. These glands are equivalent to the prostatic glands in men. They, except for the ones which form Skene's duct, regress in women. Another group of glands lined by squamous cells develops as a prolongation of the epithelium of the vaginal canal. These, too, regress before birth but may persist to give rise to paraurethral cysts. The other types of the cyst occurring at the paraurethral location are mesonephric and paramesonephric cysts, which have already been mentioned.

Cysts usually develop secondary to the blockage due to subclinical infection and trauma.

Paraurethral cysts occur both in neonates (Blaivas et al. 1976) and adults (Das 1981).

Clinically, patients may present with dysuria, dyspareunia, vaginal discharge and a vaginal mass (James 1979; Tancer 1965; Hainsworth 1956). Infection and abscess may occasionally complicate the condition.

25.1.1 Pathological Features

The cysts vary in size from 1 to 3 cm.

Microscopical features vary. The lining may be formed by transitional cell with foci of squamous cells.

25.1.2 Treatment

Marsupialisation and total excision with the presenrvation of urethral integrity is the usual method of treatment.

References

Blaivas JG, Pais VM, Retik AB (1976) Paraurethral cysts in female neonate. Urology 7:504–507

Das SP (1981) Paraurethral cysts in women. J Urol 126:41–43

Hainsworth E (1956) Cyst of Skene's gland. J Obstet Gynaecol Br Commonw 63:420–421

James ST (1979) A large cyst of Skene's duct – a rare cause of superficial dyspareunia. Aust NZ J Obstet Gynaecol 19:61–62

Tancer ML (1965) Bartholin's cyst and paraurethral lesions. Clin Obstet Gynecol 8:982–996

26 Urethral Diverticulum

The urethral diverticulum is a pouch in the urethro-vaginal septum communicating with the urethral canal (Nel 1955). The diverticulum may be congenital (Counsellor 1949; Gilbert and Cintron 1954; MacKinnon et al. 1959; Silk and Lobowitz 1969) or acquired. The congenital variety may arise from a remnant of Gartner's duct, faulty union of the primordial folds, cell rests, vaginal wall cyst of the müllerian origin or congenital dilatation of the paraurethral ducts. The acquired variety may develop as a result of trauma to the urethra commonly due to childbirth, infection and obstruction in the paraurethral glands (Edward and Beebe 1955; Coddington and Knob 1983; Ginsburg and Genadry 1984). The overwhelming majority of diverticuli are considered to be acquired, although it may be difficult to determine whether a diverticulum in the adult is congenital or acquired (Nel 1955). Some authors (Peters and Vaughan 1976) believe that all diverticuli are acquired.

26.1 Clinical Features

Urethral diverticuli are seen among parous women of 25–50 years of age (Widholm and Rynanen 1967), 75% occurring between the 3rd and 5th decades (Ginsburg and Genadry 1983). About 2%–5% of women seem to be affected (Andersen 1967; Davis and Robinson 1970; Hajj and Evans 1980). About 80% of patients are asymptomatic (Hajj and Evans 1980). The symptomatic patients complain of urinary frequency due to urinary tract infection, urgency and dysuria (Ginsburg and Genadry 1983) and, occasionally, pain radiating to the lower abdomen, inguinal folds, vagina and perineum. Pyuria and haematuria (Widholm and Ryynanen 1967) also occur. Some patients complain of dyspareunia, anterior abdominal wall mass and stress incontinence (Ginsburg and Genadry 1984). Clinical diagnosis is made by the presence of a palpable cystic mass in the urethral region which is likely to be tender to touch. Confirmation of the diagnosis is made by urethral radiography including cystourethrogram and cineradiograph.

26.2 Gross Appearance

The size of an urethral diverticulum is 2 cm with a range between 0.5 and 5 cm (Pathak and House 1970). The ostium is located in the middle third of the posterior wall. The removed sac is smooth surfaced, and the contents may be either urine, pus, grit or stones. The wall may be thin, thick and fibrous.

26.3 Microscopical Appearance

The wall of the sac may consist of all the layers of the urethral wall. There may be a break in the muscle layer, and in some cases, all the layers of the wall may show the break. The lining epithelium of the excised sac may be partially or completely replaced by abscess and granulation tissue. When the epithelium is present, it may be transitional, squamous, cuboidal, low columnar or combination. Occasionally, glandular tissue is seen in the wall.

Malignancy is an infrequent complication of urethral diverticulum, but several patients with carcinoma complicating the diverticulum have been described (Melnick and Birdsall 1960; Wishard et al. 1960; Rosenfeld and Fruchtman 1964).

26.4 Treatment

Clinical evaluation is important. Urethrogram, intravenous pyelogram, urethroscopy and urethral pressure profile are to be performed before treatment is undertaken. Antibiotics may be necessary to combat infections. The surgical procedure differs with different surgeons.

References

Andersen MJF (1967) The incidence of diverticula of the female urethra. J Urol 98:96–98

Coddington CC, Knob DR (1983) Urethral diverticulum. Obstet Gynecol Surv 38:357–364

Counsellor V (1949) Urethral diverticulum in the female: a clinical study. Am J Obstet Gynecol 57:231–236

Davis BL, Robinson DG (1970) Diverticula of the female urethra: assay of 120 caes. J Urol 104:850–853

Edward EA, Beebe RA (1955) Diverticula of the female urethra. Obstet Gynecol 5:729–738

Gilbert C, Cintron F (1954) The urethral diverticulum in the female. Am J Obstet Gynecol 67:616–627

Ginsburg D, Genadry R (1983) Suburethral diverticulum: classification and therapeutic considerations. Obstet Gynecol 61:685–688

Ginsbureg DS, Genadry R (1984) Suburethral diverticulum in the female. Obstet Gynecol Surv 39:1–7

Hajj SN, Evans MI (1980) Diverticula of the female urethra. Am J Obstet Gynecol 136:335–338

MacKinnon M, Pratt JH, Pool TL (1959) Diverticulum of the female urethra. Surg Clin North Am 39:953–962

Melnick JL, Birdsall TM (1960) Carcinoma of a diverticulum of the female urethra. Am J Obstet Gynecol 80:347–352

Nel JB (1955) Diverticulum of the female urethra. J Obstet Gynaecol Br Commonw 62:90–97

Pathak UN, House MJ (1970) Diverticulum of the female urethra. Obstet Gynecol 36:789–794

Peters WA III, Vaughan ED Jr (1976) Urethral diverticulum in the female: etiologic factors and post operative results. Obstet Gynecol 47:549–552

Rosenfeld LJ, Fruchtman B (1964) Carcinoma in diverticula of the female urethra. Obstet Gynecol 24:924–927

Silk MR, Lobowitz JM (1969) Anterior urethral diverticulum. J Urol 101:66–67

Widholm O, Ryynanen VA (1967) Diverticulum of the female urethra. Acta Obstet Gynecol Scand 46:107–117

Wishard WMN Jr, Nourse MH, Mertz JHO (1960) Carcinoma in diverticulum in female urethra. J Urol 83:409–413

27 Urethral Caruncle

Urethral caruncle is a red fleshy mass a few millimeters to a few centimeters in diameter commonly seen in the posterior part of the urethral meatus of post-menopausal women. The lesion is asymptomatic but may cause pain and bleeding if ulcerated or thrombosed.

27.1 Microscopical Appearance

Classically, three varieties have been described, namely, papillomatous, angiomatous and granulomatous. The papillomatous type appears to be the least common. In this type, the surface epithelium, which is transitional, is thrown into papillary folds which are seldom made up of more than 5–6 layers of cells. The angiomatous type consists of many capillaries and small-sized blood vessels, many of which are dilated and engorged with blood, and oedematous, loose connective tissue stroma. The granulomatous variety, in addition, displays inflammatory cells and fibrous tissue stroma. Histiocytes are usually not a conspicuous component.

27.2 Treatment

Depending on the size the lesion is removed or cauterised. The tissue should be submitted for routine histology, as neoplasms can masquerade as caruncles.

28 Benign Tumours

28.1 Urethral Papilloma

Papillomas of the urethra are usually small and less than 1 cm in size (Marshall et al. 1960). Dysuria and bleeding may be the main symptoms.

28.1.1 Microscopical Appearance

Papillomas are small masses of short filiform structures composed of a fibrovascular core covered by several layers of squamous or transitional cells. The urethral polyps can therefore be of both squamous cell and transitional cell types.

The papillary lesions of the urethra, particularly the squamous type, are now suspected to be due to HPV infections. In men, urethral condylomata acuminata is a well-recognised condition. In women, urethral condylomata are often associated with vulval condylomata acuminata. They are similar to the vulval warts in gross and histopathological appearances. Although viral proteins have been detected in the urethral lesions, the types of wart virus involved have not yet been properly worked out.

28.2 Haemangioma

Haemangioma is a rare tumour of the urethra (Radman 1965). The patients present usually with haematuria. Haemangioma may be congenital. More often, however, they represent the varicosities of urethral vessels.

Haemangiomas are red or brown, polypoid masses of average 1–2 cm in diameter protruding through the meati.

28.2.1 Treatment

These lesions may be multifocal in the urinary tract (Anderson et al. 1977). When a haemangioma is discovered, investigations should be directed to find more of these lesions along the urinary tract. They are excised under anaesthesia.

28.3 Leiomyoma

Leiomyomas are also uncommon tumours of the urethra. They are three times more frequent in women than in men (Lake et al. 1981).

Clinically, leiomyomas are generally asymptomatic, but they may produce post-void hesitancy or dribbling when they are large in size. Uncommonly, the patient may present with intermittent haematuria and obstruction (Shield and Weiss 1981).

28.3.1 Gross Appearance

The tumours are located either paraurethrally or protrude through the urethral meatus. Both sessile and pedunculated neoplasms are seen. The average size is 1 cm, but they may be larger (Herbut 1952). The cut surface is greyish-tan in colour and firm to rubbery in consistency.

28.3.2 Microscopical Appearance

The tumours are composed of interlacing bundles of smooth muscle forming whorls and irregular fascicles. They may be covered by squamous or transitional epithelium.

28.3.3 Treatment

The treatment is simple excision (Shield and Weiss 1981).

28.4 Nephrogenic Adenoma

Nephrogenic adenomas are so-called because of the close similarities of their tubular components to the renal tubules. These lesions are more common in the urinary bladder than in the urethra. Men are more commonly affected than women.

The patient may present with hematuria.

Grossly, nephrogenic adenomas are small, polypoid or papillary nodules 2–4 mm in size and grey to pink in colour.

Microscopically, nephrogenic adenomas are located in the lamina propria and are composed of tubules that vary in size and shape. Some of the tubules are dilated, containing pink amorphous material which is PAS/D positive. The tubules are lined by cuboidal, columnar and flattened epithelial cells with clear and eosinophilic cytoplasm and vesicular or hyperchromatic nuclei. Mitotic figures may be noticed but never form a conspicuous feature. In some areas, the tubules are arranged in tight clusters, and in others, they may be loosely scattered in the connective tissue background. The stroma always shows inflammatory cell infiltrations and the presence of thin-walled blood vessels.

The aetiology of the condition is not known. Nephrogenic metaplasia has been attributed to trauma, irritation and infection (Bhagavan et al. 1981). The lesion has not been reported in the fetus or neonate (Peterson and Matsumoto 1978).

28.4.1 Treatment

The condition is benign. Excision and fulguration is adequate. Occasionally, the lesion recurs.

28.5 Other Benign Tumours

Rare sub-urethral fibroma (Sered et al. 1956) and granular cell tumour have also been mentioned as arising in the urethra.

References

Papilloma

Marshall FG, Uson AC, Melicow MM (1960) Neoplasms and carucles of female urethra. Surg Gynecol Obstet 110:723–733

Haemangioma

Anderson RU, Andonian RW, Jamison RL (1977) Multiple haemangiomas involving genitourinary tract. Urology 10:246–248

Radman HM (1965) Urethral haemangioma. J Urol 94:580–581

Leiomyoma

Herbut PA (1952) Urological pathology. Lea and Febiger, Philadelphia, p 93

Lake MH, Kossow A, Bokinsky G (1981) Leiomyoma of the bladder and urethra. J Urol 125:742–743

Shield DE, Weiss RM (1981) Leiomyoma of the female urethra. J Urol 109:430–431

Nephrogenic Adenoma

Bhagavan B, Tiasmson EM, Wenk RE (1981) Nephrogenic adenoma of the urinary bladder and urethra. Hum Pathol 12:907–916

Peterson LJ, Matsumoto LM (1978) Nephrogenic adenoma in urethral diverticulum. Urology 11:193–195

Other Benign Tumours

Sered H, Phillip EA, Foss HG (1956) Suburethral fibromas. Am J Obstet Gynecol 71:1362–1365

29 Malignant Tumours

29.1 Primary Carcinoma

Primary carcinoma of the female urethra is a rare tumour accounting for less than 0.02% of all malignancies occurring in women (Fagan and Hertig 1955). In general, malignancies of the female urethra have been reported to be twice as frequent as in men (McCrea 1952).

29.1.1 Clinical Features

The age of the patients ranges from 24 (Kamat et al. 1981) to 89 years old (Peterson et al. 1973), the peak incidence being between the 5th and 7th decades (Bolduan and Farah 1981). The majority of patients are more than 50 years old (Desai et al. 1973). The symptoms are more often similar to those associated with urinary tract infections (Peterson et al. 1973). Urethral bleeding, spotting (Bracken et al. 1976), haematuria, frequency, dysuria, incontinence, urinary retention, tenesmus and pain (Desai et al. 1973) are the usual complaints. Some patients consult their physician for obstruction (Allen and Nelson 1978), tumour in the urethral orifice (Skjaeraasen 1969) and painful urethral mass (Rhamy et al. 1973). A few patients may be asymptomatic (Braken et al. 1976).

The clinical staging system proposed by Grabstald et al. (1966) and Prempree et al. (1978) have been found useful for prognosis. Staging system proposed by Grabstald et al. (1966):

Stage 0: In situ (limited to mucosa)
- Stage A: Submucosa (not beyond submucosa)
- Stage B: Muscular (infiltrating periurethal muscle)
- Stage C: Periurethral
  - i. Infiltrating muscular wall of vagina
  - ii. Infiltrating muscular wall of vagina with invasion of vaginal mucosa
  - iii. Infiltrating other adjacent structures such as bladder, labia, clitoris

Stage D: Metastases
- i. Inguinal lymph nodes
- ii. Pelvic lymph nodes below aortic bifurcation
- iii. Lymph nodes above aortic bifurcation
- iv. Distant

Modified staging system of Prempree et al. (1978):

Stage I: Disease limited to the distal one-half of the urethra
Stage II: Disease involving entire urethra with extension to the periurethral tissues but not involving the vulva or bladder neck
Stage IIIA: Disease involving the urethra and vulva
B: Disease involving the vaginal mucosa
C: Disease involving urethra and bladder neck
Stage IVA: Disease involving parametrium or paracolpium
B: Metastases
- i. Inguinal lymph nodes
- ii. Pelvic nodes
- iii. Para-aortic
- iv. Distant

29.1.2 Gross Appearance

The most common site of urethral carcinoma is the external meatus (Zeigerman and Gordon 1970). The tumour may appear as a greyish-pink thickening of the mucosa, ulcer, nodule, fungating growth or papillomatous caruncle.

29.1.3 Microscopical Appearance

The distal two-thirds of the female urethra is lined by non-keratinising squamous cell epithelium with a gradual change to transitional epithelium in the proximal third. Squamous cell carcinoma constitutes 70% of all urethral carcinomas, followed by adenocarcinoma and transitional cell carcinoma (Hopkins et al. 1983). In some series, squamous cell carcinomas constituted only about 6%–10% of all carcinomas (Ruchs et al. 1952; Skjaeraasen 1969; Benson et al. 1982). It is often difficult to determine the exact site of origin when the tumour is extensive or advanced or involves a wide area of the urethral region. Adenocarcinomas are thought to originate from the paraurethral glands or Skene's glands (Walker and Huffman 1947; De Haan and Johnson 1960; Knoblich 1960). Tiltman (1975), on the other hand, thought that they originated in glandular metaplasia, urethritis glandularis or embryonal rests of mesonephric or paramesonephric ducts. Adenocarcinomas are the most common carcinomas arising in the mucous glands of the urethral diverticulum (Ritter 1953).

Squamous cell carcinomas are histologically similar to the squamous cell carcinomas arising in other parts of the body. Histological grades vary from well differentiated with pearl formation to very poorly differentiated with pseudosarcomatous spindle cell appearance (Ampil 1985). An in situ phase of squamous cell carcinoma has been noticed in some patients (Ruchs et al. 1952).

The adenocarcinomas, which constitute from 10% (Knoblich 1960; Peterson et al. 1973) to 23% (Bracken et al. 1976) of all carcinomas, are composed of malignant glands lined by low columnar, cuboidal and columnar epithelium, which may be stratified. Areas of squamous metaplasia can occasionally be seen. Adenocarcinoma with papillary formation and clear cells have been reported (Konnack 1973; Cea et al. 1975; Assimos and O'Connor 1984), with the suggestion that they are similar to the so-called mesonephric carcinoma of the female genital tract. In one series, 9 of the 23 patients with adenocarcinoma had clear cell carcinoma (Meis et al. 1987). As the urethra is partly lined by transitional epithelium, transitional cell carcinoma also occur in the female urethra (Skjaeraasen 1969; Peterson et al. 1973; Bracken et al. 1976; Allen and Nelson 1978; Elkon et al. 1980). Both in situ and papillary types (Roberts and Melicow 1977) have been noticed. Some 10% of the adenocarcinomas are mucin secreting (Rhamy et al. 1973), containing mucus-secreting and signet ring type cells (Menville and Counseller 1935; Klotz 1974).

Urethral cancer spreads by direct extension. Metastasis from the urethral carcinoma occurs through lymphatic channels. Carcinoma of the anterior urethra spreads to the vaginal nodes, and from the posterior urethra to the pelvic nodes (Monaco et al. 1958). Distant metastasis is uncommon and occurs late (Eisenstaedt 1951). In one series (Grabstadt 1966), the incidence of distant metastasis was 14%.

29.1.4 Prognosis

Prognosis depend on the stage of the tumour. An anterior urethral carcinoma has a better prognosis than a posterior one (Levine 1980; Ali et al. 1988). Carcinoma of the proximal urethra or involvement of the entire urethra carry grave prognosis (Antoniades 1969; Blath and Boehm 1973). Metastasis to the inguinal nodes is prognostically bad. Involvement of the bladder neck signifies a poor outlook. The overall survival rate is about 30%.

29.1.5 Treatment

Various modalities of treatment have been tried. Radiotherapy appears to be the mainstay of treatment for urethral carcinoma (Taggart et al. 1972). Surgery and radiotherapy in various combinations have also been employed. Good results have been achieved with local excision and interstitial irradiation in the carcinoma limited to the distal third (anterior) of the urethra (Desai et al. 1973). Interstitial radiation is the treatment of choice in stage I and IIIa lesions (Pointon and Pole-Wilson 1968). For deeper tumours, external beam therapy is used (Turner and

Hendry 1980). Prempree et al. (1984), employing various modes of radiotherapy, achieved a good 5-year, disease-free survival in a series of 14 patients. In advanced disease, pre-operative external irradiation followed by anterior exenteration should be considered (Bracken et al. 1976).

References

Ali MM, Klein FA, Hazra TA (1988) Primary female urethral carcinoma: a retrospective comparison of different treatment techniques. Cancer 62:54–57

Allen R, Nelson RP (1978) Primary urethral malignancy: review of 22 cases. South Med J 71:547–550

Ampil FL (1985) Primary malignant neoplasms of the female urethra. Obstet Gynecol 66:799–804

Antoniades J (1969) Radiation therapy in carcinoma of the female urethra. Cancer 24:70–76

Assimos DG, O'Connor VJ Jr (1984) Clear cell adenocarcinoma of the urethra. J Urol 131:540–541

Benson RC Jr, Tunca JC, Buchler DA et al. (1982) Primary carcinoma of female urethra. Gynecol Oncol 14:313–318

Blath RA, Boehm FH (1973) Carcinoma of female urethra. Surg Gynecol Obstet 136:574–576

Bolduan JP, Farah RN (1981) Primary urethral neoplasms: review of 30 cases. J Urol 125:198–200

Bracken RB, Johnson DE, Miller LS et al. (1976) Primary carcinoma of the female urethra. J Urol 116:188–192

Cea PC, Ward JN, Lavengood RW Jr et al. (1975) Mesonephric adenocarcinoma in urethral diverticula. Urology 10:583–589

Chu AM (1973) Female urethral carcinoma. Radiology 107:627–630

De Haan QC, Johnson CG (1960) Adenocarcinoma of the paraurethral glands: report of a case. Am J Obstet Gynecol 80:1108–1110

Desai S, Libertino JA, Zinman L (1973) Primary carcinoma of female urethra. J Urol 110:693–695

Eisenstaedt JS (1951) Primary carcinoma of female urethra with metastases. Am J Surg 81:612–617

Elkon D, Kim JA, Huddleston AL et al. (1980) Primary carcinoma female urethra. South Med J 73:1439–1442

Fagan GE, Hertig AT (1955) Carcinoma of the female urethra: a review of the literature: report of eight cases. Obstet Gynecol 6:1–11

Grabstald H (1973) Tumors of the urethra in men and women. Cancer 32:1236–1255

Grabstald H, Hilaris B, Henschke U et al. (1966) Cancer of female urethra. JAMA 197:835–842

Hopkins SC, Vider M, Nag SK et al. (1983) Carcinoma of the female urethra: reassessment of modes of therapy. J Urol 129:958–961

Kamat MR, Kulkarni JN, Dhumale RG (1981) Primary carcinoma of female urethra: review of 20 cases. J Surg Oncol 16:105–109

Klotz PG (1974) Carcinoma of Skene's gland associated with urethral diverticulum. J Urol 112:487–488

Knoblich R (1960) Primary adenocarcinoma of the female urethra: a review and report of 3 cases. Am J Obstet Gynecol 80:353–364

Konnack JW (1973) Mesonephric carcinoma involving the urethra. J Urol 110:76–78

Levine RL (1980) Urethral cancer. Cancer 45:1965–1972

McCrea LE (1952) Malignancy of the female urethra. Urol Surv 2:85–149

Meis JM, Ayala AG, Johnson DE (1987) Adenocarcinoma of the urethra in women. Cancer 60:1038–1052
Menville JG, Counseller Vs (1935) Mucoid carcinoma of female urethra. J Urol 33:76–81
Monaco AP, Murphy GB, Dowling WB (1958) Primary cancer of female urethra. Cancer 11:1215–1221
Peterson DT, Dockerty MB, Utz DC et al. (1973) Primary carcinoma of the female urethra. J Urol 110:72–75
Pointon RCS, Pole-Wilson DS (1968) Primary carcinoma of the urethra. Br J Urol 40:682–693
Prempree T, Wigenberg MJ, Scotts RM (1978) Radiation treatment of primary carcinoma of female urethra. Cancer 42:1177–1184
Prempree T, Amornmarn R, Patanaphan V (1984) Radiation therapy in primary carcinoma of female urethra: II An update on results. Cancer 54:729–733
Rhamy RK, Boldus RA, Allison RC et al. (1973) Therapeutic modalities in adenocarcinoma of the female urethra. J Urol 109:638–640
Ritter DW (1953) Primary malignancy of the female urethra. West J Surg Obstet Gynecol 61:420–429
Roberts TW, Melicow MM (1977) Pathology and natural history of urethral tumours in females. Urology 10:583–589
Ruchs RM, Frerichs JB, Arneson AN (1952) Cancer of female urethra. Cancer 5:748–753
Skjaeraasen E (1969) Cancer of the female urethra: a clinical study of 25 cases. Acta Obstet Gynecol Scand 48:589–597
Taggart CG, Castro JR, Rutledge FN (1972) Carcinoma of the female urethra. Am J Roentgenol Radium Ther Nucl Med 114:145–151
Tiltman AJ (1975) Primary adenocarcinoma of female urethra. J Pathol 117:97–99
Turner AG, Hendry WF (1980) Primary carcinoma of female urethra. Br J Urol 52:549–554
Walker LM, Huffman JW (1947) Adenocarcinoma of the female urethra: a review. Q Bull Northwest Univ Med Sch 21:115–125
Zeigerman JH, Gordon SF (1970) Cancer of the female urethra: a curable disease. Obstet Gynecol 36:785–789

29.2 Melanoma

Malignant melanoma of the female urethra is seen infrequently. Until 1981, only about three dozen patients had been described (Godec et al. 1981).

29.2.1 Clinical Features

The patients are between 32 and 80 years old (Block and Hotchkiss 1971) and present commonly with terminal haematuria (Das Gupta and Grabstald 1965) and occasionally with non-specific symptoms such as dysuria, perineal pain, vaginal discharge or urethral incompetence (Block and Hotchkiss 1971).

29.2.2 Pathological Features

Urethral melanoma appears as a haemorrhagic or pigmented polyp, black ulcerated area or papillary mass 2.5–4 cm in size.

The tumour is composed of nests, cords, groups and sheets of hyperchromatic and pleomorphic cells with round, oval and spindle-shaped nuclei and prominent nucleoli. Bizarre giant cells may be scattered within the tumour. Melanin pigments are usually abundant but may be sparse in an occasional tumour. Immunoperoxidase examination for S-100 and ultrastructural demonstration of melanosomes help in establishing the diagnosis. The presence of junctional activity in the adjacent epithelium is an important clue in the differential diagnosis between primary urethral and metastatic melanoma.

29.2.3 Prognosis

The prognosis of urethral melanoma is uniformly poor. Delay in the diagnosis is a major factor which influences the ultimate outcome (Katz and Grabstald 1976). Urethral melanoma spreads early to neighbouring tissues and regional lymph nodes and haematogenously later to distant sites. Metastases to the deep pelvic nodes are also an ominous sign (Godec et al. 1918).

29.2.4 Treatment

The rarity of urethral melanomas has precluded establishment of a definite modality of treatment. Radical surgery, radiation and chemotherapy have been tried without much success. Aggressive ablative surgery including prophylactic node dissection should be the initial course of choice (Block and Hotchkiss 1971). One of the two patients with 5-years' survival was treated by local excision, sub-total urethrectomy and bilateral lymph node dissection, and the other by cystectomy and urethrectomy with uretero-ileal anastomoses (Katz and Grabstald 1976).

References

Block NL, Hotchkiss RS (1971) Malignant melanoma of the female urethra: report of a case with 5 year survival and review of the literature. J Urol 105:251–255

Das Gupta T, Grabstald H (1965) Melanoma of the genitourinary tract. J Urol 93:607–614

Godec CJ, Cass AS, Hitchcock R et al. (1981) Melanoma of the female urethra. J Urol 126:553–555

Katz JI, Grabstald H (1976) Primary malignant melanoma of the female urethra. J Urol 116:454–457

29.3 Sarcoma

Sarcoma of the female urethra is extremely rare. Roberts and Melicow (1977) mentioned 1 patient with leiomyosarcoma in 65 cases of urethral tumours.

29.4 Secondary Tumours

The female urethra is commonly affected by the direct extension of malignant lesions of the vulva and vagina. Deposit from distant primary sites such as bronchial carcinoma, lymphoma (Roberts and Melicow 1977) and colonic carcinoma (Graf et al. 1962) has occasionally been mentioned.

References

Graf EC, Callahan DH, Sozer I (1962) A study of tumors of female urethra. J Urol 88:64–70

Roberts TW, Melicow MM (1977) Pathology and natural history of urethral tumors in females. Urology 10:583–589